Multiple Sclerosis

Butterworths International Medical Reviews

Neurology

Published titles

1 **Clinical Neurophysiology**
   Erik Stålberg and Robert R. Young

2 **Movement Disorders**
   C. David Marsden and Stanley Fahn

3 **Cerebral Vascular Disease**
   Michael J. G. Harrison and Mark L. Dyken

4 **Peripheral Nerve Disorders**
   Arthur K. Asbury and R. W. Gilliatt

5 **The Epilepsies**
   Roger J. Porter and Paolo L. Morselli

Next title

Movement Disorders 2
C. David Marsden and Stanley Fahn

Multiple Sclerosis

Edited by

W. I. McDonald, PhD, FRACP, FRCP
Professor of Clinical Neurology, Institute of Neurology; Honorary Consultant Physician,
The National Hospitals, Queen Square and Maida Vale, and Moorfields Eye Hospital,
London, UK

and

Donald H. Silberberg, MD
Professor and Chairman, Department of Neurology, University of Pennsylvania School of
Medicine, Philadelphia, Pennsylvania, USA

Butterworths
London   Boston   Durban   Singapore   Sydney   Toronto   Wellington

First published 1986

© **Butterworth & Co. (Publishers) Ltd, 1986**

British Library Cataloguing in Publication Data

Multiple sclerosis.—
  (Butterworths international medical reviews)
  1. Multiple sclerosis
  I. McDonald, W. Ian   II. Silberberg, D. H.
  616.8′34   RC377

  ISBN 0-407-00411-4

Photoset by Butterworths Litho Preparation Department
Printed and bound in England by Robert Hartnoll Ltd., Bodmin, Cornwall

Foreword

For almost a quarter of a century (1951–1975), subjects of topical interest were written about in the periodic volumes of our predecessor, *Modern Trends in Neurology*. Although both that series and its highly regarded editor, Dr Denis Williams, are now retired, the legacy continues in the present Butterworths series in Neurology. As was the case with *Modern Trends*, the current volumes are intended for use by physicians who grapple with the problems of neurological disorder on a daily basis, be they neurologists, neurologists in training, or those in related fields such as neurosurgery, internal medicine, psychiatry, and rehabilitation medicine.

Our purpose is to produce annually a monograph on a topic in clinical neurology in which progress through research has brought about new concepts of patient management. The subject of each monograph is selected by the Series Editors using two criteria: first, that there has been significant advance in knowledge in that area; and second, that such advances have been incorporated into new ways of managing patients with the disorders in question.

This has been the guiding spirit behind each volume, and we expect it to continue. In effect we emphasize research, both in the clinic and in the experimental laboratory, but principally to the extent that it changes our collective attitudes and practices in caring for those who are neurologically afflicted.

C. D. Marsden
A. K. Asbury
Series Editors

Preface

Multiple sclerosis, the major cause of neurological disability among young and middle-aged adults, is attracting increased attention from specialists in neurology, neurosurgery, ophthalmology, urology, orthopaedics, physical medicine and psychiatry, as well as the family physician who is often the mainstay of care for the afflicted patient. Investigators from many disciplines have increased our understanding of the phenomena which characterize multiple sclerosis, and this is beginning to modify the clinical care which we provide for the patient. Our purpose in this volume is to provide a framework for a better understanding of the disease process and for current and future clinical management.

The volume is organized so as to lead from the process of diagnosis, incorporating modern methods of assessment, through descriptions of aetiological and pathogenetic factors and the pathophysiology of the disease to specific information about the management of patients with multiple sclerosis. We are indebted to our distinguished coauthors who have provided their view of the current conclusions which can be reached within their areas of expertise. Our secretaries, Miss Jane Cook and Miss Lori Buell, have been of the greatest help and we have enjoyed most constructive support from the Butterworths staff for which we are grateful.

W. Ian McDonald
Donald H. Silberberg

Contributors

Mindy L. Aisen, MD
Department of Neurology, Albert Einstein College of Medicine, Bronx, New York, USA

G. H. du Boulay
Professor, Lysholm Radiological Department, The National Hospital, London, UK

Alastair Compston, PhD, MRCP
Consultant Neurologist, University Hospital of Wales, Cardiff, UK

George W. Ellison, MD
Department of Neurology, Reed Neurological Research Center, UCLA, Los Angeles, California, USA

Francisco Gonzalez-Scarano, MD
Department of Neurology, School of Medicine, University of Pennsylvania, Philadelphia, Pennsylvania, USA

Igor Grant, MD, FRCP(C)
Professor of Psychiatry, UCSD School of Medicine; Assistant Chief of Psychiatry, Veterans Administration Hospital, San Diego, California, USA

Robert P. Lisak, MD
Department of Neurology, School of Medicine, University of Pennsylvania, Philadelphia, Pennsylvania, USA

W. I. McDonald, PhD, FRACP, FRCP
Professor of Clinical Neurology, Institute of Neurology; Honorary Consultant Physician, The National Hospitals, Queen Square and Maida Vale, and Moorfields Eye Hospital, London, UK

Neal Nathanson, MD
Professor and Chairman, Department of Microbiology, School of Medicine, University of Pennsylvania, Philadelphia, Pennsylvania, USA

I. E. C. Ormerod, MB, MRCP
Institute of Neurology, The National Hospital, London, UK

Labe Scheinberg, MD
Department of Neurology, Albert Einstein College of Medicine, Bronx, New York, USA

Donald H. Silberberg, MD
Professor and Chairman, Department of Neurology, University of Pennsylvania School of Medicine, Philadelphia, Pennsylvania, USA

Charles R. Smith, MD
Department of Neurology, Albert Einstein College of Medicine, Bronx, New York, USA

Richard S. Spielman, PhD
Department of Human Genetics, School of Medicine, University of Pennsylvania, Philadelphia, Pennsylvania, USA

Contents

1
The diagnosis of multiple sclerosis

W. I. McDonald and D. H. Silberberg

INTRODUCTION

The implications of the diagnosis of multiple sclerosis are profound. The prospect of future disability, financial hardship and the disruption of personal and family life crowd in on the patient when it is made. The physician must therefore be clear in his own mind about the relative certainty of the diagnosis, and he must be careful not to overstate the position when presenting it to the patient. In the absence of an effective treatment, early diagnosis has been of comparatively little importance but the need is changing as the therapeutic prospects improve with the performance of increasing numbers of rationally based and carefully controlled clinical trials. The trials themselves demand early and precise diagnosis within recognized limits of confidence so that like can be compared with like in treated and control groups.

The diagnosis of multiple sclerosis remains fundamentally clinical and requires, in essence, the demonstration that a patient of an appropriate age has had at least two episodes of neurological disturbance implicating necessarily distinct sites in the central white matter. In recent years clinical assessment has been supplemented by a number of investigations which facilitate the identification of multiple sites of damage in the central nervous system (especially evoked potentials and imaging) or demonstrate the existence of characteristic immunological abnormalities (especially cerebrospinal fluid electrophoresis). None of these tests, however, is specific for multiple sclerosis and the data they provide have to be interpreted in the light of the clinical picture. Even the finding at post-mortem of unsuspected plaques or demyelination is not in itself diagnostic of multiple sclerosis unless the histological characteristics of the lesion indicate unmistakably that the lesions are of different ages.

In this chapter we review the criteria for the diagnosis of multiple sclerosis, discuss the place of various diagnostic techniques and deal with some particular problems encountered in clinical practice.

DIAGNOSTIC CRITERIA

A number of schemes have been formulated over the years in attempts to define diagnostic categories of varying certainty. All are based on the clinico-pathological definition of the disease established by Charcot (1868). Until recently the criteria have been based exclusively on clinical features. In the past decade the reliability of various investigative techniques has been established and the frequency with which the results are abnormal in multiple sclerosis as defined on the basis of clinical criteria has also been established. Since clinical criteria themselves are not specific there is no inherent reason why the results of investigations should not be included, and this has been done in the criteria formulated by the Poser Committee (Poser *et al.*, 1983). However, we wish to emphasize that the diagnosis finally depends on the clinical behaviour of the disorder in the individual patient over time. In order to permit comparisons between the results of research based on these criteria and earlier studies, a distinction has been kept between categories based exclusively on clinical features and those incorporating the results of investigation.

The criteria of the Poser Committee (like those of the Schumacher Committee, 1965) were designed for the conduct of research and therefore exclude monosymptomatic patients. Since certain isolated abnormalities of the nervous system (e.g. optic neuritis) commonly represent the first clinical expression of multiple sclerosis it is necessary that these episodes be defined too. It is obvious that there would be many advantages if the diagnostic criteria used in research and clinical practice were uniform. For this reason we have abandoned the use of the classifications applied earlier and have adopted the Poser Committee's criteria, supplemented by the definitions of individual episodes.

The Poser Committee's criteria

The background to the formulation of these criteria and guidelines for their application are given in the original publications (Poser *et al.*, 1983, 1984). The following summary is based on these publications.

Definitions

Appropriate age
The Poser Committee restricted the acceptable age of onset to 10–59 years because the criteria were designed for use in research protocols and there was a need to minimize the risk of contaminating patient groups with patients suffering from other diseases. It is important to realize, however, that cases can present rarely outside this range (Noseworthy *et al.*, 1983). We have personally seen cases of clinically definite disease presenting for the first time at the ages of 7 and 74 years.

Attack (bout, episode, exacerbation, relapse)
The occurrence of a symptom or symptoms of neurological dysfunction, with or without objective confirmation, lasting more than 24 hours constitutes an attack. Certain individual symptoms may, however, last only a matter of seconds (e.g. the surge of paraesthesiae following neck flexion – Lhermitte's symptom), or a minute or two (e.g. tonic seizures or episodic dysarthria (Matthews, 1975), *see* Chapter 10). These brief symptoms individually do not constitute an 'attack' but the period of days or weeks during which they recur does.

Clinical evidence of a lesion

This is provided by the demonstration of abnormal signs on examination. Such evidence is of course acceptable in the formulation of the diagnosis even if no longer present when the patient is first seen, provided they were elicited and recorded by a competent examiner in the past. A common source of difficulty in diagnosis is the inability to demonstrate abnormalities in the routine physical examination related to parts of the nervous system other than that implicated by the symptoms with which the patient has presented. Certain clinical tests may be helpful in particular circumstances. It is helpful, for example, to be able to demonstrate abnormalities in the optic nerve in patients presenting with symptoms referrable to the spinal cord or brainstem: useful observations in these circumstances include slits in the nerve fibre layer of the retina (Frisén and Hoyt, 1974), unilateral loss of colour vision, Pulfrich's effect (the illusion that a pendulum swinging in one plane is describing an ellipse (Frisén *et al.*, 1973) and a relative afferent pupillary defect. In patients with optic neuritis the observation of abnormally jerky eye movements or relative slowing of adduction on abrupt recentring from the deviated position are useful. In all these circumstances, however, the demonstration of the additional signs at presentation does not *per se* constitute grounds for diagnosing clinically definite multiple sclerosis (*see below*).

Paraclinical evidence of a lesion

This is provided by procedures additional to the physical examination, e.g. evoked potential techniques and imaging of the central nervous system (*see* Chapter 2). The lesion may or may not have produced symptoms or signs in the past; in the latter case the lesion is said to be subclinical.

Typical of multiple sclerosis

In making the diagnosis only those clinical features *characteristic* of multiple sclerosis should be used. These features are those which derive from the known sites of predilection for plaques, e.g. optic neuritis, paraesthesiae or weakness in the limbs, vertigo, and urinary urgency or incontinence. Exceptionally, certain other sites may be involved, producing symptoms or signs which are compatible with the diagnosis but should not be used in making it. Examples in this category are muscular wasting, progressive visual failure, major epilepsy and aphasia. The presence of such features in an otherwise typical case does not constitute grounds for rejecting the diagnosis, but it is in such circumstances that it is particularly desirable to have other supporting evidence, in particular CSF oligoclonal bands or multiple lesions detected by evoked potentials or imaging.

Remission

A definite improvement of signs and/or symptoms that has been present for at least 24 hours is called a remission for the purpose of these criteria. A remission must last at least 1 month to be considered significant.

Separate lesions

Separate signs and/or symptoms must not be explicable on the basis of a single lesion. Difficulty is often encountered clinically when patients present, for example, with an undoubted brainstem lesion producing acute vertigo but associated a week or two later with sensory or motor disturbance in the limbs which could be due to an extension of the original lesion, or to the development of a separate lesion in the spinal cord. In these circumstances, loss of a tendon jerk (provided there is no evidence of a peripheral cause) indicating involvement of the intramedullary portion of the afferents may be helpful. Difficulty may be encountered with optic neuritis when the second eye is affected: if this occurs within 2 weeks of the first, convention has it that there is then only a single lesion. Sequential involvement of the optic nerves at longer intervals constitutes multiple lesions, but since occasional patients are seen who have many attacks of optic neuritis without developing clinical evidence of more widely disseminated lesions even after many years, multiple sclerosis is not diagnosed under these circumstances (Parkin, Hierons and McDonald, 1984).

Laboratory support
In the classification which follows this term is used to refer only to evidence, obtained from the cerebrospinal fluid, of immunological abnormality in relation to the central nervous system, i.e. oligoclonal bands in the absence of such bands in the serum, and increased production of IgG. Assays of myelin basic protein in cerebrospinal fluid have some place in the assessment of activity of disease, but the abnormalities are not specific to demyelination (Palfreyman *et al.*, 1978, 1979; Thompson *et al.*, 1985). Other procedures such as evoked potential studies and imaging are regarded as an extension of the clinical examination.

The criteria

There are two groups of cases, *definite* and *probable*, each with two subgroups, *clinical* and *laboratory-supported* (*Table 1.1*). As already stressed, these criteria were designed for research protocols and therefore exclude the less definite cases which are discussed below. It is self evident that under all circumstances there must be no other cause for the symptoms, signs or abnormal results of investigations.

Table 1.1 New diagnostic criteria for multiple sclerosis (Poser *et al.*, 1983, 1984)

Category	Attacks	Clinical evidence	Paraclinical evidence		Cerebrospinal fluid OB/IgG
Clinically definite multiple sclerosis					
1	2	2			
2	2	1	and	1	
Laboratory supported definite multiple sclerosis					
1	2	1	or	1	+
2	1	2			+
3	1	1	and	1	+
Clinically probable multiple sclerosis					
1	2	1			
2	1	2			
3	1	1	and	1	
Laboratory supported probable multiple sclerosis					
1	2				+

OB: oligoclonal bands

CLINICALLY DEFINITE MULTIPLE SCLEROSIS
(1) Two attacks and clinical evidence of two separate lesions.
(2) Two attacks, clinical evidence of one and paraclinical evidence of another separate lesion.

Comment
The two attacks must involve different parts of the central nervous system, must each last a minimum of 24 hours and be separated by a period of at least 1 month.

Certain symptoms provide clear evidence of anatomical localization, and provided the information is deemed to be reliable, they may be substituted for evidence obtained from physical examination for one of the lesions. Examples include trigeminal neuralgia in a patient under the age of 40 years, and Lhermitte's symptom in a patient under the age of 50 years, provided there is no evidence of an independent local cause. Other possible substitutions are discussed by Poser *et al.* (1984) but extreme caution must be used in making them.

Paraclinical evidence of lesions may be provided from electrophysiological procedures including evoked potentials and stimulation of motor cortex (Cowan *et al.*, 1984) and imaging procedures (*see* Chapter 2).

LABORATORY-SUPPORTED DEFINITE MULTIPLE SCLEROSIS
(1) Two attacks, either clinical or paraclinical evidence of one lesion and cerebrospinal fluid oligoclonal bands.
(2) One attack, clinical evidence of two separate lesions and cerebrospinal fluid oligoclonal bands.
(3) One attack, clinical evidence of one and paraclinical evidence of another separate lesion, and cerebrospinal fluid oligoclonal bands.

Comment
The two attacks must involve different parts of the central nervous system, each have lasted at least 24 hours and be separated by a minimum of 1 month. One of the episodes must involve a part of the central nervous system distinct from that demonstrated on clinical examination or on paraclinical evidence. Historical information cannot be substituted for clinical evidence. Whether the evidence is clinical or paraclinical both lesions must not have been present at the time of the first examination and must be separated in time by a period of at least 1 month. This separation in time is designed to minimize the risk of including cases of acute disseminated encephalomyelitis.

Patients with steadily progressive symptoms from onset may be included in this category provided that the evidence (clinical or paraclinical) of the second lesion (e.g. a delayed visual evoked potential in a patient with progressive spastic paraplegia) was not present at presentation. If it was present then, the case is acceptable as multiple sclerosis only if progression has taken place for at least 6 months. The problem of progressive spastic paraplegia is further discussed below.

CLINICALLY PROBABLE MULTIPLE SCLEROSIS
(1) Two attacks and clinical evidence of one lesion.
(2) One attack and clinical evidence of two separate lesions.
(3) One attack, clinical evidence of one lesion and paraclinical evidence of another, separate lesion.

Comment

The two attacks must involve separate parts of the central nervous system. Historical information cannot be substituted for abnormal physical signs. The restrictions discussed under laboratory-supported definite multiple sclerosis also apply.

LABORATORY-SUPPORTED PROBABLE MULTIPLE SCLEROSIS
(1) Two attacks and CSF oligoclonal bands.

Comment

The two attacks must involve different parts of the central nervous system, each have lasted at least 24 hours and be separated by a minimum of 1 month.

Experience with nuclear magnetic resonance imaging (NMR or NMRI) has already made it clear that the detection of new lesions by serial scanning (with the precautions discussed in Chapter 2) promises to make a substantial difference to the confidence with which patients can be classified, and the length of time for which they need be followed before being reclassified into a more definite category.

SPECIAL PROBLEMS

A significant number of patients whom the neurologist sees is not covered by the Poser criteria. The proper handling of such patients requires a knowledge of the risk of developing the clinically disseminated disease.

Optic neuritis

Acute unilateral optic neuritis in adults is one of the commonest manifestations of demyelinating disease. It is characterized clinically by the rapid development of visual loss, usually accompanied by pain which is increased by eye movement. The visual impairment usually progresses over a matter of a few days or a week or two, persists for 3–4 weeks and then resolves over a period of 2–3 months. Recovery to 6/9 (20/30) or better occurs in 90% of patients (Gould *et al.*, 1977; McDonald, 1983). A central scotoma at the height of the visual loss is usual but a variety of other defects including sectorial loss and arcuate scotomata may be found, especially during the earlier stages and during resolution. The optic disc is swollen in rather less than 50% of patients and haemorrhages are rare. These features help to distinguish optic neuritis from other conditions with which it may be confused (such as ischaemic optic neuropathy, central serous retinopathy, and tumour) which must be carefully excluded.

The risk of developing multiple sclerosis after optic neuritis has been better studied than after other isolated lesions. Optic neuritis is the presenting feature in approximately 20% of cases of multiple sclerosis and occurs during the course of the illness in about 75% (*see* review by Shibasaki, McDonald and Kuroiwa, 1981). Estimates of the risk of developing multiple sclerosis vary widely, being influenced, among other things, by latitude (*see* review by McDonald, 1983). A recent estimate in Massachusetts puts the overall risk at 35%. In the UK the risk is higher, probably reaching at least 75% (McDonald, 1983; D. Francis *et al.*, unpublished observations). There is evidence for the existence of several factors influencing the risk of developing multiple sclerosis. They include age and sex (Cohen, Lessell and Wolf, 1979), the presence of HLA-DR2*, and winter onset in HLA-DR2 positive individuals (Compston *et al.*, 1978). Since the HLA effect is not absolute, however, routine typing is not indicated. The presence of oligoclonal bands in the cerebrospinal fluid also increases the risk of subsequent development of multiple sclerosis (Moulin *et al.*, 1983).

Acute simultaneously bilateral optic neuritis is uncommon in adult life. Some cases undoubtedly do go on to develop the clinically disseminated disease but most do not, even after 30 years (Parkin, Hierons and McDonald, 1984).

Progressive visual failure is usually due to tumour, but is occasionally the presenting feature of multiple sclerosis (Ormerod and McDonald, 1984). It should not, however, be regarded as such without careful exclusion of compression and long-term follow-up.

In childhood, acute bilateral optic neuritis is more often recognized than unilateral optic neuritis, partly perhaps because young children may show no behavioural deficit with visual loss confined to one eye. Long-term follow-up of bilateral cases shows that the risk of developing multiple sclerosis is low, though it may be higher after unilateral optic neuritis (Kennedy and Carter, 1961; Parkin, Hierons and McDonald, 1984).

The finding of other neurological abnormalities (clinical or paraclinical) at presentation raises the question of multiple sclerosis. The yield from somato-sensory and brainstem auditory evoked potentials is generally rather low (Matthews, 1978; Sanders, Roylan and Hogenhuis, 1984; Matthews, 1985). The yield from NMRI is higher (Ormerod *et al.*, 1985; Chapter 2) but until follow-up has established the risk of developing the clinically disseminated disease in patients with multiple lesions at presentation, such cases should not be classified as multiple sclerosis unless serial follow-up has provided unequivocal evidence for the development of new lesions. Opinion is divided over the need for lumbar puncture in isolated optic neuritis. We do not perform it routinely, the decision depending on the clinical picture in the individual patient.

Acute brainstem lesions

Symptoms of acute brainstem disturbance such as vertigo, diplopia and trigeminal neuralgia occur in the course of multiple sclerosis in the majority of patients and are the presenting feature in about 15% (Shibasaki, McDonald and Kuroiwa, 1981). The time course of evolution and the prognosis for remission are similar to those for optic neuritis. There has been neither a prospective study of the risk of developing multiple sclerosis after lesions of this kind, nor an assessment of risk factors. However, Fielder *et al.* (1981) found a significant association with HLA-DR2 when groups of patients with isolated brainstem or spinal cord lesions were analyzed together. As in optic neuritis, the incidence of evoked potential abnormalities at remote sites (spinal cord and optic nerve) is low and the incidence of supratentorial abnormalities at NMRI high – approximately 68% (*see* Chapter

---

*Our investigation was carried out before international agreement on HLA nomenclature was reached. The association that we observed was with a locally definite antigen named BT101. This proved to be equivalent to DR2, but with some cross reaction with DRw1 and DRw6. For our present purpose, however, the two can be regarded as equivalent.

2). It therefore seems likely that the risk of developing multiple sclerosis following an acute brainstem lesion may be similar to that following optic neuritis, but the point is not established and the caveats about interpretation of additional lesions at presentation of optic neuritis apply.

Spinal cord syndromes

Acute or sub-acute sensory, motor or sphincter disturbances similar in time course and outcome to that of optic neuritis and attributable to partial lesions of the spinal cord are the presenting feature in at least one-third of patients with multiple sclerosis (Shibasaki, McDonald and Kuroiwa, 1981). Again there has been no satisfactory assessment of the risks of developing multiple sclerosis after such episodes. The HLA association is discussed under acute brainstem lesions. Visual and auditory evoked potentials and NMRI may provide evidence of additional lesions, but as in the case of optic neuritis the significance of their existence at presentation still has to be determined by systematic follow-up.

The situation appears to be rather different for cases of acute transverse myelitis in which a more or less complete cord lesion is accompanied by reflex loss and a high cell count in the CSF. The incidence of multiple sclerosis in such cases appears to be much lower – 10% (*see* review by Poser, 1984). The association of such a syndrome with acute bilateral optic neuritis is sometimes referred to as Devic's disease, although the evidence that it is pathologically distinct from multiple sclerosis is unconvincing (Allen, 1984).

Progressive spastic paraplegia of middle life presents a special problem. Multiple sclerosis is a common cause of this syndrome (Marshall, 1955; Poser, 1984) and the demonstration of abnormalities in the visual evoked potential, oligoclonal bands in the cerebrospinal fluid and multiple lesions at NMRI all provide strong support for the diagnosis, particularly when clear evidence is obtained for the appearance of new lesions after the first assessment. This evidence cannot however exclude cord compression, and when there is evidence of a fairly circumscribed level of abnormality, or when the results of any of the investigations have atypical features, myelography should be performed. We have seen a patient with undelayed but nevertheless abnormal visual evoked potentials who had an Arnold Chiari malformation. Improvement in NMRI technology can be expected to reduce the number of myelograms which are necessary.

APPROACH TO THE PATIENT SUSPECTED OF HAVING MULTIPLE SCLEROSIS

Several principles should influence the plan of action when the neurologist is confronted by a patient suspected of having multiple sclerosis. First, an attempt should be made to reach a diagnosis on clinical grounds. When the criteria for clinically definite multiple sclerosis are fulfilled and all the features are characteristic of the disease, laboratory investigation is unnecessary except in those patients who wish to have the added confidence that it may bring. Second, when there is insufficient evidence to make a definite diagnosis on clinical grounds alone additional lesions should be sought by electrophysiological and imaging techniques, and the presence or absence of an immunological abnormality in relation to the central nervous system established by cerebrospinal fluid electrophoresis. Third, elaborate and expensive investigations should be avoided unless there are clear indications for them. That said, the neurologist should not shrink from appropriate contrast studies if compression or angioma are a material possibility.

In patients with acute isolated lesions evidence of asymptomatic affection of other parts of the central white matter may be sought along the lines described above. Since as already mentioned the finding of additional lesions, or of oligoclonal bands in the cerebrospinal fluid, does not carry therapeutic implications and the data cannot at present lead to a definite prognosis in the individual patient, we do not fully investigate all such patients routinely. The same can be said of tests to confirm the presence of the isolated lesion, e.g. the visual evoked potential in optic neuritis. However, because the risk of misdiagnosis is appreciable in the monosymptomatic patient, we do usually carry out these confirmatory procedures. If the findings are atypical, then further investigation is indicated.

The chronically progressive isolated lesion always requires systematic investigation to exclude compression, and even if the results are negative the patient should be followed until the diagnosis is established.

Timing of investigation

The timing of investigation is influenced by a number of factors. The patient with an isolated lesion should be assessed in the acute stage, although in optic neuritis the visual evoked potential is more usefully recorded when acuity is recovering. Some patients are more comfortable, however, with a full investigation even after an isolated episode. As far as patients with recurring episodes of neurological disturbance are concerned, the appropriate time for full investigation is usually when it is clear to the patient that the illness is continuing and requires explanation.

References

ALLEN, I. M. (1984) Demyelinating diseases. In *Greenfield's Neuropathology*, 4th edn., edited by J. H. Adams, J. A. N. Corselis and L. W. Duchen, pp. 338–384. London: Edward Arnold

CHARCOT, J.-M. (1868) Histologie de la sclérose en plaques. *Gazette Hôpital, Paris*, **41**, 554–555, 557–558, 566

COHEN, M. M., LESSELL, S. and WOLF, P. A. (1979) A prospective study of the risk of developing multiple sclerosis in uncomplicated optic neuritis. *Neurology* (Minneapolis), **29**, 208–213

COMPSTON, D. A. S., BATCHELOR, J. R., EARL, C. J. and McDONALD, W. I. (1978) Factors influencing the risk of multiple sclerosis developing in patients with optic neuritis. *Brain*, **101**, 495–511

COWAN, J. A., ROTHWELL, J. C., DICK, J. P. R., THOMPSON, P. D., DAY, B. L. and MARSDEN, C. D. (1984) Abnormalities in central pathway conduction in multiple sclerosis. *Lancet*, **2**, 304–307

FIELDER, A. H. L., BATCHELOR, J. R., NASON VAKARELIS, B., COMPSTON, D. A. S. and McDONALD, W. I. (1981) Optic neuritis and multiple sclerosis: do factor B alleles influence progression of disease? *Lancet*, **1**, 1246–1248

FRISÉN, L. and HOYT, W. F. (1974) Insidious atrophy of retinal nerve fibres in multiple sclerosis. *Archives of Ophthalmology*, **92**, 91–97

FRISÉN, L., HOYT, W. F., BIRD, A. C. and WEALE, R. A. (1973) Diagnostic uses of the Pulfrich phenomenon. *Lancet*, **2**, 385

GOULD, E. S., BIRD, A. C., LEAVER, P. K. and McDONALD, W. I. (1977) Treatment of optic neuritis by retrobulbar injection of triamcinolone. *British Medical Journal*, **1**, 1495–1497

KENNEDY, C. and CARTER, S. (1961) Relation of optic neuritis to multiple sclerosis in children. *Pediatrics*, **28**, 377–387

McDONALD, W. I. (1983) The significance of optic neuritis. *Transactions of the Ophthalmological Societies of the United Kingdom*, **103**, 230–246

MARSHALL, J. (1955) Spastic paraplegia of middle age. A clinicopathological study. *Lancet*, **1**, 643–646

MATTHEWS, W. B. (1975) Paroxysmal disorders in multiple sclerosis. *Journal of Neurology, Neurosurgery and Psychiatry*, **38**, 617–623

MATTHEWS, W. B. (1978) Somatosensory evoked potentials in retrobulbar neuritis. *Lancet*, **1**, 443

MATTHEWS, W. B. (1985) Laboratory diagnosis. In *McAlpine's Multiple Sclerosis*, 4th edn. by W. B. Matthews, E. D. Acheson, J. R. Batchelor and R. O. Weller, edited by W. B. Matthews, pp. 167–209. Edinburgh: Churchill Livingstone

MOULIN, D., PATY, D. W. and EBERS, G. C. (1983) The predictive value of cerebrospinal fluid electrophoresis in 'possible' multiple sclerosis. *Brain*, **106**, 809–816

NOSEWORTHY, J., PATY, D. W., WONNACOTT, T., FEASBY, T. and EBERS, G. (1983) Multiple sclerosis after age 50. *Neurology*, **33**, 1537–1544

ORMEROD, I. E. C. and McDONALD, W. I. (1984) Multiple sclerosis presenting with progressive visual failure. *Journal of Neurology, Neurosurgery and Psychiatry*, **47**, 943–946

ORMEROD, I. E. C., McDONALD, W. I., DU BOULAY, G. H. *et al.* (1985) Disseminated lesions at presentation in patients with optic neuritis. *Journal of Neurology, Neurosurgery and Psychiatry* (in press)

PALFREYMAN, J. W., JOHNSTON, R. V., RATCLIFF, J. G., THOMAS, D. G. T. and FORBES, C. D. (1979) Radioimmunoassay of serum myelin basic protein and its application to patients with cerebrovascular accident. *Clinica Chimica Acta*, **92**, 403–409

PALFREYMAN, J. W., THOMAS, D. G. T. and RATCLIFF, J. G. (1978) Radioimmunoassay of human myelin basic protein in tissue extract, cerebrospinal fluid and serum and its clinical application to patients with head injury. *Clinica Chimica Acta*, **82**, 259–270

PARKIN, P. J., HIERONS, R. and McDONALD, W. I. (1984) Bilateral optic neuritis. A long-term follow up. *Brain*, **107**, 951–964

POSER, C. M. (1984) Taxonomy and diagnostic parameters in multiple sclerosis. *Annals of the New York Academy of Sciences*, **436**, 233–245

POSER, C. M., PATY, D. W., McDONALD, W. I., SCHEINBERG, L. and EBERS, G. C. (EDS) (1984) *The Diagnosis of Multiple Sclerosis*. New York: Thieme-Stratton Inc.

POSER, C. M., PATY, D. W., SCHEINBERG, L. *et al.* (1983) New diagnostic criteria for multiple sclerosis: guidelines for research proposals. *Annals of Neurology*, **13**, 227–231

SANDERS, E. A. C. M., ROYLAN, J. P. H. and HOGENHUIS, L. (1984) Central nervous system involvement in optic neuritis. *Journal of Neurology, Neurosurgery and Psychiatry*, **47**, 241–249

SCHUMACHER, G. A., BEEBE, G. W., KIBLER, R. F. *et al.* (1965) Problems of experimental trials of therapy in multiple sclerosis. *Annals of the New York Academy of Sciences*, **122**, 552–568

SHIBASAKI, H., McDONALD, W. I. and KUROIWA, Y. (1981) Racial modification of clinical picture of multiple sclerosis: comparison between British and Japanese patients. *Journal of the Neurological Sciences*, **49**, 253–271

THOMPSON, A. J., BRAZIL, J., FEIGHERY, C. *et al.* (1985) Cerebrospinal fluid myelin basic protein in multiple sclerosis. *Acta Neurologica Scandinavica* (in press)

2
Imaging of multiple sclerosis
I. E. C. Ormerod, G. H. du Boulay and W. I. McDonald

The primary purpose of imaging the central nervous system (CNS) in multiple sclerosis (MS) has been to assist in the diagnosis. At first, only secondary changes such as cerebral or spinal cord atrophy could be demonstrated, but the introduction of scanning methods has permitted imaging of the lesions themselves. A variety of techniques has been used, the most sensitive being nuclear magnetic resonance imaging (NMRI). Problems of specificity and quantitation remain to be solved, but already the form and distribution of abnormalities observed in an appropriate clinical setting may be decisive in reaching a diagnosis of MS.

In this chapter we review the role of the various imaging techniques available in the assessment of patients with MS, and indicate future developments which may be of value.

EARLY TECHNIQUES

Pneumoencephalography

Prior to the introduction of scanning techniques the ability to demonstrate abnormalities in the CNS of patients with MS was limited. X-ray techniques relying on air or iodine-containing contrast media were unable to demonstrate the presence of individual lesions. Pneumoencephalography was used to demonstrate ventricular enlargement and cortical atrophy in MS (Freeman and Cohen, 1945), but it did not permit a distinction between the many causes of cerebral atrophy. It now has no place in the assessment of patients with MS.

Myelography

Myelography can similarly demonstrate atrophy of the cord in established MS. Acute lesions, for example those producing the clinical syndrome of transverse myelitis, may be associated with expansion of the cord (Haughton, Ho and Boe-Decker, 1979) which may be confused with an intramedullary mass lesion due to tumour or haemorrhage. Such acute swelling, in which oedema presumably plays an important part, may be shown to subside subsequently by myelography. Reversible spinal cord swelling can also be seen occasionally in subacute progressive spinal paraparesis in patients who later develop clinically definite MS (Feasby *et al.*, 1981).

RADIO-NUCLIDE BRAIN SCANNING

The first method of imaging the brain itself in MS was isotopic brain scanning and the first abnormal scan was published in 1954 (Seaman, Ter-Pogossian and Schwartz, 1954). A review of 160 patients reported in 1974 (Antunes, Schlesinger and Michelsen, 1974) showed positive scans in only three. The low spatial resolution of the technique partly explains this. In addition, leakage of isotope through the blood–brain barrier (upon which the visible abnormality of the scan depends), may only occur in the acute phase, a suggestion supported by the finding of abnormal isotope scans in three patients who also had contrast enhancing areas on CT scanning (Aita, 1978). Further confirmation was obtained by serial scanning of patients, when return to a normal appearance occured with time (Cohan, Fermaglich and Auth, 1975), presumably as the damaged blood–brain barrier regained its integrity. *Figure 2.1* shows an abnormal isotope scan in MS, with a region of uptake in the cerebral hemisphere.

POSITRON EMISSION TOMOGRAPHY (PET)

Recently, metabolic data have been obtained from the application of sophisticated developments of radio-nuclide brain scanning, for example PET.

PET has been used to obtain images of the brain in MS employing the positron emitting isotope ^{15}O. Brooks *et al.* (1984) recently applied this technique (Ter-Pogossian *et al.*, 1969; Frackowiak *et al.*, 1980) to obtain images of regional cerebral blood flow, oxygen extraction fraction and oxygen utilization in 15 patients with MS, comparing their findings with an age-matched control group (*Figure 2.2*). They found that cerebral blood flow and oxygen utilization in both cerebral cortex and deep cerebral white matter were reduced in their patients and that this generalized reduction correlated well with CT evidence of atrophy. However, the oxygen extraction fraction was the same in both groups, suggesting that, within the limit of the spatial resolution of the technique, there were no zones of focal cerebral ischaemia in the MS group. No correlation was found with locomotor dysfunction, but a significant association existed between cognitive function and cortical oxygen utilization. The lowest levels of oxygen utilization were associated with the greatest deterioration in IQ.

The absence of evidence of regional ischaemia and the association of cerebral atrophy with abnormalities in the PET scans led the authors to conclude that their results reflected an increased volume of 'non-functioning brain tissue' rather than a reduction in oxygen usage by intact neurons and that cerebral function, as assessed by this method, would be the same in both groups if equal volumes of intact neuronal tissue were to be compared.

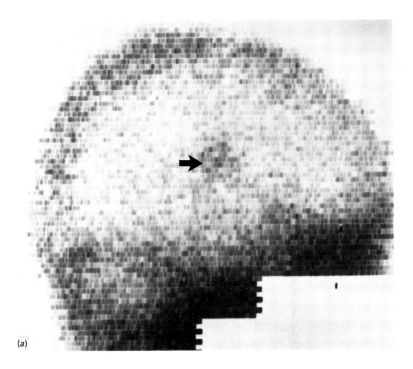

(a)

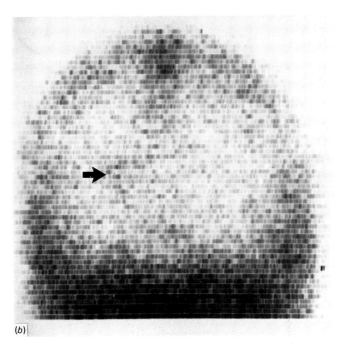

(b)

Figure 2.1 Isotope scan showing an area of abnormal uptake (arrowed) in the right cerebral hemisphere, on the (*a*) lateral and (*b*) antero-posterior images

14

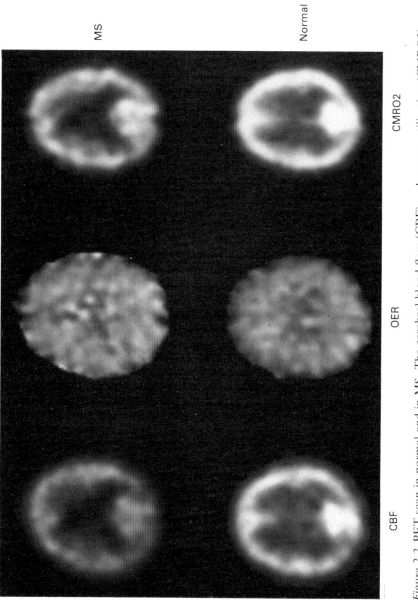

Figure 2.2 PET scan in normal and in MS. The cerebral blood flow (CBF) and oxygen utilization (CMRO2) are reduced in MS, but the oxygen extraction fraction (OER) is unchanged. There is no evidence of regional ischaemia. (From Brooks *et al.*, 1984, courtesy of the Editor and Publisher *Journal of Neurology, Neurosurgery and Psychiatry*)

While this technique offers some insight into the metabolic function of the brain, the present resolution of 1.7 cm limits its use since many individual plaques within the white matter will remain undetected. Moreover, as the authors pointed out, interpretation of data from cerebral cortex (approximately 5 mm thick) is hampered by inevitable partial volume effects from the adjacent white matter.

X-RAY CT SCANNING

It was not immediately accepted that MS could produce alterations in the brain detectable by computerized tomography (CT) scanning and general agreement on the type and frequency of abnormalities had to wait until high resolution, high efficiency CT scanners were widely available. The initial reports of cerebral atrophy, manifested as enlargement of the lateral ventricles in severe chronic MS, corresponded with what was already known of the disease from autopsy studies and from pneumoencephalography. The first report describing focal lesions in CT scans appeared in 1976 (Cala and Mastaglia, 1976); 19 patients with probable or definite disease were examined. Four showed atrophy and, in seven, discrete low attenuation lesions were seen in the deep cerebral white matter, around the ventricles, or both. It was subsequently reported that the margin of the lateral ventricles appeared somewhat ragged and irregular either focally or diffusely. In a large review, Gyldensted (1976) reported cerebral atrophy in more than three-quarters of his patients and found lesions, predominantly periventricular, in more than one-third.

Improved scanners and more sophisticated interpretation, aided by selective windowing of the images, showed that part of what had been thought at first to be lateral ventricular enlargement actually consisted of a 'halo' where the attenuation values were not quite as low as those of CSF. The halo consisted of numerous more or less rounded lesions of different sizes, together with more homogeneous amorphous regions — something in fact very like, though not generally as extensive as, the white areas now familiar from the spin-echo scans of nuclear magnetic resonance imaging. These changes around the lateral ventricles on CT scans could be confluent areas penetrating deep into the surrounding white matter, and were often strikingly symmetrical. Such an appearance, seen in over 20% in one series (Delouvrier *et al.*, 1980), was observed more often around the occipital horns than the frontal horns, in keeping with the known pathological distribution of lesions.

Some individual small rounded lesions were also seen well away from the lateral ventricles, most noticeably in the region of the corona radiata. Though a few of these isolated areas of low attenuation were large, many were small, no more than a few pixels (the smallest units from which the image is formed) in diameter. To confirm their existence, to try to provide further differential diagnostic information (usually fruitlessly) or because it is often routine, organic iodine contrast enhanced scans were made after the plain scans. Initial reports described no enhancement of the regions of low attenuation nor of the apparently normal brain (Gyldensted, 1976). However, in a few cases, sometimes when the patient was experiencing an acute neurological episode, one or more of these low attenuation regions were found to enhance (*Figure 2.3*), to be surrounded by enhancement (*Figure 2.4*), or both (Lindegaard *et al.*, 1983). In one series (Delouvrier *et al.*, 1980), 78% of the localized areas of contrast enhancement appeared in previously isodense areas of

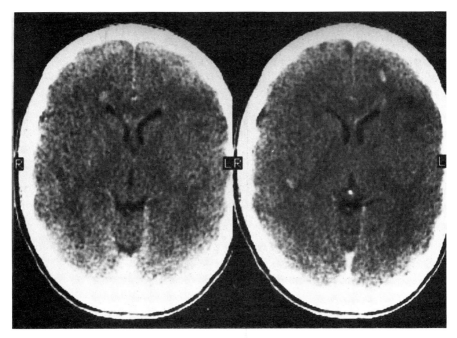

Figure 2.3 CT scan after iodine-containing contrast medium, demonstrating several areas of abnormal enhancement

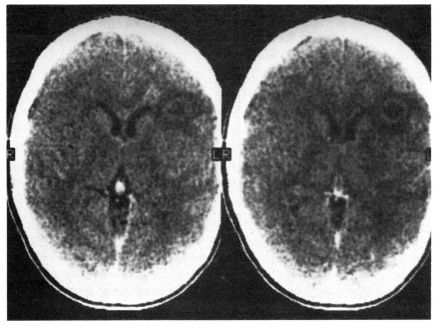

Figure 2.4 CT scan showing ring enhancement, after intravenous iodine-containing contrast medium

the brain. The pattern of contrast enhancement was also found to be variable, with a peripheral type of ring enhancement seen in some lesions, but in others a central area of enhancement was observed in a previously isodense region. These observations, together with those on radio-nuclide scanning, suggested that there was a reversible breakdown in the blood–brain barrier in the acute lesion. This interpretation was in keeping with an earlier report of staining of plaques by trypan blue injected post-mortem (Broman, 1964). A further report (Aita, 1978) established that contrast enhancement was reversible over a matter of days, or a week or two.

A recent development in CT scanning of MS has been the use of high-dose iodine-containing contrast medium and delayed scanning. The high volume delayed (HVD) scan was originally introduced for use in other intracranial diseases (Hayman, Evans and Hinck, 1979) but subsequent clinical studies in MS have shown the detection of enhancing lesions to be significantly increased. The previous studies on enhancing lesions in the white matter had shown an incidence of 9% (Hershey, Gado and Trotter, 1979) to 25% (Haughton *et al.*, 1979) but the cases in these series were not particularly selected to show acute lesions. Using the HVD technique and selecting patients with a high probability of acute lesions, nearly 75% (Vinuela *et al.*, 1982) demonstrated abnormal contrast enhancement. In addition, by this technique, lesions have been demonstrated not only in the cerebral white matter but also at the grey/white matter junction and in the cortical grey matter itself. These findings probably reflect not only the superiority of HVD technique but also the improvement in spatial resolution with the latest generation of CT scanning machines. A direct comparison of the delayed high dose iodine scan with a conventional low dose immediate scanning technique has also been made, with the two scans being performed on the same group of patients (Sears *et al.*, 1982). In total over twice as many lesions were demonstrated with the delayed technique and the size of the lesions and intensity of contrast enhancement of the lesions appeared significantly greater.

The increase in attenuation values after injection of intravenous contrast medium has been used to provide a measure of cerebral blood volume (Zilkha *et al.*, 1976). Change from normal is just detectable in some forms of cerebral atrophy, but the technique has not been used in MS. Another contrast agent is stable non-radioactive xenon gas, administered by inhalation. Xenon is highly soluble in fat and is also radiopaque. It can therefore be used both to map the distribution of lipid and to provide a CT scan based measurement of blood flow. As a lipid marker xenon has been employed in suspected MS to increase the visibility of lesions (Radue and Kendall, 1978), which appear as negative low-attenuation regions against the background of relatively high-attenuation white matter (*Figure 2.5*). The development of stable xenon CT blood flow maps is still in progress.

Most CT scans are made as axial sections: computer reformatting of contiguous thin axial sections into a sagittal or coronal plane has recently been practised, but with lesions so difficult to see such projections have not been widely used. For organizational as well as these technical reasons the distribution of lesions on sagittal and coronal CT reformatted sections has not been the subject of a detailed study. CT scanning of the cerebellar hemispheres is almost as satisfactory as that of the cerebrum and lesions have been seen there but the brainstem is almost always partly obscured by artefact so that only gross abnormalities can be detected reliably and CT scanning has thrown no light on the frequency or distribution of brainstem plaques.

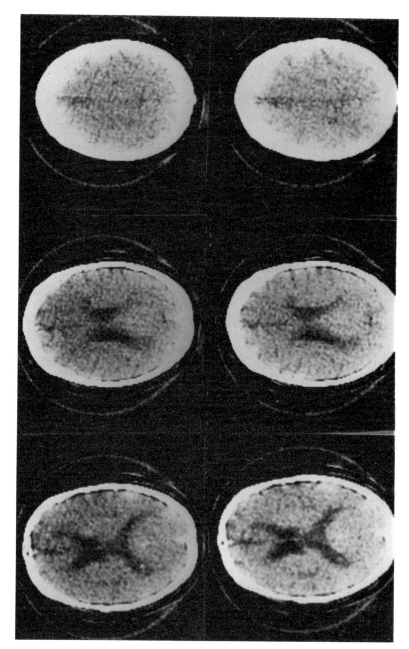

Figure 2.5 CT scans plain (above) and after xenon (below). In the xenon-enhanced scan the low attenuation areas around the ventricles are seen more clearly

There have been several reports of CT scanning in optic neuritis. An earlier report of low attenuation lesions in the optic nerves accompanying or following optic neuritis, or in established MS (Cala and Mastaglia, 1976) was received with some scepticism because of the problems that the partial volume effect must impose on optic nerve imaging. There is no agreement that isolated 'plaques' can be demonstrated in the optic nerve. Diffuse enlargement and contrast enhancement of the optic nerve in acute optic neuritis have been described in two patients (Osher and Tomsak, 1980). However, such changes are a non-specific finding and have been observed in a number of conditions, including tumours of the optic nerve sheath, papilloedema, Graves' disease, central retinal vein occlusion and acute Leber's optic neuropathy (Cabanis *et al.*, 1978).

Differential diagnosis and CT scanning

The CT changes in MS are not specific and can be seen in a variety of other disorders although the pattern and distribution of the abnormalities may give a guide to the diagnosis. The small isolated lesions in MS are difficult or impossible to distinguish from the lacunae of vascular disease. Occasionally the lesion of MS may resemble a tumour. Van der Valden, Bots and Endtz (1979) and Nelson *et al.* (1981) reported cases in which the scan demonstrated a single large low density area in the cerebral hemisphere, with ring enhancement, surrounding low attenuation suggestive of oedema and displacement of midline structures. In both instances a diagnosis of tumour was made initially, although biopsy of the lesion subsequently revealed the pathological changes of MS.

Rarely, poorly-defined low attenuation areas may be found around the ventricles in patients with increased cerebrospinal fluid pressure in the absence of other manifestations of hydrocephalus (Moseley and Radue, 1979).

The subcortical arteriosclerotic leukomalacia often associated with hypertension (which when associated with dementia is referred to as Binswanger's disease) (Rosenberg *et al.*, 1979) causes more evenly distributed white matter low attenuation, especially in the frontal lobes.

The familial leukoencephalopathies usually present in childhood. CT scans show diffuse, symmetrical low attenuation with cerebral atrophy (Kendall and Kingsley, 1980). The radiological features are not diagnostic but there are characteristics of distribution of maximum degeneration which are reflected in the CT scan appearances. In Krabbe's disease the white matter changes are diffuse. In adrenoleukodystrophy the occipital lobes are predominantly affected. Spongiform degeneration (Canavan's disease) may spare the internal capsules. In Alexander's disease the abnormalities are markedly frontal. In several of these conditions there may be abnormal enhancement, usually in bands around the margins of the most affected white matter. In Alexander's disease the enhancement may surround the ventricles but, unlike the pattern of MS, the basal ganglia enhance prominently. Alexander's and Canavan's diseases cause macrocephaly. Many of the mucopoly-saccharidoses and lipidoses result in diffuse low attenuation of the white matter.

Metachromatic leukodystrophy (which may first present in adult life) tends to affect first the frontal white matter. A diffuse leukoencephalopathy with correspondingly diffuse CT changes may accompany malignant neoplasia elsewhere in the body. A disseminated necrotizing leukoencephalopathy accompanies the treatment of conditions such as acute lymphatic leukaemia with methotrexate or other antimetabolic drugs with or without additional radiotherapy. This multifocal coagulative necrosis is maximal in the periventricular regions and if survival is prolonged, calcifications may be seen in the deepest parts of the white matter.

Spinal cord manifestations

CT scanning of the spinal cord is of little clinical value in MS because of the limited detail obtainable from the images. In severe and chronic cases plain CT, or CT myelography, show cord atrophy. In cases of transverse myelitis in the acute phase the cord may be swollen.

Summary

CT scanning provides a good technique for the assessment of overall atrophy and ventricular enlargement in patients with MS and also for the detection of specific focal lesions. That the latter do indeed correspond to MS plaques has been confirmed by biopsy and post-mortem examination (Lebow *et al.*, 1978; Haughton *et al.*, 1979). On the plain scans lesions appear as areas of low attenuation, irrespective of their age. However, using contrast agents, enhancement may be seen in acute lesions. Using higher doses of contrast media and delayed scanning times the incidence of such enhancing areas is increased. Enhancement probably represents breakdown of the blood–brain barrier. The CT scan abnormalities in MS thus have essentially three forms – atrophy, low attenuation areas and localized contrast enhancement – which may occur alone or in combination. CT scanning has become a recognized adjunctive diagnostic method for MS. A positive finding may aid diagnosis in difficult cases but a negative finding is unhelpful.

MS AND NUCLEAR MAGNETIC RESONANCE IMAGING (NMRI) (MAGNETIC RESONANCE IMAGING, MRI)

Although improvements in CT scanning have increased the ability to detect the lesions in MS, even the more advanced CT systems remain rather insensitive. Recently published criteria for the diagnosis of MS (Poser *et al.*, 1983) include investigative evidence of asymptomatic lesions. It is here that NMRI has shown itself to be a powerful new technique. The first report of its use in MS came from Hammersmith Hospital, London (Young *et al.*, 1981). Ten patients with MS were studied, eight of whom were clinically definite and two probable. CT scans were performed with and without intravenous contrast; a total of 19 lesions was apparent. The NMRI scans revealed not only these 19 lesions but 112 more. These important findings have since been widely confirmed (e.g. Crooks *et al.*, 1982).

NMR technique

Clinical NMRI is mainly based on the study of hydrogen nuclei (protons) because of their natural abundance and their high NMR signal. The principle can in theory be applied to any nuclei with an odd number of either protons or neutrons or both, because such nuclei have magnetic properties. When nuclei of this kind are placed in a magnetic field they align themselves with it. If electromagnetic radiation of appropriate frequency (in the radiofrequency range for clinically useful systems) is introduced, the nuclei are displaced from their alignment with the magnetic field. Having been disturbed the nuclei generate a signal which can be detected in a receiver coil. When the radiofrequency (RF) pulse ends, the nuclei return to their initial positions, the rate of return being determined by two time constants, T_1 and T_2. T_1 is the longitudinal (spin-lattice) relaxation time and reflects the rate of loss of energy of excited nuclei to the surrounding atoms. T_2 is the transverse relaxation time and is dependent on the rate at which the excited nuclei exchange energy with each other and in so doing become dephased, thereby causing the RF signal to decay. The signal obtained is determined by the number of protons present (proton density) and the values of T_1 and T_2. The pulse sequences used in NMRI are designed to exploit differences between T_1 and T_2 to generate contrast between different tissues in normal and pathological states. In normal brain, white matter has a shorter T_1 and T_2 than grey matter and, in addition, has a lower proton density. CSF has a longer T_1 and T_2 than either white or grey matter of brain.

Pulse sequences

A number of different types of images can be produced by the various pulse sequences. The two main sequences are inversion recovery (IR) and spin-echo (SE). Both are dependent on the proton density but the pulse-timing intervals are arranged to emphasize differences in T_1 in the former and, in the latter, differences in T_2 (*Figure 2.6*). The use of one of these sequences with inappropriate pulse-timing intervals will reduce or even abolish its ability to detect lesions by diminishing the contrast between normal and abnormal tissue. Recent experience has led to some agreement on the appropriate pulse-timing intervals at particular field strengths.

The initial report of the NMRI findings in MS (Young *et al.*, 1981) was based only on the IR technique. The lesions were of increased T_1 relative to brain and appeared as areas of low signal intensity (black). However, with the IR sequence the CSF within the ventricles is also of low signal and this can lead to diagnostic confusion between small lesions around the ventricles (a common site) and partial volume effects. SE sequences were subsequently introduced (*Figure 2.7*) and were found to be particularly useful (Brant-Zawadski *et al.*, 1983; Lukes *et al.*, 1983).

Ideally, with the SE sequences, the pulse intervals should be timed to make CSF of lower signal than brain, and lesions of higher signal than either brain or CSF. When this is done the lesions appear as white areas around black ventricles, making discrimination between normal and abnormal tissue easier. It was also found that in many instances the SE sequence was more sensitive than the IR in detecting the lesions of MS, although the SE sequence in general revealed less anatomical detail. The detection of lesions with the SE sequences is mainly due to the increased T_2 of the lesions relative to the surrounding brain, although there are accompanying increases in measured proton density which also influence the signal.

Abnormalities in MS

The abnormalities have a different appearance with the two main pulse sequences now in use; they appear black with IR, and usually as white areas with SE. The

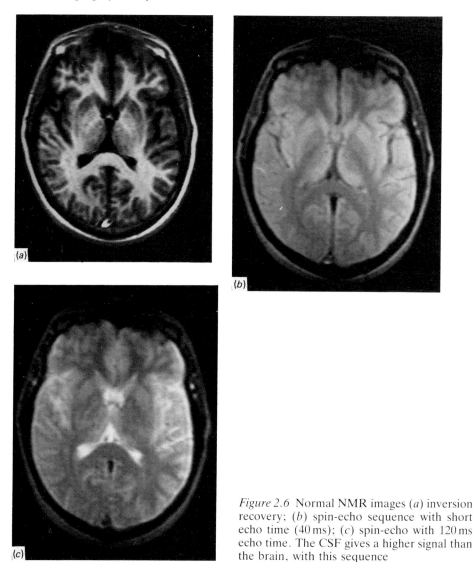

Figure 2.6 Normal NMR images (*a*) inversion recovery; (*b*) spin-echo sequence with short echo time (40 ms); (*c*) spin-echo with 120 ms echo time. The CSF gives a higher signal than the brain, with this sequence

distribution of the lesions seen on scans in living patients has not yet been confirmed at necropsy in an individual case but the pattern is similar to that described pathologically (Lumsden, 1970), and following Stewart *et al.* (1984) we have scanned brains at post-mortem and found a similar distribution of abnormalities which have been confirmed as typical of MS histologically (Scaravilli, Ormerod and McDonald, unpublished observations).

Periventricular lesions are almost universally found and are most marked at the occipital horns and trigones, but also are present along the bodies of the ventricles and around the frontal and temporal horns. We have observed these lesions in 69 out of 70 patients with clinically definite MS and in a recent review of 41 patients (Runge *et al.*, 1984) they were present in all. In the latter studies the trigones were

23

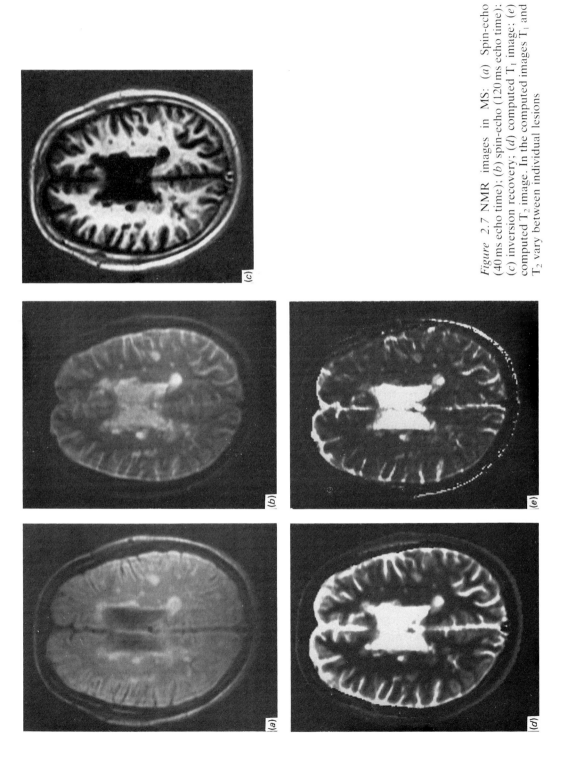

Figure 2.7 NMR images in MS: (*a*) Spin-echo (40 ms echo time); (*b*) spin-echo (120 ms echo time); (*c*) inversion recovery; (*d*) computed T_1 image; (*e*) computed T_2 image. In the computed images T_1 and T_2 vary between individual lesions

involved in every patient and the ventricular bodies and the frontal and occipital horns were involved in the majority (86%, 97% and 92% respectively); the temporal horns were affected in only 32%. Discrete lesions within the white matter were also frequently seen, most commonly in the supraventricular region (84%). Brainstem lesions were seen in 30% and cerebellar lesions were seen in 7%. The lesions in general appear more clearly defined with the IR technique, particularly around the ventricles, but are often more extensive on the SE sequences. This study and others (Lukes *et al.*, 1983) confirmed the increased sensitivity of the SE images over IR for demonstrating the abnormalities in the cerebrum and cerebellum in MS, although brainstem lesions may be better visualized with IR sequences. As previously mentioned, however, the appearance is influenced by the pulse-timing intervals used (Johnson *et al.*, 1984).

There is a wide variation in measured T_1 and T_2 of lesions in any one subject which may be so great that examination by a single set of pulse-timing intervals, particularly when SE sequences are being used, may result in some lesions being missed. If an attempt is being made to determine the distribution of lesions throughout the brain, a range of sequences may be necessary, particularly when quantitation of the amount of abnormal tissue is needed, for example in monitoring therapy (*see below*). The pathological significance of this variation in T_1 and T_2 is not yet established. It may reflect the age of lesions, as in general an increase in T_1 and T_2 would be expected to occur in association with an increased amount of unbound water, corresponding to the oedema of the more acute lesions. Some evidence for this view has been obtained recently from a comparison of serial observations on patients with acute and chronic brainstem lesions (Ormerod and Rudge, unpublished observations) and from a study of the evolution of cold-induced lesions in the cerebral hemispheres of the cat (Barnes, McDonald and Landon, unpublished observations).

NMRI is particularly useful in imaging in the posterior fossa (*Figure 2.8*) where the absence of bone artefact and the ability to scan directly in axial, sagittal (*Figure 2.9*) and coronal planes, combined with its inherent sensitivity in detecting abnormalities in MS make it superior to X-ray CT. In 70 patients with MS, we found cerebellar lesions in 32 and brainstem lesions in 41, a higher incidence than that found by Runge *et al.* (1984), but in keeping with the clinical picture of MS (Shibasaki, McDonald and Kuroiwa, 1981). The brainstem lesions are commoner in the pons than in the medulla or mid-brain and are often contiguous with the fourth ventricle or aqueduct, sometimes extending the whole length of these structures.

Examination of the cervical spinal cord has been rather more difficult, due in part to its relatively small size and the higher resolution required. However, the low signal from cortical bone and capacity for direct imaging in different planes are advantageous. Surface coils have been of some value in improving the signal to noise ratio on the images within a defined volume. Maravilla *et al.* (1984) have reported abnormalities in the cervical cord similar in distribution to the lesions reported in the classical pathological descriptions of Cruveilhier (1835–1842). They studied 21 patients with MS, all of whom had abnormalities in the cervical spinal cord. The use of thinner 'sections' and surface coils may increase the detection rate of lesions. The longitudinal arrangement of the lesions at post-mortem suggests that sagittal or coronal cuts would be more likely to be helpful than axial cuts. Imaging of the thoracic cord is considerably more difficult because of its even smaller size and the presence of artefact produced by respiratory and cardiac movement.

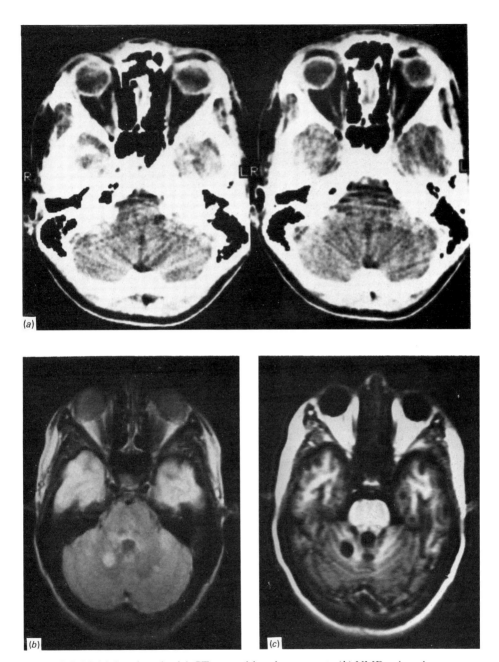

Figure 2.8 Multiple sclerosis. (*a*) CT scan with enhancement; (*b*) NMR spin-echo sequence; (*c*) NMR inversion recovery sequence; all the images are from the same patient. The CT scan is normal. The NMR scans shows a large lesion in the right cerebellar hemisphere

26

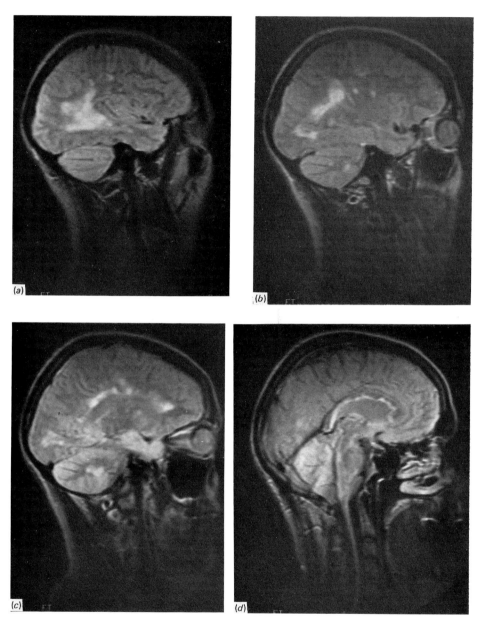

Figure 2.9 NMR scans in MS. A series of images in the sagittal plane from left (*a*) to the midline (*d*). There is extensive periventricular involvement with the lesions extending into the cerebral white matter. The corpus callosum is diffusely affected

Studies on 'isolated' neurological lesions

When patients present with acute, apparently isolated, lesions of the type seen in MS, e.g. optic neuritis, it is of considerable interest to know whether the abnormalities are truly isolated or whether there are additional, asymptomatic lesions elsewhere in the central white matter. That such lesions occur is indicated by the presence of abnormal evoked potentials elicited by stimulation of pathways other than those implicated by the patients' symptoms (Sanders *et al.*, 1984).

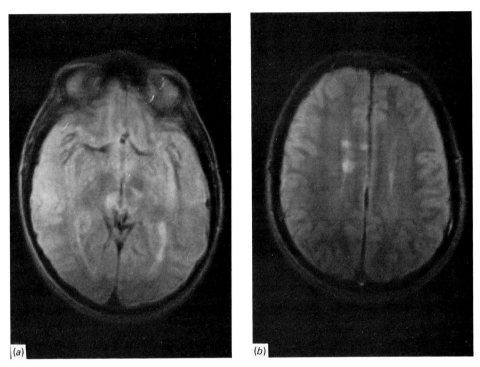

Figure 2.10 An abnormal NMR scan (spin-echo) in a patient with isolated acute unilateral optic neuritis. There are abnormalities around the trigone, occipital horn (*a*) and on the roof of the lateral ventricle (*b*)

Optic neuritis

We have scanned 28 adult patients with isolated unilateral optic neuritis, and three with bilateral simultaneous optic neuritis. In these 31 patients additional abnormalities were found in 19. The periventricular regions (*Figure 2.10*) were abnormal in 18 and additional isolated lesions were seen in 13, with discrete white matter lesions alone being seen in one case. The overall incidence of multiple lesions (61%) is substantially higher than that reported for CT scanning in optic neuritis (Feasby and Ebers, 1982; Sanders *et al.*, 1984).

Isolated brainstem lesions

In the study by Rudge already referred to, 25 patients with isolated brainstem lesions were investigated and additional lesions were found in 17 (*Figure 2.11*). As in the case of optic neuritis, periventricular changes were the most frequent finding, being present alone in three cases and with other lesions in a further 12. In the remaining two patients discrete cerebral lesions were seen without any accompanying abnormalities around the ventricles.

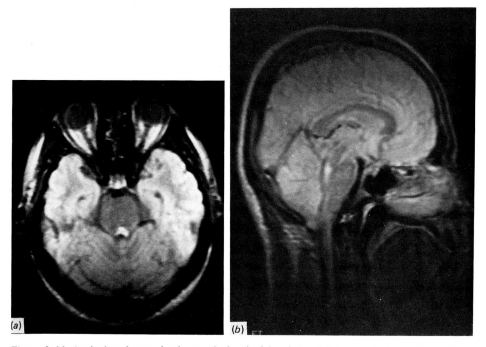

Figure 2.11 An isolated acute brainstem lesion in (*a*) axial and (*b*) sagittal plane. The patient presented with a bilateral internuclear ophthalmoplegia

Spinal cord lesions

Twenty patients with a clinically isolated spinal cord syndrome have also been examined by NMRI. Seven had presented acutely and the remainder had a recurrent or progressive picture clinically. No patient had clinical evidence of neurological abnormalities outside the spinal cord. In only three patients were we able to demonstrate unequivocally a lesion within the spinal cord and in all cases it was in the upper cervical region. Eight of the 20 had normal cerebral scans, 11 showed evidence of periventricular changes with or without additional lesions. In one patient there was a single brainstem lesion identified, with no other abnormalities around the ventricles.

In all three groups of isolated lesions that we have studied the distribution of asymptomatic lesions resembles that of MS and in the optic neuritis group the incidence, 61%, is in keeping with that of the known risk of developing clinically evident multiple sclerosis in the UK (McDonald, 1983). It is, however, premature to conclude that the cases with disseminated lesions already have MS. The frequency with which an isolated syndrome such as optic neuritis is the only clinical expression of a more disseminated but nevertheless monophasic pathological process (i.e. an acute disseminated encephalomyelitis) is unknown. There is clinical evidence that such an event is not infrequent in cases of optic neuritis in childhood, following which MS is very uncommon, and a similar picture is occasionally seen in adults without the development of MS even after three decades (Parkin, Heirons and McDonald, 1984). The presence of oligoclonal bands in isolated optic neuritis is associated with an increased risk of subsequent development of MS (Moulin, Paty and Ebers, 1983) and it would be of considerable interest to know whether the presence of such bands correlates with the presence of multiple lesions on NMRI scans. Follow-up is required to establish the prognostic significance of finding multiple lesions at presentation.

NMR changes in other diseases

Before NMRI can be used in differential diagnosis it is important to know not only the range and pattern of abnormalities in MS, but also in other conditions with which it may be confused clinically, pathologically or radiologically. It is also important to know the frequency with which abnormalities may be found in apparently normal individuals.

Cerebral vascular disease

The diffuse periventricular changes and focal lesions seen in CT scans of patients with MS resemble those found in patients with evidence of diffuse cerebral vascular disease (Rosenberg *et al.*, 1979) and comparable changes have been reported with NMRI in both conditions (Ormerod *et al.*, 1984). We therefore investigated 23 patients with cerebral vascular disease, aged 23–80 years, including patients with late onset epilepsy and CT scan evidence of lesions consistent with lacunae, acute stroke, transient global amnesia, and Binswanger's disease (*Figure 2.12*). All showed focal lesions, some small and indistinguishable from the focal lesions seen in MS, and others larger and corresponding with the territory of medium or large cerebral vessels. Nineteen of the 23 showed periventricular changes which in some patients were smoother in outline than those observed in MS. In other cases, however, the changes in the two conditions were indistinguishable.

Cerebellar degeneration

Progressive ataxia in middle life is a common source of difficulty in diagnosis. We have examined 11 such cases fulfilling the criteria for the diagnosis of cerebellar degeneration (Harding, 1984) and without other features, either clinical or investigative, of MS. All showed evidence of cerebellar atrophy with or without

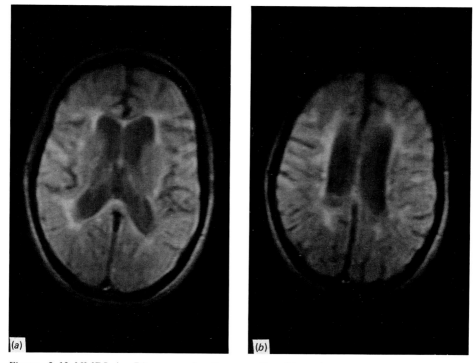

Figure 2.12 NMRI in Binswanger's disease. On this spin-echo sequence there are periventricular abnormalities and discrete lesions in the cerebral white matter

brainstem atrophy and one showed gross cerebral cortical atrophy. Two had periventricular lesions resembling those seen in MS: one of these patients had retinitis pigmentosa. One patient showed focal cerebellar abnormalities and one showed evidence of focal lesions in the cerebral hemispheres (*Figure 2.13*).

Other conditions

Periventricular changes have been reported in association with hydrocephalus, post-irradiation damage to the central nervous system, dementia of unspecified type and following infections of the CNS (Bradley *et al.*, 1984). Older subjects (over 60 years) who are neurologically normal may also show changes in signal from the periventricular region (*Figure 2.14*) resembling those seen in cerebral vascular disease and MS (Bradley, 1984). In a study of 37 apparently healthy individuals aged 19–62 (mean 38 years), we found 34 to be without blemish with the sequences in current use. Two individuals had a few small isolated lesions in the hemispheres and one patient had extensive periventricular changes indistinguishable from those in MS (*see Figure 7.7*). This apparently healthy volunteer subject gave no history of previous neurological illness in response to a general screening questionnaire, but the circumstances of recruitment precluded a detailed neurological assessment. The occasional finding of abnormalities in normal

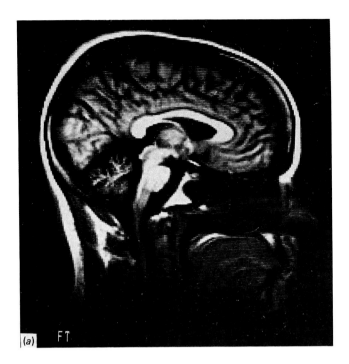

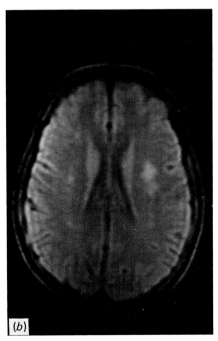

Figure 2.13 (*a*) A patient with a late onset cerebellar degeneration showing atrophy of the cerebellum and brainstem in sagittal section. (*b*) Another patient with cerebellar degeneration, showing lesions in the cerebral white matter

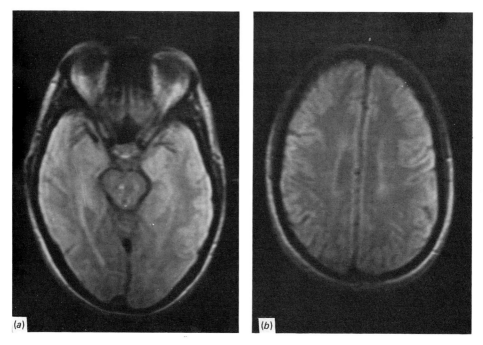

Figure 2.14 NMR scan of a normal subject aged 63 years. There are areas of increased signal (*a*) around the occipital horn and trigone, and (*b*) along the body of the lateral ventricles

individuals is in keeping with the observations of Gilbert and Sadler (1983) who found evidence of unsuspected MS at post-mortem in five of 2450 brains examined at routine necropsy.

NMR and the diagnosis of multiple sclerosis

It is obvious that, sensitive though NMRI is in detecting abnormalities in the central nervous system in MS, it cannot of itself provide a diagnosis. The position is similar to that of the evoked potential techniques – it can reveal abnormalities in the parts of the nervous system which have been examined, but the interpretation of their significance depends on the rest of the clinical and investigative picture. NMRI is not necessary in order to establish the diagnosis of clinically definite MS, but it may give added confidence when there is clinical uncertainty. Its particular value is in providing objective evidence of multiple lesions in patients with a relapsing and remitting history but with physical signs or evoked potential abnormalities indicative of only a single lesion. In patients with a history of a single episode the presence of multiple lesions inevitably raises the question of MS, but as we have already discussed we cannot provide conclusive evidence for it. In patients with progressive ataxia the absence of periventricular lesions makes the diagnosis of MS unlikely but the converse, on our present rather limited experience, is not true. NMRI is particularly helpful in the patient with rather vague symptoms and no abnormal physical signs in whom an organic basic is in doubt.

Origin of the abnormal NMR signals in MS

Any hypothesis about the origin of the abnormal signals in MS must take into account their similarity to those of vascular disease in which the pathological process is different. As already mentioned, it is obvious that the signal in proton NMRI will be altered by a change in water content of the tissue. Thus oedema could readily account for at least some of the changes seen in the acute lesions of both MS and ischaemia. Two other factors might contribute to the abnormalities in chronic lesions. Myelin loss *per se* is unlikely to play a significant part since the protons in myelin contribute little to the normal signal from brain (Pykett and Rosen, 1983; Bottomley *et al.*, 1984). It is important to stress that the periventricular lesions in Binswanger's disease are *not* demyelinating in nature (although the term is sometimes loosely used to describe them) but are characterized by complete degeneration of axons as well as myelin (Janota, 1981). The morphological feature common to the focal and diffuse periventricular lesions of cerebral vascular disease and MS is astrocytic gliosis (McDonald, 1985). The replacement of myelin by astrocyte processes would be expected to increase the amount of water per unit volume. It is also conceivable that the signal from protons is modified by the macro-molecular environment provided by the glial fibrils.

Future applications of NMRI

One of the promising applications of NMRI is in monitoring therapy. Our recent experience suggests that a reduction in the rate of appearance of new lesions in treated patients compared with controls might be detected more quickly than alterations in the clinical progress of the disease. The disappearance of lesions which have been shown to be stable would also be helpful. However, before NMRI can be used effectively in monitoring therapy, several problems have to be overcome.

First, the natural history of the lesions must be ascertained and the time taken to achieve stability of size, T_1, T_2 and proton density, and the NMRI characteristics of stable as opposed to unstable lesions must be established. Second, it must be possible accurately to re-scan the same portion of the brain on successive occasions. Controlling head position by determining the antero-posterior angulation relative to the orbito-meatal line (using a laser light source) and selection of the level of axial cuts from an inital sagittal scan is helpful, though not ideal. Third, a standard set of sequences must be used in serial studies. Sometimes lesions poorly visible with a short echo time (e.g. SE 30) become more apparent with a longer echo time (e.g. SE 60) and the apparent size of a visible lesion may change with changing sequences. Fourth, as much of the brain as possible should be surveyed at each examination. The use of sequential single slices with a range of echo time makes the scanning time unacceptably long for the patient, but multi-slice or volume imaging techniques promise to overcome this limitation. Fifth, a method for quantitation of the amount of abnormal tissue detectable with the chosen sequences and resolution of the individual machine is required. Runge *et al.* (1984) proposed a system of grading in which the changes are divided into four groups based on the size, number and distribution of lesions. Although this system has some merit, it has the drawback that it depends essentially on the actual position of lesions and the assumption of some fixed order of progression of the disease, an assumption which it is known from clinical and pathological studies is not valid. Despite these limitations NMRI is already potentially useful, although at a fairly crude level, in monitoring therapy and so rapid is the technical progress at present that its usefulness is likely to increase swiftly in the next year or two.

Finally, it is reasonable to anticipate that NMRI will contribute to the analysis of the pathogenesis of MS. If, as seems probable from the work on tumours (Carr *et al.*, 1984). changes in the blood–brain barrier can be demonstrated it should be possible to define more clearly the early stages of the development of lesions. Combination of imaging with proton shift spectroscopy may make it possible to characterize the sequence of metabolic changes in lesions during life.

Acknowledgements

We are grateful to the physicians and surgeons of the Moorfields Eye Hospital and The National Hospitals, Queen Square and Maida Vale, London for referring patients to us. The NMRI facility was established by the MS Society of Great Britain and Northern Ireland. The work is in addition supported by grants from The Medical Research Council.

References

AITA, J. F. (1978) Cranial CT and multiple sclerosis: contrast enhancing lesions. *Archives of Neurology*, **35**, 185

ANTUNES, J. L., SCHLESINGER, E. B. and MICHELSEN, W. J. (1974) The abnormal brain scan in demyelinating diseases. *Archives of Neurology*, **30**, 269–271

BOTTOMLEY, P. A., HART, H. R., EDELSTEIN, W. A. *et al.* (1984) Normal human brain studied by magnetic resonance at 1.5 Tesla. *Radiology*, **150**, 441–446

BRADLEY, W. G. (1984) Patchy periventricular white matter lesions in the elderly: a common observation during NMR imaging. *Non-invasive Medical Imaging*, **1**, 35–41

BRADLEY, W. G., WALUCH, V., WYCOFF, R. R. and YADLEY, R. A. (1984) Differential diagnosis of periventricular abnormalities in MRI of the brain. In *Program and Book of Abstracts of the Society of Magnetic Resonance in Medicine, 3rd Annual Meeting*, New York, 1984, pp. 81–82. San Francisco: The Society of Magnetic Resonance in Medicine

BRANT-ZAWADSKI, M., DAVIS, P. L., CROOKS, L. E. *et al.* (1983) NMR demonstration of cerebral abnormalities: comparison with CT. *American Journal of Roentgenology*, **140**, 847–854

BROMAN, T. (1964) Blood-brain barrier damage in multiple sclerosis. Supra-vital test – observations. *Acta Neurologica Scandinavica*, **40** (Suppl. 10), 21–24

BROOKS, D. J., LEENDERS, K. L., HEAD, G., MARSHALL, J., LEGG, M. J. and JONES, T. (1984) Studies on regional cerebral oxygen utilization and cognitive function in multiple sclerosis. *Journal of Neurology, Neurosurgery and Psychiatry*, **47**, 1182–1191

CABANIS, E. A., SALVOLINI, U., RODALLEC, A., MERICHELLI, F., PASQUINI, U. and BONNIN, T. (1978) Computed tomography of the optic nerve. 2. Size and shape modifications of papilloedema. *Journal of Computer Assisted Tomography*, **2**, 150

CALA, L. A. and MASTAGLIA, F. L. (1976) Computerized axial tomography in multiple sclerosis. *Lancet*, **1**, 689

CARR, D. H., BROWN, J., BYDDER, G. M. *et al.* (1984) Intravenous chelated gadolinium as a contrast agent in NMR imaging of cerebral tumours. *Lancet*, **1**, 484–485

COHAN, S. L., FERMAGLICH, J. and AUTH, T. L. (1975) Abnormal brain scans in multiple sclerosis. *Journal of Neurology, Neurosurgery and Psychiatry*, **38**, 120–122

CROOKS, L. E., MILLS, C. M., DAVIS, P. L. *et al.* (1982) Visualization of cerebral and vascular abnormalities by NMR imaging. The effects of imaging parameters on contrast. *Radiology*, **144**, 843–852

CRUVEILHIER, J. (1835–1842) *Atlas d'anatomie pathologique*. Paris: Ballière

DELOUVRIER, J. J., TRITSCHLER, J. L., DESBELDES, M. T., CAMBIER, J. and NAHUM, H. (1980) Computerized tomography in multiple sclerosis. In *Choices and Characteristics in Computerized Tomography*. Proceedings of the Eighth Congress of the European Society of Neuroradiology, Strasbourg, 1979, edited by H. Wackenheim and G. H. du Boulay, pp. 81–91. Amsterdam: Kugler

FEASBY, T. E. and EBERS, G. C. (1982) Risk of multiple sclerosis in isolated optic neuritis. *Canadian Journal of Neurological Sciences*, **9**, 269

FEASBY, T. E., PATY, D. W., EBERS, G. C. and FOX, A. J. (1981) Spinal cord swelling in multiple sclerosis. *Canadian Journal of Neurological Sciences*, **8**, 151–153

FRACKOWIAK, R. S. J., LENZI, G.-L., JONES, T. and HEATHER, J. D. (1980) Quantitative measurement of regional cerebral blood flow and oxygen metabolism in man using ^{15}O and positron emission tomography: theory, procedure and normal values. *Journal of Computer Assisted Tomography*, **4**, 727–736

FREEMAN, W. and COHEN, R. (1945) Electroencephalographic and pneumoencephalographic studies of multiple sclerosis. *Archives of Neurology and Psychiatry*, **53**, 246–247

GILBERT, J. J. and SADLER, M. (1983) Unsuspected multiple sclerosis. *Archives of Neurology*, **40**, 533–536

GYLDENSTED, C. (1976) Computed tomography of the cerebrum in multiple sclerosis. *Neuroradiology*, **12**, 33–42

HARDING, A. E. (1984) *The Hereditary Ataxias and Related Disorders*. Edinburgh: Churchill Livingstone

HAUGHTON, V. M., HO, K. C. and BOE-DECKER, R. A. (1979) The contracting cord sign of multiple sclerosis. *Neuroradiology*, **17**, 207–209

HAUGHTON, V. M., HO, K. C., WILLIAMS, A. and ELDERIK, O. K. (1979) CT detection of demyelinated lesions in MS. *American Journal of Radiology*, **132**, 213–215

HAYMAN, L. A., EVANS, R. A. and HINCK, V. C. (1979) Rapid high dose contrast computed tomography of isodense subdural haematoma and cerebral swelling. *Radiology*, **131**, 381–383

HERSHEY, L. A., GADO, M. H. and TROTTER, J. L. (1979) Computerised tomography in the diagnostic evaluation of multiple sclerosis. *Annals of Neurology*, **5**, 32–39

JANOTA, I. (1981) Dementia, deep white matter damage and hypertension: 'Binswanger's disease'. *Psychological Medicine*, **11**, 39–48

JOHNSON, M. A., LI, D. K. B., BRYANT, D. J. and PAYNE, J. A. (1984) Magnetic resonance imaging: serial observation in multiple sclerosis. *American Journal of Neuroradiology*, **5**, 495–499

KENDALL, B. E. and KINGSLEY, D. P. E. (1980) The diagnostic and prognostic significance of CT in neuro-degenerative, metabolic and leucodystrophic disease in childhood. In *Choices and Characteristics in Computerised Tomography*. Proceedings of the Eighth Congress of the European Society of Neuroradiology, Strasbourg, 1979, edited by A. Wackenheim and G. H. du Boulay, pp. 65–80. Amsterdam: Kugler

LEBOW, S., ANDERSON, D. C., MAESTRI, A. and LARSON, D. (1978) Acute multiple sclerosis with contrast-enhancing plaques. *Archives of Neurology*, **35**, 435–439

LINDEGAARD, O., GYLDENSTED, C., JUHLER, M. and ZEEBERG, A. (1983) CT findings in acute MS. *Acta Neurologica Scandinavica*, **68**, 77–83

LUKES, S. A., CROOKS, L. E., AMINOFF, M. J. et al. (1983) Nuclear magnetic resonance imaging in multiple sclerosis. *Annals of Neurology*, **13**, 592–601

LUMSDEN, C. E. (1970) The neuropathology of multiple sclerosis. In *The Handbook of Clinical Neurology*, Volume 9, edited by P. J. Vinken and G. W. Bruyn, pp. 217–309. Amsterdam: North Holland

McDONALD, W. I. (1983) The significance of optic neuritis. *Transactions of the Ophthalmological Societies of the United Kingdom*, **103**, 230–246

MARAVILLA, K. R., WEINRET, J. C., SUSS, R. and NUNNALLY, R. (1984) Magnetic resonance demonstration of multiple sclerosis plaques in the cervical cord. *American Journal of Neuroradiology*, **5**, 685–689

MOSELEY, I. F. and RADUE, E. W. (1979) Factors influencing the development of periventricular lucencies in patients with raised intracranial pressure. *Neuroradiology*, **17**, 65–69

MOULIN, D., PATY, D. W. and EBERS, G. C. (1983) The predictive value of cerebrospinal fluid electrophoresis in 'possible' multiple sclerosis. *Brain*, **106**, 809–816

NELSON, M. J., MILLER, S. L., McLAIN, L. W. and GOLD, L. H. A. (1981) Multiple sclerosis: large plaque causing mass effect and ring sign. *Journal of Computer Assisted Tomography*, **5**, 892–894

ORMEROD, I. E. C., ROBERTS, R. C., DU BOULAY, E. P. G. H. et al. (1984) NMR in multiple sclerosis and cerebral vascular disease. *Lancet*, **2**, 1334

OSHER, R. H. and TOMSAK, R. L. (1980) Computed tomographic features in optic neuritis. *American Journal of Ophthalmology*, **89**, 699–702

PARKIN, P. J., HEIRONS, R. and McDONALD, W. I. (1984) Bilateral optic neuritis. A long-term follow-up. *Brain*, **107**, 951–964

POSER, C. M., PATY, D. W., SCHEINBERG, L. et al. (1983) New diagnostic criteria for multiple sclerosis: guidelines for research protocols. *Annals of Neurology*, **13**, 227–231

PYKETT, I. L. and ROSEN, B. (1983) Nuclear magnetic resonance; *in vivo* proton chemical shift imaging. *Radiology*, **149**, 197–201

RADUE, E. W. and KENDALL, B. E. (1978) Iodine and xenon enhancement of computed tomography in multiple sclerosis. *Neuroradiology*, **15**, 153–158

ROSENBERG, G. A., KORNFELD, M.,STOVRING, J. and BICKNELL, J. M. (1979) Subcortical arteriosclerotic encephalopathy (Binswanger): computerised tomography. *Neurology*, **29**, 1102–1106

RUNGE, V. M., PRICE, A. C., KIRSCHNER, H. S., ALLEN, J. H., PARTAIN, C. L. and JAMES, A. E. (1984) Magnetic resonance imaging of multiple sclerosis: a study of pulse-technique efficiency. *American Journal of Roentgenology*, **143**, 1015–1026

SANDERS, E., REULEN, J. P. H. and HOGENHUIS, L. A. H. (1984) Central nervous system involvement in optic neuritis. *Journal of Neurology, Neurosurgery and Psychiatry*, **47**, 241–249

SEAMAN, W. B., TER-POGOSSIAN, M. M. and SCHWARTZ, H. G. (1954) Localisation of intracranial neoplasms with radioactive isotope. *Radiology*, **62**, 30–36

SEARS, E. S., McCAMMAN, A., BIGELOW, R. and HAYMAN, A. (1982) Maximising the harvest of contrast enhancing lesions in multiple sclerosis. *Neurology (NY)*, **32**, 815–820

SHIBASAKI, H., McDONALD, W. I. and KUROIWA, Y. (1981) Racial modification of clinical picture of multiple sclerosis: comparison between British and Japanese patients. *Journal of the Neurological Sciences*, **49**, 253–271

STEWART, W. A., HALL, L. D., BERRY, K. and PATY, D. W. (1984) Correlation between NMR scan and brain slice data in multiple sclerosis. *Lancet*, **1**, 412

TER-POGOSSIAN, M. M., EICHLING, J. O., DAVIES, B. O., WELCH, M. J. and METZGER, J. M. (1969) The determination of regional cerebral blood flow by means of water labelled with radioactive oxygen-15. *Radiology*, **93**, 31–40

VAN DER VALDEN, M., BOTS, G. T. A. M. and ENDTZ, L. J. (1979) Cranial CT in multiple sclerosis showing a mass effect. *Surgical Neurology*, **12**, 307–310

VINUELA, F. V., FOX, A. J., DEBRUN, G. M., FEASBY, T. E. and EBERS, G. C. (1982) New perspectives in computed tomography of multiple sclerosis. *American Journal of Radiology*, **139**, 123–127

YOUNG, I. R., HALL, A. S., PALLIS, C. A., LEGG, N. J., BYDDER, G. M. and STEINER, R. E. (1981) Nuclear magnetic resonance imaging of the brain in multiple sclerosis. *Lancet*, **2**, 1063–1066

ZILKHA, E., LADURNER, G., LINETTE, M. D., DU BOULAY, G. H. and MARSHALL, J. (1976) Computer subtraction in regional cerebral blood volume measurements using the EMI scanner. *British Journal of Radiology*, **49**, 330–334

3
Epidemiology

Francisco Gonzalez-Scarano, Richard S. Spielman and
Neal Nathanson

INTRODUCTION

The aetiology and pathophysiology of multiple sclerosis (MS) have been the subject
of a number of theories which have collapsed under careful scrutiny. Very few
findings have been as reproducible as the uneven geographical distribution of MS,
and few issues have remained as interesting and provocative. Any theory that
attempts to define the aetiology of MS must account for its unusual distribution.
Yet the epidemiological data by themselves can only suggest avenues for research,
and alone they are unlikely to provide the solution to this biological puzzle. In spite
of the large number of studies which have been published, and the general
acceptance of many of the major findings, there are no underlying theories that can
fully explain the epidemiological patterns.

   In this chapter we review the major epidemiological features of MS and discuss
their importance. We will assume that most readers are not familiar with
epidemiological techniques and therefore a brief outline of the most common
methodologies and their relative merits will be presented first.

METHODOLOGICAL CONSIDERATIONS

There are a number of methodological problems which impinge on epidemiological
studies of MS (Kurtzke, 1983). These are briefly noted below to indicate the
limitations of published studies.

   The diagnosis of MS is notoriously difficult in some instances (Hallpike, Adams
and Tourtellotte, 1983). Even experienced neurologists may disagree on the
classification of cases, and there are different views as to the minimum criteria
required for diagnosis. Furthermore, until recently, there have been few laboratory
tests that can be used to confirm the diagnosis while the patient is living. Because of
these problems it is usual to categorize cases in two groups; either probable or
possible. In some classifications these categories are referred to as clinically definite
and probable (*see* Chapter 1). In theory, diagnosis at death should be more
accurate because of the pathological examination, but in practice death certificates
are often incomplete and underestimate the number of cases of MS (Malmgren *et*

al., 1983). Since MS may not become manifest until age 50 or over, many cases may not have developed at the time of a single survey (Kurtzke, 1983). When comparing surveys of different populations the prevalence rate must be age-standardized (Alter, Leibowitz and Speer, 1966).

MS is not a routinely reported disease in any country, and there are only a few countries where official MS registers exist. This means that most epidemiological studies involve a major effort for the collection of the most elementary data. Since registers and clinic rosters usually do not correspond with geographically defined populations, a listing of cases may be impossible to relate to a well-defined population base.

There are two types of population-based rates which may be obtained for a disease: incidence or prevalence. Incidence, that is the number of newly occurring cases per unit time and unit population, is difficult to determine directly for MS because the insidious appearance of symptoms makes it hard to date onset accurately; in some cases the diagnosis may be assigned with confidence only after several years of follow-up. Therefore, prevalence is the more common measure. Point prevalence, that is the number of cases existing at a given point in time, is ascertained in most studies. It should be noted that prevalence is the algebraic product of incidence and duration; thus prevalence reflects survival time as well as true incidence (Clark *et al.*, 1984). In other words, doubling of survival time would double prevalence at a constant incidence rate. An increase in survival time may have accounted for the increased prevalence of MS in some regions (Acheson, 1972).

The low frequency of MS also makes population-based studies very cumbersome and expensive, since a large population must be used, or a smaller population must be followed for a long time, in order to collect adequate numbers of cases. The only practical alternative is the use of case-control (or retrospective) studies in which each case is matched by one or several controls. This is a powerful approach which has yielded important information for many chronic diseases. It is particularly suited for testing hypotheses regarding factors proposed to be either causal or risk-determining. However, there may be bias in case-control studies, since under-matching of controls can produce false correlations while over-matching can obscure important risk factors.

GENERAL FINDINGS

Prevalence studies

The observation that MS does not occur in a uniform pattern worldwide began in the 1920s, about a half-century after the initial descriptions of the disease by Charcot (1872), but at a time when clinical neurology was still in its infancy and many relatively developed countries did not have any well-trained practitioners. Differences in prevalence were frequently attributed to the lack of uniform standards of health care and to poor recognition of the disease. Over the past 25 years it has become clear that the distribution of the disease is regional with a distinct predilection for temperate climates and for economically developed countries. The general pattern holds true whether one looks at the incidence, the prevalence, or the mortality due to MS (Acheson, 1972; Kurtzke, 1983), although the rates vary with different methodologies.

MS is seen with greater frequency as the distance from the equator is increased. This applies primarily to the northern hemisphere (*Tables 3.1* and *3.2*), where the great majority of the studies have been performed, but studies in Australia (McCall, Sutherland and Acheson, 1969) and New Zealand (Hornabrook, 1971; Cuningham, 1972) suggest there is higher prevalence in countries with increasing distance south of the equator as well. Some investigators have divided the world

Table 3.1 The prevalence of multiple sclerosis at various latitudes of Europe[a]

Country	Region	Latitude (°N)	Rate per 100 000	Year of study	Reference
Iceland		64	58	1974	Kurtzke, Gudmundsson and Bergmann (1982)
Finland		63	40	1971	Wikstrom and Palo (1975)
Scotland	Shetlands Orkneys	60	309	1974–1977	Poskanzer *et al.* (1980)
	Northeast	57	178	1980	Downie and Phadke (1984)
England	Northumberland	55	42	1958	Poskanzer, Schapira and Miller (1963)
Ireland		53	66	1971	Brady *et al.* (1977)
Germany	Hamburg	54	57	1960	Behrend (1966)
Netherlands	Groningen	53	58	1959	Dassel (1960)
England	Cornwall	51	63	1958	Hargreaves (1969)
Switzerland		47	52	1957	Georgi *et al.* (1960, 1961)
Italy	Varese	46	15	1971	Cazzullo *et al.* (1973)
	Novara	45	20	1976	Caputo *et al.* (1979)
France	Marseille	43	14	1960	Behrend *et al.* (1963)
Spain	Cataluna	42	6	1968	Oliveras *et al.* (1968)
Italy	Bari	41	13	1975	Amprino *et al.* (1977)
	Sardinia	39	12	1964	Caruso, Uras and Coni (1968)

[a] Modified from Kurtzke, 1975, 1980

Table 3.2 The prevalence of multiple sclerosis at various latitudes of North America[a]

Country	Region	Latitude (°N)	Rate per 100 000	Year of study	Reference
Canada	Winnipeg	50	35	1960	Stazio, Paddison and Kurland (1967)
USA	Seattle	47	69	1977	Visscher *et al.* (1977)
USA	Missoula	47	59	1958	Siedler, Nicholl and Kurland (1958)
Canada	Halifax	45	21	1955	Alter *et al.* (1960)
USA	Rochester, Minnesota	44	60	1965	Percy *et al.* (1971)
USA	Los Angeles	34	22	1977	Visscher *et al.* (1977)
USA	Charleston	33	9	1956	Alter *et al.* (1960)
USA	Houston	30	7	1959	Chipman (1966)
USA	New Orleans	30	10	1962	Stazio *et al.* (1964)

[a] After Kurtzke, 1975, 1980

into three large clusters with low, medium and high prevalence of MS (Acheson, 1972; Kurtzke, 1975, 1980). In such a paradigm, tropical countries and Asia are classified as areas of low incidence, the southern region of the USA as a zone of medium incidence and the northern USA as a high incidence zone. Northern European countries also fall into the high incidence region. Others interpret the same data as evidence of a continuum of disease, ranging from very low to very high, and view the clustering as an artefact of the studies available and of the arbitrary division into low and medium zones of countries and regions south of the 37th parallel.

Longitude must also be taken into account, since regions at the same latitude (Rochester, Minnesota (44°N) and Marseille, France (43°N) for example, *Table 3.1*) may have widely differing prevalences of MS. A country like Israel (32°N), with a small but heterogeneous population and a relatively high incidence of disease (Alter, Leibowitz and Speer, 1966), considering its position relative to the equator, is another example of the problem of generalizing about equatorial distance and MS distribution. Japan, another northern country, has a low incidence of MS, as do most oriental countries. Other factors, such as degree of economic development, number of hours of sunshine and climate in general, have been related to MS, with the correlations being nearly as strong as the correlation with latitude (Norman, Kurtzke and Beebe, 1983).

Table 3.1 presents a sample of the prevalence of MS in several countries of Europe obtained from various original studies and reviews. It clearly shows a variety of prevalence rates, ranging from a high of more than 300 cases per 100 000 to less than 10 per 100 000 in several subtropical regions. One could argue that comparing rates of any disease between diverse societies is likely to lead to artefactual distortions. Nevertheless, even among relatively well-developed countries with similar diagnostic facilities there are considerable differences in prevalence, and the data document a definite correlation with latitude.

United States

Many of the vagaries of different health systems, demographics and racial characteristics, can be obviated by studying disease rates in a large transcontinental country like the USA. While in comparison with most western European countries the American population is ethnically heterogeneous, this heterogeneity is widely distributed among different geographical regions.

A large study attempted to identify and enumerate every individual with MS living in the conterminous USA in January, 1976 (Baum and Rothschild, 1981). The prevalence of MS was 58 per 100 000. There were significant differences in the prevalence of MS above and below the 37th parallel, but detailed regional breakdowns were not available. When high quality prevalence studies for localized regions in North America are compared (*see Table 3.2*), it is clear that prevalence increases with latitude (Kurtzke, 1975, 1980).

VETERANS STUDIES

The studies of Beebe, Kurtzke and collaborators (Beebe *et al.*, 1967; Kurtzke, 1978; Kurtzke, Beebe and Norman, 1979, 1985), begun with the US veteran population from World War II, have now been extended to study populations from later conflicts. The advantages of this extensive group of studies are: (1) the availability of complete sets of vital statistics, including birthplace and residence;

(2) relatively complete data regarding health prior to as well as after induction; (3) the presence of sociological and intelligence data; and (4) the availability of health records so that the diagnosis could be corroborated. Most of the studies have used the case-control methodology, with each case matched with random controls according to age and month of induction into the service. The data are thus expressed as ratios of cases of MS to controls (MS/C) for each variable, geographical or otherwise, that was studied. A ratio greater than one implies a greater number of MS cases related to that variable.

Table 3.3 MS case/control ratios among white United States veterans, according to residence at birth and at entry in active duty (EAD)[a]

Residence at birth	Residence at EAD			
	North	*Middle*	*South*	*Totals*
North	1.48	1.27	0.74	1.44
Middle	1.40	1.03	0.73	1.04
South	0.70	0.65	0.56	0.57
Totals	1.46	1.03	0.58	1.06

[a] After Kurtzke, Beebe and Norman (1985). Cases are compared with military controls matched for age and date of EAD. This table is based on 4980 cases and 4709 controls. North: states north of latitude 41–42°; South: states south of latitude 37°.

The essential findings are:

(1) The MS/C ratios for whites, based on either place of birth or residence at induction, moved from high values in the northern USA to low values in the south (*Table 3.3*).
(2) The MS/C ratio was higher for induction from a metropolitan area, and correlated positively with socioeconomic status.
(3) There was no relationship between climatic conditions (other than temperature) and the development of disease.
(4) The differences in the risk of development of MS from north to south has been extended to black Americans, although the total prevalence among blacks is still much lower than that of their white counterparts (Kurtzke, Beebe and Norman, 1985).

Most recently the veterans cohorts have been looked at from the standpoint of migration, and these data will be discussed below.

Migration studies

Geographical variation in MS prevalence suggests that the risk of disease is determined, at least in part, by residence. However, there are alternative explanations, such as genetic differences, so that additional confirmation is needed. For this reason there has been great interest in the influence of migration, particularly between two areas with different MS prevalence, upon the risk of disease.

Methodological problems

Migrant studies involve special methodological problems which must be noted. First, in many studies MS prevalence has not been accurately measured in both the countries of origin and of destination. Second, the migrant population is difficult to quantitate because many countries do not keep accurate or accessible records on numbers of emigrants or immigrants. Since migration can occur at any age, it is necessary to have age-specific data according to the country of origin and year of migration. Assembling reliable population data poses a major problem and is a key to a well-executed migration study. Third, migrants do not always have access to optimal medical care, so it may be difficult to ascertain all cases of MS in a defined migrant population. Finally, it is informative to compute the rates of MS among children born to migrants after reaching the country of destination. However, this is best done in settings where there is relatively little intermarriage between migrants and other ethnic groups with a different risk of MS. Because of these difficulties there are few studies of the children of migrants. The following summary is based on selected migration studies which are generally accepted as among the best in design and analysis.

South Africa

There has been a regular stream of migration from the UK and Europe, a high risk area, to South Africa, a low risk area. It is clear that migrants from England have a relatively high risk (prevalence of 49 per 100000) similar to that in the UK. In

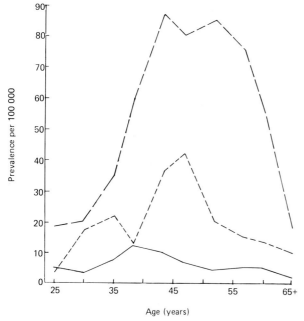

Figure 3.1 Age-specific prevalence rates for multiple sclerosis in white South-Africans, 1960. (Adapted from Dean, 1967) — — — — immigrants; -------- SA English; ——— SA Afrikaans

contrast, the rate among English-speaking whites (the descendants of immigrants) was 11 per 100 000 (Dean, 1967; Dean and Kurtzke, 1971). The pattern of age-specific prevalence (*Figure 3.1*) showed that indigenous English-speaking whites had a higher risk than Afrikaans-speaking whites, but one which was less than one-third of immigrants. Cases of MS were then tabulated according to age at migration; when this distribution was compared to an expected distribution (based on population data), there was a paucity of cases migrating under the age of 15 (Dean and Kurtzke, 1971). It was concluded that the risk of MS was lower for Europeans migrating at ages 0–14 than for those migrating as adults.

Israel

Israel receives two streams of immigration, from Europe, a high risk area, and from Afro-Asia, a low risk area. Several findings have emerged from a series of studies of MS by Alter and his collaborators (Alter, Leibowitz and Speer, 1966; Leibowitz, Kahana and Alter, 1973; Alter, Kahana and Loewenson, 1978). MS rates among immigrants are markedly higher in Europeans than in Afro-Asians. However,

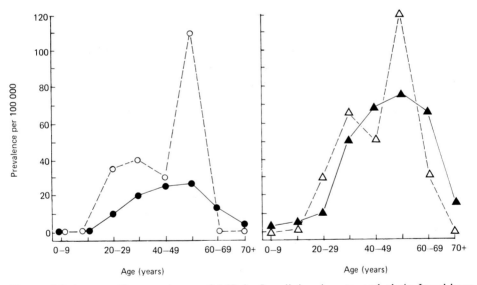

Figure 3.2 Age-specific prevalence of MS in Israeli immigrants and their Israel-born children, according to region of origin. (After Leibowitz, Kahana and Alter, 1973) ●–● Afro-Asians; ○–○ father born in Afro-Asia; ▲–▲ Europeans; △–△ father born in Europe

children of immigrants showed similar, relatively high, rates regardless of the origin of their fathers. Rates were markedly higher among Israel-born children of Afro-Asian immigrants than in the immigrants themselves (*Figure 3.2*). Consistent with this, Afro-Asian immigrants arriving at age 0–4 appeared to have a much higher risk than did immigrants arriving at age 15 or older (Alter, Kahana and Loewenson, 1978), but this conclusion is based on very small numbers and must be interpreted with caution.

United States

The well-documented stratification of MS prevalence according to latitude within the continental USA has already been presented (*see Tables 3.2* and *3.3*). It is therefore possible, within a single country with fairly uniform standards of medical care and diagnostic criteria, to examine the effects of migration. Visscher, Detels and collaborators (Visscher *et al.*, 1977; Detels *et al.*, 1978) have conducted a massive study of MS in Seattle, Washington (a high risk area) and Los Angeles, California (a low risk area). They found that immigrants from the northern USA to Seattle had a prevalence of MS which was twice that of immigrants from the northern USA to Los Angeles. However, immigrants from the southern USA to either city had a prevalence of MS which was much lower than immigrants from the northern USA, but which was similar for migrants to Seattle and Los Angeles.

The other major study of migration within the USA is that of veterans (*see Table 3.3*). Here a comparison is made of place of birth and residence at entry into active duty. Clearly, a move from north to south, or the reverse, had a significant influence on the risk of subsequent MS.

United Kingdom

A study of immigrants to the Greater London region (Dean *et al.*, 1976) reported the incidence of admission to hospital for probable MS. Immigrants from Ireland and Europe had a rate similar to that for persons born in the UK, while the incidence was much lower (about one-quarter) for immigrants from the Indian subcontinent and the West Indies. This study, unfortunately, had some major methodological shortcomings (Kurtzke, 1976), and it is unclear what the long-term age-specific incidence was for migrants from low risk regions, relative to the rates in their countries of origin.

France

A study of half-Vietnamese children migrating to France (Kurtzke and Bui, 1980) reported that these migrants had an MS prevalence of 89 per 100 000, similar to that estimated for Denmark and much in excess of expectation for Asians. Since the rate was based on only three cases, and since no data were collected for Vietnam, this study must be interpreted with caution.

EPIDEMICS IN ISOLATED POPULATIONS

Faroe Islands

Unusual concentrations of MS cases offer potential leads regarding aetiology or risk factors. Therefore, the report (Kurtzke and Hyllested, 1975; Nathanson and Miller, 1978) of an 'epidemic' of MS in the Faroe Islands excited considerable interest. A meticulous collection of cases by Kurtzke and Hyllested (1979) indicated that 24 cases of MS had onsets from 1943 to 1960, with no cases in the

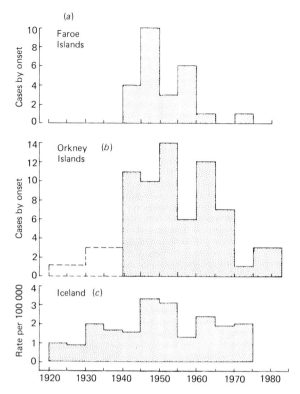

Figure 3.3 Incidence of MS in three North Atlantic island populations, to show post World War II rise in cases. (*a*) Probable cases of MS by year of onset, Faroe Islands 1920–1977, plotted by 5-year periods. During this interval the population of the Faroe Islands rose gradually from over 20 000 to over 40 000 (Data from Kurtzke and Hyllested, 1979). (*b*) Probable cases of MS by year of onset, Orkney Islands, 1940–1982, plotted by 5-year periods. During this period the population was quite constant being about 24 000 in 1941 and about 19 000 in 1982. Cases for 1920–1940 are incomplete and are shown with a dashed line. (Data from Poskanzer *et al.*, 1980 and Cook *et al.*, 1985). (*c*) Probable cases of MS by year of onset, Iceland, 1920–1974. Annual incidence rates per 100 000 are plotted for 5-year periods. (Data from Kurtzke, Gudmundsson and Bergmann, 1982).

decade 1933–1942 and only one case in the decade 1961–1970 (*Figure 3.3*). This outbreak was preceded by the occupation of the Faroe Islands by British troops in the years 1940–1945. An epidemic of canine distemper (Cook, Dowling and Russell, 1978) was reported to have lasted throughout the British occupation, with no disease prior to 1940 nor after 1956–1957.

Orkney and Shetland Islands

The Orkney and Shetland Islands, situated North of Scotland, have the highest rates of MS in the world (Poskanzer *et al.*, 1977, 1980). For the period 1940–1969 the annual incidence was estimated at 7.5 per 100 000 for Shetland and 9.3 per

100 000 for Orkney, in comparison with incidence rates in other high risk areas of no greater than 2 per 100 000 (Kurtzke, 1983). A recent study (Cook *et al.*, 1985) reported a drop in incidence for the period 1965–1983, compared with the 25 years 1941–1964. A record of cases by onset (*Figure 3.3*) suggests a similar pattern to that described above for the Faroe Islands and Iceland (that is, an elevated incidence for 1941–1965). A major occupation by British troops also took place in Shetland and Orkney from 1939–1945.

Iceland

Iceland, an island with a population of about 200 000, is too small to perpetuate certain viruses, such as measles of humans and distemper of dogs (Nathanson, Palsson and Gudmundsson, 1978). A detailed study (Kurtzke, Gudmundsson and Bergmann, 1982) has been carried out to search for evidence of an epidemic similar to that seen in the Faroe Islands. The data clearly indicate that the incidence of MS was very low from 1900–1920 and increased during the period 1920–1930 to a rate of about 2 per 100 000. This rate has remained constant from 1930 to 1975, except for the period 1945–1954 when the rate was about 3 per 100 000 or 50% higher (*see Figure 3.3*). Both Kurtzke *et al.* (1982) and Cook *et al.* (1980) have interpreted the higher incidence for 1945–1954 as an 'epidemic' superimposed on a background incidence. Iceland was occupied by Allied troops during World War II and there was an epidemic of distemper during 1941–1942. These observations have led to the speculation (Cook *et al.*, 1980) that MS in Iceland exhibits the same chronological pattern that is described above for the Faroe Islands.

Comment

Data on MS in these three island populations have now been collected and reviewed with great care. Therefore, credence must be given to the pattern of elevated incidence for a period of 15–25 years beginning around the onset of World War II. Furthermore, it is clear that these populations, because of their small size and isolation, are subject to a pattern of disappearance, reintroduction, and epidemic spread for certain viral diseases, for instance measles (Cook *et al.*, 1985).

  These observations suggest the hypothesis that a viral agent was introduced about 1940 and spread through the indigenous population for several years. Assumption of incubation periods of 2–20 years would explain cases with onset from the early 1940s to the early 1960s. This hypothetical explanation is derived, in part, from the well-documented fact (Yorke *et al.*, 1979) that many virus infections cannot be perpetuated in small human or animal populations, which therefore are highly susceptible; introduction of a virus previously absent then leads to rapid spread and an epidemic. Furthermore, it is clear that the wartime occupation resulted in the epidemic introduction of at least one virus disease, canine distemper, in both Iceland and the Faroe Islands. Thus, it is plausible that the pattern of rise and fall of MS in these three populations reflects the introduction of a causal virus around 1940. We have argued elsewhere (Nathanson, Palsson and Gudmundsson, 1978) that it is unlikely that this agent is the distemper virus itself.

GENETIC EPIDEMIOLOGY: PREVALENCE OF MULTIPLE SCLEROSIS IN RELATIVES

Background

The hypothesis of a viral agent suggests a specific environmental cause of MS, but individuals differ genetically in their responses to environmental agents. This interaction between genetic make-up and environment complicates the genetic analysis considerably.

In the classical analysis of a genetic disease the first step is the determination of the segregation ratio, that is the frequency of the disease in offspring and sibs of patients. When these frequencies turn out to be the familiar values of 25% (recessive) or 50% (dominant), the inheritance pattern is straightforward and the disease is recognized as a Mendelian trait. It has long been known that MS occasionally occurs in several members of the same family. These familial cases occur much more frequently than expected from the population prevalence (*see below*), which suggests a role for genetic determinants in MS. However, the segregation ratio is much lower than the ratio expected for a Mendelian disease and the genetic interpretation is still not certain. In this section we summarize the kinds of family data that have been collected in MS and discuss briefly the problems in interpreting the data from the standpoint of genetics.

It has been customary, until recently, to report the relevant data as the percentage of cases that are 'familial', that is those index cases who have at least one affected close relative. Defined in this way, the occurrence of MS in relatives is useless for genetic analysis. The frequency of familial cases depends in part on the number of relatives of the index case and therefore on family size. For proper genetic analysis it is necessary to calculate a true prevalence for each class of first degree relatives (sibs, parents, and offspring). These frequencies are then analogous to the segregation ratios (25%, 50%) that are standard statistics for genetic studies of Mendelian disorders. In the genetics literature such prevalences are called 'recurrence' risks. It is particularly interesting to compare the recurrence risks for sibs, parents and offspring with the prevalence in the general population, as well as with the simple Mendelian ratios noted above.

Recurrent risk data from the literature

Summaries of recurrence risk data for MS have appeared in several recent reviews (Spielman and Nathanson, 1982; Haile, Hodge and Iselius, 1983). *Table 3.4* summarizes data pooled from available studies. Within each class of first degree relatives, the individual estimates for recurrence from different studies vary by a factor of about three, with the more recent studies in general yielding the higher estimates. The general population prevalence in the high-incidence geographical areas that are the site of the family studies is about 0.0004–0.0006 (40–60 per 100 000), so the risk to relatives in *Table 3.4* appears to be increased about 10–30 fold. This is the evidence for familial aggregation.

Of course, familial aggregation is not necessarily evidence for genetic causation, since the excess of affected relatives could in principle be due to some entirely non-genetic environmental cause. It is extremely difficult to rule out this possibility with conventional family data alone. The effects of shared genes and shared environments, especially for sibs, are confounded in the recurrence data, unless

Table 3.4 Prevalence of MS in first-degree relatives
(recurrence rate) and twins (concordance) of multiple
sclerosis patients[a]

First-degree relatives	Recurrence rate[b]
Parents	41/ 6521 = 0.0063
Sibs	125/10 682 = 0.0117
Offspring	9/ 1521 = 0.0059
Twins	*Concordance*
Monozygotic (MZ)	31/107 = 0.29
Dizygotic (DZ)	13/101 = 0.13

[a] From Spielman and Nathanson, 1982.
[b] The corresponding population prevalence of MS is around
    0.0004–0.0006.

relatives raised apart (e.g. after adoption) can be studied. However, experience
with other non-Mendelian diseases (schizophrenia, diabetes mellitus) makes it
likely that there is some substantial genetic contribution.

Concordance for MS in twins

One classical approach to the genetics of disease is through twin studies.
Furthermore, conclusions from these data serve to supplement those based on
recurrence rates in first degree relatives. In our previous review (Spielman and
Nathanson, 1982), we tabulated published data on concordance of monozygotic
(MZ) and dizygotic (DZ) twins for MS. These data are summarized in *Table 3.4*.
Recent observations (Xu and McFarlin, 1984) suggest that the clinically unaffected
MZ twin often has laboratory findings associated with MS. Here, however, we
confine our attention to overt clinical MS. It is well known that twin concordance
rates, especially when based on a small number of personally observed twins, are
likely to suffer from ascertainment bias; that is, twins are more likely to be reported
if both are affected than if only one is affected with the disease under study. As a
result it seems likely that the concordance frequencies in *Table 3.4* are
overestimates, but one key conclusion may be drawn confidently. The prevalence
of MS in genetically identical MZ twins of patients with MS is only about 30%; and
because of the probable bias this should be considered an upper limit. Thus even
when the entire genotype of an MS patient is duplicated, the probability of
developing the disease phenotype is still much less than 100%. This observation is
the strongest evidence for the presence of non-genetic determinants in MS,
although it provides no indication of what those determinants might be. But it
implies that what the patient with MS inherits is only *susceptibility* to the disease;
other influences are needed to produce overt MS.

Genetic interpretation of family data

Although the recurrence rates for relatives are clearly an order of magnitude higher
than the prevalence in the general population, they reach an absolute value of only

about 0.5%–1%, far below the values expected for ordinary Mendelian inheritance. If MS does in fact have a large genetic component, the very low recurrence rates call for some explanation. There are two main requirements for classical Mendelian inheritance: the trait must be determined by alleles at a single locus, and there must be complete penetrance of genotypes, that is the disease genotype must always result in the disease phenotype. It is likely that MS fails to meet both of these requirements. First, alleles at several genetic loci may be required for the disease phenotype, so that MS is a polygenic trait. This situation is well known in studies of animal breeding. But even if multiple loci contribute to MS, this cannot be the entire explanation, since MZ twins, who have *all* their genetic loci identical, also have low recurrence (concordance) rates for MS. This suggests the additional possibility, already described above, that the genetic component confers only *susceptibility* to MS, and does not always result in disease. In this situation, the gene or genes are said to show 'incomplete penetrance'. The two explanations are not mutually exclusive; the genetic component could still consist of several genes contributing to susceptibility. In any case, it is probably impossible to determine the nature and even the number of such genes involved, in the absence of biochemical or other genetic markers for them. (One such marker has been established in the form of HLA system, and some other possibilities exist, *see* Chapter 4.)

From the viewpoint of genetic interpretation, the main importance of the recurrence rates is that they can yield information about 'mode of inheritance' of susceptibility, and these conclusions can be drawn regardless of incomplete penetrance or number of genes involved. As a rule of thumb, if a disease is dominant (appearing in heterozygotes as well as homozygotes), the recurrence rate in sibs will be approximately equal to that in parents or offspring. If, however, the disease is recessive (appearing only in homozygotes), the sib recurrence will in general be much greater (10- to 50-fold greater for rare genes) than that in parents or offspring. Therefore, if the recurrence data in *Table 3.4* are taken at face value the small excess of sib recurrence suggests only a modest degree of recessiveness.

However, this conclusion is complicated by two further considerations. First, the rule of thumb described above does not take into account the effect of differences and similarities in environment. If sibs experience more similar environments than do parents and offspring, and if environmental 'triggers' are essential for MS, the recurrence rates for sibs are likely to be inflated, compared with their true genetic values. Thus the effects of shared sib environments and genetic recessiveness are confounded in the comparison of sib versus parent–offspring recurrence rates, and conventional family data cannot separate the two. The second consideration is the variable age of onset of MS. Since a substantial fraction of MS cases have onset in late adulthood (Kurtzke, 1983), two groups which differ in average age cannot be compared directly with respect to prevalence. Some form of age-adjustment is needed, and this is best accomplished by calculating age-specific prevalences for each group.

We are not aware of any published age-specific recurrence rates for MS. However, Spielman and Lisak (unpublished observations, 1985) have begun to collect and tabulate the necessary data. Here we shall simply summarize the preliminary results to illustrate the problem. The index cases are 400 patients with a positive diagnosis of MS seen at the Hospital of the University of Pennsylvania between 1981 and 1985 and are unselected with respect to positive family history. A detailed genetic questionnaire was obtained from each patient by interview. All reports of affected first degree relatives were confirmed by examination or by obtaining unequivocal hospital records. The results, summarized in *Table 3.5*, show a crude prevalence of 0.010 for the parents of patients with MS. The corresponding prevalence among sibs is 0.008. It thus appears at first that the recurrence rate in parents is higher than that in sibs. However, when the different average ages of

Table 3.5 Comparison of crude and age-specific prevalence for parents and sibs of multiple sclerosis patients[a]

	Prevalence among	
	Parents	*Sibs*
All ages	0.010 (8/776)	0.008 (8/953)
Cumulative prevalence[b] to age:		
50	0.008 (696)[c]	0.011 (319)
60	0.010 (481)	0.011 (128)
70	0.012 (251)	0.011 (34)

[a] Spielman and Lisak, unpublished observations, 1985.
[b] Calculated by the life-table method of Cutler and Ederer (1953).
[c] Numbers in parenthesis are sample sizes at specified age. Standard errors are 0.004 for all age-specific estimates.

parents and sibs (64 vs 44) are taken into account using a life-table approach (Cutler and Ederer, 1953), the cumulative risk at age 50 is *lower* in parents than sibs, but increases in succeeding decades. The apparent constancy of the rate in sibs is probably an artefact of the small number of sibs who have reached age 60 or 70; as the sib cohort ages, it is likely that the estimate of the sib recurrence rate will increase more than the parent recurrence rate. These results, though preliminary, illustrate concretely the importance of obtaining age-specific recurrence rates.

Interpretation of twin concordance data

In the discussion of twin data above, we drew only the most cautious and unexceptionable inferences, restricting our attention to the MZ data and ignoring the DZ twins. The classical twin method, however, relies on the comparison of MZ and DZ corcordance rates. If applied to the twin data in *Table 3.4* this approach supports a genetic contribution to MS, since DZ twins, with only half their genes in common, are concordant about half as frequently (13%) as MZ twins (29% concordance). This method of course assumes that the environments of MZ twins are no more similar than those of DZ twins. Furthermore, this sort of analysis does not help to discriminate between polygenic inheritance with an environmental contribution or single locus inheritance acting in dominant fashion (but with incomplete penetrance). We earlier expressed doubts about any such conclusions (Spielman and Nathanson, 1982) because twin concordance rates are likely to be biased upwards, by an amount that is possibly not equal for MZ and DZ twins. These same reservations apply to another particularly striking aspect of the twin data. In *Table 3.4* the DZ concordance rate (13%) appears to be about 10-fold higher than the sib recurrence rate, but this excess may also represent ascertainment bias. For example, in very carefully ascertained twin material from Denmark, Heltberg and Holm (1982) found only one (4%) affected among 28 DZ twins of patients with MS.

Nevertheless, it is possible that the DZ concordance rate is truly higher than the sib recurrence, and this point of view has been argued forcefully by James (1985). (Ideally the comparison should be carried out with age-specific rates, but these are rarely available.) Since DZ twins are genetically no more similar than ordinary sibs, this excess of DZ concordance would strongly implicate environmental influences ('triggers'), shared to a greater extent by twins than by other sibs. These influences would most likely operate at a time when twins are still together, presumably in (early) childhood. As discussed in other parts of this review, these putative triggering events are not at all well identified. But it is possible that careful scrutiny of the various exposures *shared* by affected sibs or twins could point to the relevant environmental features.

CONCLUSIONS AND SUMMARY

The epidemiological and genetic observations which have been reviewed do not fit neatly into a consistent theory of the aetiology and pathogenesis of MS. Nevertheless, we believe that certain conclusions can be drawn with some certainty.

(1) A vast number of studies has now established geographic patterns of MS risk, particularly north of the equator, with higher rates associated with colder climates. However, there appear to be major exceptions, such as Japan, a low risk country with a temperate climate. Furthermore, it is still quite unclear what the geographic pattern means (Nathanson and Miller, 1978). It seems likely that these broad differences will never provide direct evidence bearing on the aetiology of MS, simply because the worldwide patterns are a very indirect reflection of the immediate cause of MS.

(2) Migration between regions of high and low incidence of MS appears to influence the risk of subsequent generations. However, most migration studies deal with the migrating generation and here the observations are considerably less clear. Often the rates in the country of origin and of destination are incompletely defined, and analysis of the migrating population is complicated by difficulty in stratifying migrants according to age at migration. The general conclusion from these studies has been that individuals migrating in childhood (under age 15) take on the risk of the country of destination. Attempts to draw inferences about the critical age of migration are probably not justified, in view of the limitations and inconsistencies in the data. Therefore, studies of the migrating generation mainly reinforce the conclusion that the risk of MS is influenced by place of residence.

(3) Family studies strongly suggest that there is a major genetic influence upon susceptibility to MS. The number of genetic loci involved and the mode of inheritance cannot be determined from the available data. However, it appears that individuals bearing the susceptible genotype have at least a ten-fold increase in the risk of developing MS.

(4) Genetic studies also provide the strongest evidence that an exogeneous or environmental 'trigger' is required to produce disease, since apparently no more than 30% of MZ twins develop MS. (The significance of laboratory abnormalities in otherwise unaffected family members is unknown at the present time.) The fact that concordance for DZ twins (0.13) is considerably higher than the recurrence rate for sibs (0.01) may also reflect the influence of a similar environment.

(5) There has been a wide expectation that epidemiological studies will lead to identification of the environmental event postulated to initiate the pathogenesis of MS. Probably the most intriguing lead is the apparent occurrence of 'outbreaks' of MS in North Atlantic island populations, particularly in the Faroe Islands (*see Figure 3.3*). These patterns are compatible with the introduction and epidemic spread of an infectious aetiological agent. Unfortunately, no systematic serological search has been made for specific viral agents.

(6) Undoubtedly, the central question in MS research is the definition of the exogenous environmental event which initiates the disease. Epidemiological studies have made a major contribution to establishing the existence of an environmental determinant in MS. But it is unlikely that further population-based studies will focus more precisely upon the identity of the postulated 'trigger' event.

Several approaches offer the possibility of more precisely defining the exogenous initiating event in MS. (a) Special epidemiological occurences, such as the apparent MS epidemic on the Faroe Islands, should be exploited. Age-specific serological profiles could be used to search for a viral pandemic which preceded the epidemic. (b) Family and twin studies could be used to search for dissimilarities in the environmental experience which may be associated with initiation of MS. (c) Alternatively, it is very possible that identification of a candidate event will emerge from non-epidemiological investigations. Crucial tests of a new aetiological hypothesis will then be provided by epidemiological studies.

Acknowledgments

This work was supported in part by a Weaver Fellowship from the National Multiple Sclerosis Society (to Francisco Gonzalez-Scarano), grant RG 1441 from the National Multiple Sclerosis Society (to Richard S. Spielman), a teacher–investigator development award NS 00717 from NINCDS (to Francisco Gonzalez-Scarano), and a Javits award NS 20904 from NINCDS (to Neal Nathanson). We thank Laura D. Pastore for outstanding secretarial service.

References

ACHESON, E. D. (1972) The epidemiology of multiple sclerosis. In *Multiple Sclerosis: A Reappraisal*, edited by M. Douglas, C. E. Lumsden and E. D. Acheson, pp. 3–80. London: Churchill Livingstone

ALTER, M., ALLISON, R. S., TALBERT, O. R. and KURLAND, L. T. (1960) Geographic distribution of multiple sclerosis. A comparison of prevalence in Charleston County, South Carolina, USA, and Halifax County, Nova Scotia, Canada. *World Neurology*, **1**, 55–70

ALTER, M., KAHANA, E. and LOEWENSON, R. (1978) Migration and risk of multiple sclerosis. *Neurology*, **28**, 1089–1093

ALTER, M., LEIBOWITZ, U. and SPEER, J. (1966) Risk of multiple sclerosis related to age at immigration to Israel. *Archives of Neurology*, **15**, 234–237

AMPRINO, D., BARNABA, A., DELLAROSA, A., LISANTI, F. and MEGNA, G. (1977) Ricerca epidemiologica sulla sclerosi multipla nella provincia di Bari. *Acta Neurologica* (Napoli), **32**, 818–832

BAUM, H. M. and ROTHSCHILD, B. B. (1981) The incidence and prevalence of reported multiple sclerosis. *Annals of Neurology*, **10**, 420–428

BEEBE, G. W., KURTZKE, J. F., KURLAND, L. T., AUTH, T. L. and NAGLER, B. (1967) Studies on the natural history of multiple sclerosis. 3. Epidemiologic analysis of the Army experience in World War II. *Neurology*, **17**, 1–17

BEHREND, R. CH. (1966) Prevalence of multiple sclerosis in Hamburg and Marseille. *Acta Neurologica Scandinavica*, **42** (Suppl. 19), 27–42

BEHREND, R. CH., SUHR, A., ROUCH, J. and ROGER, J. (1963) Etude statistique sur la sclerose en plaques à Marseille. *Revue Neurologique*, **109**, 630–634

BRADY, R., DEAN, G., SECERBEGOVIC, S. and SECERBEGOVIC, A.-M. (1977) Multiple sclerosis in the Republic of Ireland. *Journal of the Irish Medical Association*, **70**, 500–506

CAPUTO, D., GHEZZI, A., MARFORIO, S., ZIBETTI, A. and PALESTRA, A. (1979) Epidemiological study of multiple sclerosis in the province of Novara. *Acta Neurologica* (Napoli), **34**, 133–141

CARUSO, G., URAS, A. and CONI, A. (1968) La sclerosi a placche in Sardegna: sua prevalenza e distribuzione in rapporto alle variazioni altimetriche del suolo. *Acta Neurologica* (Napoli), **23**, 381–392

CAZZULLO, C. L., MONTANINI, R., MARFORIO, S. and ZIBETTI, A. (1973) Studio epidemiologico della sclerosi multipla: esempio di ricerca epidemiologica in neurologia. *Riversta Neurobiologica*, **19**, 165–174

CHARCOT, J. M. (1872) *Lecons sur les Maladies du Systeme Nerveux*. Paris: Delahaye

CHIPMAN, M. (1966) Multiple sclerosis in Houston, Texas, 1954–1959. A study of the methodology used in determining a prevalence rate in a large southern city. *Acta Neurologica Scandinavica*, **42** (Suppl. 19), 77–82

CLARK, V. A., VISSCHER, B. R., DETELS, R., VALDIVIEZO, N. L., MALMGREN, R. M. and DUDLEY, J. P. (1984) Application of simulation techniques for estimating duration of multiple sclerosis from prevalence-formed cohorts. *American Journal of Epidemiology*, **119**, 445–455

COOK, S. D., CROMANTY, J. I., TAPP, W., POSKANZER, D., WALKER, J. D. and DOWLING, P. C. (1985) Declining incidence of multiple sclerosis in the Orkney Islands. *Neurology*, **35**, 545–551

COOK, S. D., DOWLING, P. C. and RUSSELL, W. C. (1978) Multiple sclerosis and canine distemper. *Lancet*, **1**, 605–606

COOK, S. D., GUDMUNDSSON, G., BENEIKZ, J. and DOWLING, P. C. (1980) Multiple sclerosis and distemper in Iceland, 1966–1978. *Acta Neurologica Scandinavica*, **61**, 244–257

CUNINGHAM, J. A. K. (1972) The prevalence of disseminated sclerosis in Christchurch. *New Zealand Medical Journal*, **76**, 417–418

CUTLER, S. J. and EDERER, F. (1953) Maximum utilization of the life table method in analyzing survival. *Journal of Chronic Diseases*, **8**, 699–712

DASSEL, H. (1960) A survey of multiple sclerosis in a northern part of Holland. *Acta Psychiatrica et Neurologica Scandinavica*, **35** (Suppl. 147), 64–72

DEAN, G. (1967) Annual incidence, prevalence, and mortality of multiple sclerosis in white South African born and in white immigrants to South Africa. *British Medical Journal*, **2**, 724–730

DEAN, G. and KURTZKE, J. F. (1971) On the risk of multiple sclerosis according to age at immigration to South Africa. *British Medical Journal*, **3**, 725–729

DEAN, G., McLOUGHLIN, H., BRADY, R., ADELSTEIN, A. M. and TALLETT-WILLIAMS, J. (1976) Multiple sclerosis among immigrants in Greater London. *British Medical Journal*, **1**, 861–864

DETELS, R., VISSCHER, B. R., HAILE, R. W., MALMGREN, R. M., DUDLEY, J. P. and COULSON, A. H. (1978) Multiple sclerosis and age at migration. *American Journal of Epidemiology*, **108**, 386–393

DOWNIE, A. W. and PHADKE, J. D. (1984) Multiple sclerosis in Northeast Scotland. *Health Bulletin*, **42**, 151–156

GEORGI, F. and HALL, P. (1960) Studies on multiple sclerosis frequency in Switzerland and East Africa. *Acta Psychiatrica et Neurologica Scandinavica*, **35** (Suppl. 147), 75–84

GEORGI, F., HALL, P. and MULLER, H. R. (1961) Zur Problematik der Multiple Sklorese. Geomedizinische Studien in der Schweiz und in Ost-Afrika und ihre Bedeutung fur Aetiologie und Pathogenese. *Bibliografie Psychiatrie Neurologie* (Basel), **114**, 1–123

HAILE, R. W., HODGE, S. E. and ISELIUS, L. (1983) Genetic susceptibility to multiple sclerosis: a review. *International Journal of Epidemiology*, **12**, 8–16

HALLPIKE, J. F., ADAMS, C. W. M. and TOURTELLOTTE, W. W. (eds.) (1983) *Multiple Sclerosis. Pathology, Diagnosis and Management*. Baltimore: Williams and Wilkins

HARGREAVES, E. R. (1969) Epidemiological studies in Cornwall. *Proceedings of the Royal Society of Medicine*, **54**, 209–216

HELTBERG, A. and HOLM, N. V. (1982) Concordance in twins and recurrence in sibships in multiple sclerosis. *Lancet*, **1**, 1068

HORNABROOK, R. W. (1971) The prevalence of multiple sclerosis in New Zealand. *Acta Neurologica Scandinavica*, **47**, 426–438

JAMES, W. H. (1985) Sib risk and the dizygotic twin concordance rate for multiple sclerosis. *Journal of Epidemiology and Community Health*, **39**, 39–43

KURTZKE, J. F. (1975) A reassessment of the distribution of multiple sclerosis. Part one, part two. *Acta Neurologica Scandinavica*, **51**, 110–136, 137–157

KURTZKE, J. F. (1976) Multiple sclerosis among immigrants. *British Medical Journal*, **1**, 1527–1528

KURTZKE, J. F. (1978) Data registries on selected segments of the population: veterans. *Advances in Neurology*, **19**, 55–67

KURTZKE, J. F. (1980) Geographic distribution of multiple sclerosis: an update with special reference to Europe and the Mediterranean region. *Acta Neurologica Scandinavica*, **62**, 65–80

KURTZKE, J. F. (1983) Epidemiology of multiple sclerosis. In *Multiple Sclerosis*, edited by J. F. Hallpike, C. W. M. Adams and W. W. Tourtellotte, pp. 47–95. Baltimore: Williams and Wilkins

KURTZKE, J. F., BEEBE, G. W. and NORMAN, J. E. JR (1979) Epidemiology of multiple sclerosis in United States veterans. I. Race, sex, and geographic distribution. *Neurology*, **29**, 1228–1235

KURTZKE, J. F., BEEBE, G. W. and NORMAN, J. E. (1985) Epidemiology of multiple sclerosis in United States veterans. III. Migration and the risk of MS. *Neurology*, **35**, 672–678

KURTZKE, J. F. and BUI, Q.-H. (1980) Multiple sclerosis in a migrant population: 2. Half-orientals immigrating in childhood. *Annals of Neurology*, **8**, 256–260

KURTZKE, J. F., GUDMUNDSSON, K. R. and BERGMAN, S. (1982) Multiple sclerosis in Iceland. I. Evidence of post war epidemic. *Neurology*, **32**, 143–150

KURTZKE, J. F. and HYLLESTED, K. (1975) Multiple sclerosis: an epidemic disease in the Faroes. *Transactions of the American Neurological Association*, **100**, 213–215

KURTZKE, J. F. and HYLLESTED, K. (1979) Multiple sclerosis on the Faroe Islands. I. Clinical and epidemiological features. *Annals of Neurology*, **5**, 6–21

LEIBOWITZ, U., KAHANA, E. and ALTER, M. (1973) The changing frequency of multiple sclerosis in Israel. *Archives of Neurology*, **29**, 107

MALMGREN, R. M., VALDIVIEZO, N. L., VISSCHER, B. R. *et al.* (1983) Underlying cause of death as recorded for multiple sclerosis patients' associated factors. *Journal of Chronic Diseases*, **10**, 699–705

McCALL, M. G., SUTHERLAND, J. M. and ACHESON, E. D. (1969) The frequency of multiple sclerosis in Western Australia. *Acta Neurologica Scandinavica*, **45**, 151–165

NATHANSON, N. and MILLER, A. (1978) Epidemiology of multiple sclerosis: critique of the evidence for a virus etiology. *American Journal of Epidemiology*, **107**, 451–461

NATHANSON, N., PALSSON, P. A. and GUNDMUNDSSON, G. (1978) Multiple sclerosis and canine distemper in Iceland. *Lancet*, **2**, 1127–1129

NORMAN, J. E., KURTZKE, J. F. and BEEBE, G. W. (1983) Epidemiology of multiple sclerosis in United States veterans. II. Latitude, climate and the risk of multiple sclerosis. *Journal of Chronic Diseases*, **8**, 551–559

OLIVERAS, DE LA RIVA, C., ARAGONES OLLE, J. M. and MERCADE SOBREQUES, J. (1968) Estudio de la incidencia relativa y absoluta de la esclerosis multiple en nuestra region. *Annali Medicina Cirurgia* (Barcelona), **54**, 13

PERCY, A. K., NOBREGA, F. T., OKAZAKI, H., GLATTRE, E. and KURLAND, L. T. (1971) Multiple sclerosis in Rochester, Minnesota – a 60-year appraisal. *Archives of Neurology* (Chicago), **25**, 105–111

POSKANZER, D. C., PRENNEY, L. B., SHERIDAN, J. L. and KUNDY, J. Y. (1980) Multiple sclerosis in the Orkney and Shetland Islands. I. Epidemiology, clinical factors, and methodology. *Journal of Epidemiology and Community Health*, **34**, 229–239

POSKANZER, D. C., SCHAPIRA, K. and MILLER, H. (1963) Epidemiology of multiple sclerosis in the counties of Northumberland and Durham. *Journal of Neurology, Neurosurgery and Psychiatry*, **26**, 368–376

POSKANZER, D. C., TERASAKI, P. I., PARK, M. S., SHERIDAN, J. L. and PRENNEY, L. B. (1977) Multiple sclerosis in the Orkney and Shetland Islands. I. Prevalence and tissue antigens. *Neurology*, **27**, 371–372

SHEPHERD, D. J. and DOWNIE, A. W. (1978) Prevalence of multiple sclerosis in north-east Scotland. *British Medical Journal*, **2**, 314–316

SIEDLER, H. D., NICHOLL, W. and KURLAND, L. T. (1958) The prevalence and incidence of multiple sclerosis in Missoula County, Montana. *Journal-Lancet* (*Minneapolis*), **78**, 358–360

SPIELMAN, R. S. and NATHANSON, N. (1982) The genetics of susceptibility to multiple sclerosis. *Epidemiologic Reviews*, **4**, 45–65

STAZIO, A., KURLAND, L. T., BELL, L. G., SAUNDERS, M. G. and ROGOT, E. (1964) Multiple sclerosis in Winnipeg, Manitoba: methodological considerations of epidemiologic survey. Ten year follow-up of a community wide study, and population re-survey. *Journal of Chronic Diseases*, **17**, 415–438

STAZIO, A., PADDISON, R. M. and KURLAND, L. T. (1967) Multiple sclerosis in New Orleans, Louisiana, and Winnipeg, Manitoba, Canada: follow-up of a previous survey in New Orleans, and comparison between the patient populations in the two communities. *Journal of Chronic Diseases*, **20**, 311–332

VISSCHER, B. R., DETELS, R., COULSON, A. H. *et al.* (1977) Latitude, migration, and the prevalence of multiple sclerosis. *American Journal of Epidemiology*, **106**, 470–475

WIKSTROM, J. and PALO, J. (1975) Studies on the clustering of multiple sclerosis in Finland. I. Comparison between the domiciles and places of birth in selected subpopulations. *Acta Neurologica Scandinavica*, **51**, 88–98

XU, X.-H. and McFARLIN, D. E. (1984) Oligoclonal bands in cerebrospinal fluid: twins with multiple sclerosis. *Neurology*, **34**, 769–774

YORKE, J. A., NATHANSON, N., PIANIGIANI, G. and MARTIN, J. (1979) Seasonality and the requirements for perpetuation and eradication of viruses in populations. *American Journal of Epidemiology*, **109**, 103–123

4

Genetic factors in the aetiology of multiple sclerosis

Alastair Compston

INTRODUCTION

The importance of genetic susceptibility to multiple sclerosis (MS) was appreciated in the 19th century accounts which first described the clinical features and pathology of the disease. Epidemiological methods for investigating the aetiology of MS depend on accurate ascertainment during life and progress has been limited by lack of a diagnostic test for the disease. The findings of Gilbert and Sadler (1983), in which five cases of unsuspected MS were found at autopsy in 2450 individuals in whom neuropathological examination was undertaken, confirm previous estimates that up to 20% of cases are not recognized during life (Mackay and Hirano, 1967) and therefore are excluded from epidemiological studies. Special difficulties arise in deciding whether to include patients with isolated demyelinating lesions in genetic and epidemiological studies; Ebers *et al.* (1981) emphasized the increased incidence of mono-symptomatic demyelination, especially optic neuritis, in the families of individuals with MS. Despite these methodological difficulties, it is clear that the aetiology of MS is multifactorial, involving environmental, genetic and immunological abnormalities. These may interact in a cascade of events, none of which is necessarily abnormal in itself, but which lead to the development of MS when they occur together.

RACIAL SUSCEPTIBILITY

Some racial groups are resistant and others susceptible to MS, irrespective of latitude-related prevalence rates. Sutherland (1956) suggested that the main factor determining the distribution of MS in northern Scotland is genetic by comparing the prevalence in Nordic ($103/10^5$) and Celtic ($50/10^5$) descendents. Davenport (1922) showed that the prevalence rate for MS in army recruits was highest in the Great Lakes areas of the USA where Finns and Scandinavians lived. Beebe *et al.* (1967) showed that the observed number of non-white cases of MS (19) in World War II army recruits fell short of the expected number by 61%.

Taking latitudinal changes into account, the present evidence indicates that the prevalence of MS is consistently and inappropriately high in individuals of Fenno-Scandian origin, whereas Orientals, American Indians, US blacks, Eskimos, Lapps, Hutterites and Hungarian gypsies show racial protection from developing the disease.

FAMILIAL MULTIPLE SCLEROSIS

Estimates of the number of patients with MS who have an affected relative vary depending on the method of ascertainment; population-based studies are most reliable. Ebers (1983) found that 12.9% of 1000 patients derived from a population study in Ontario, Canada, had an affected relative; Sadovnick and McLeod (1981) reported that 73/416 (17.5%) of their patients living in British Columbia, Canada, had at least one relative with proven or clinically definite MS and an additional 21/416 (5%) had at least one relative with possible MS. These and other published studies indicate that the incidence of a family history in patients with MS is approximately 15%. In most such instances only two individuals are affected, and pedigrees containing a greater number of cases occur in only 15% of multiplex families. There are many individuals at increased risk of developing MS through having an affected relative in each multiplex family and considerably less than 15% of these individuals are eventually also affected by the disease.

The Canadian studies and pedigrees collected from various other published sources, which are not derived from a population base, each indicate that the commonest relationship between affected individuals is sibship (31%); parent–child combinations occur in 20% of multiplex families, uncles/aunts share the disease in a further 22%, cousins in 23% and more distant relationships account for the remainder.

Sadovnick and McLeod (1981) have calculated empirical recurrence risks for first, second and third degree relatives of index patients; as expected, these show that the risk is highest for siblings (2.8%) and decreases thereafter in parents (2.3%), aunts/uncles (1.8%), cousins (1.4%), children (1%) and nephews/nieces (0.2%). No significant difference in risk is seen when comparing male and female relatives of index patients.

Pedigree analysis has also been carried out to determine whether birth order affects the probability of developing MS and there is some evidence that cases are more likely to occur in early birth ranks but the results are inconsistent, possibly for methodological reasons (James, 1984).

MULTIPLE SCLEROSIS IN TWINS

There have been two recent studies of twins, in which one of each pair is already known to have MS, testing the hypothesis that a genetically influenced disease is more likely to affect both of a monozygotic than dizygotic pair. Williams *et al.* (1980) collected 30 twin pairs; six were excluded because the diagnosis was uncertain, 12 of the remaining 24 were monozygotic and 12 dizygotic (*Table 4.1*). Concordance for MS in the monozygotic pairs was six (50%) and in the dizygotic pairs two (17%). Two out of the three monozygotic twin pairs aged 50 and over, but neither of the dizygotic pairs who had reached this age, were concordant for MS. Oligoclonal bands, similar to those found in the concordant pairs and other patients with MS, were subsequently detected by iso-electric focusing in four monozygotic and eight dizygotic unaffected twin partners (Xu and McFarlin, 1984). Once again, this finding stresses the problem of diagnosis and interpretation of laboratory abnormalities in individuals who are clinically normal. Although these estimates for concordance may be spuriously high in both monozygotic and dizygotic pairs because of the method of ascertainment by advertisement, which could have introduced a selection bias favouring concordance, the difference between monozygotic and dizygotic twin pairs in this study was also seen in the more recent investigation of twins from Canada.

Table 4.1 Concordance and CSF abnormalities in 30 twin pairs with multiple sclerosis (adapted from Williams *et al.* (1980); Xu and McFarlin (1984))

	Monozygotic		*Dizygotic*	
	No.	*Concordance*	*No.*	*Concordance*
All twin pairs	12	6 (50%)	12	2 (17%)
Both twins aged >50 years	3	2 (76%)	2	0 (0%)
		CSF abnormality		
Unaffected twin in non-concordant pairs	6	4 (67%)	9	8 (88%)
Number of individuals with uncertain diagnosis (MZ pairs = 4; DZ pairs = 2)	8	5 (63%)	4	3 (75%)

MZ = monozygotic; DZ = dizygotic

Ebers *et al.* (1984) identified each patient with a twin from 5000 cases with MS throughout Canada. The incidence of twinning (1/80) conformed to the normal twin frequency and indicated that the sample was not biased. Each twin partner was examined; seven of 25 monozygotic pairs were concordant (28%) compared with one out of 40 (2.5%) dizygotic pairs. These two studies contain one important difference: the concordance in dizygotic twin pairs identified by Williams *et al.* (1980) is significantly higher than the empirical recurrence risk for other siblings (2.8%). This suggests an important environmental factor in determining the incidence of multiplex MS in these families since dizygotic twins and other siblings are genetically similar but differ in their environmental exposure. The Canadian study showed no difference in concordance between dizygotic twins and other siblings. However, the results in monozygotic twins from both studies provide strong evidence for a genetic contribution to the aetiology of MS.

ESTIMATES OF HERITABILITY

An overall assessment of the genetic contribution to susceptibility can be calculated from pedigree analysis in a familial disease where inheritance does not conform to a Mendelian pattern and susceptibility is influenced by multiple interacting genes whose expression is affected by environmental factors. Estimates of heritability in MS (52%) based on documenting 7255 relatives of 206 patients (Roberts and Bates, 1982) indicate an appreciable hereditary component to the disease and confirm the tendency for the number of affected relatives to decrease with kinship. The evidence from pedigree analysis indicating that susceptibility to MS is probably under polygenic control has now been supplemented by laboratory studies using specific genetic markers, especially those encoded within the major histocompatibility complex.

THE HISTOCOMPATIBILITY SYSTEM (HLA) AND MS

Early attempts to identify markers of susceptibility to MS were limited by the few genetic systems which could be studied. There is no consistent disturbance in the distribution of blood groups; Beebe *et al.* (1967) included a comparison of biological variables in their study of World War II army recruits, but found no significant differences in anthropometrics or blood groups between patients and matched controls. The report of an association between the HLA antigens A3/B7 and MS (Jersild *et al.*, 1973a) stimulated detailed investigation of the relationship between the HLA system and MS. It should be remembered that knowledge of the structure, complexity and biological function of the major histocompatibility complex (MHC) and the serological, cellular and recombinant DNA techniques which have been developed for investigating the system have changed since 1973 and many early findings have not been repeated using these more sophisticated reagents and techniques.

The HLA system consists of several closely placed genetic loci on the short arm of the sixth human chromosome. Each of the main HLA loci (HLA-A, -B, -C and -D) shows considerable polymorphism so one of many alternative gene forms may be found at each locus in any individual. So far, 23 HLA-A, 47 HLA-B and 8 HLA-C specificities have been defined serologically. The HLA-D locus was originally identified using mixed lymphocyte culture (MLC) or similar techniques; subsequently, products of the HLA-D related (DR) locus which have a restricted tissue distribution were identified serologically. But more recent analyses using these and other methods indicate that the HLA-D region consists of at least four main sub-loci (DP, formerly SB; DQ, formerly DC; DR and DZ) (Bodmer and Bodmer, 1984). There are 16 provisional DR alleles, three at DQ and six at the DP locus. Direct evidence and analogies with the murine histocompatibility system (H-2) (*Figure 4.1*) indicate that HLA gene products exert a restricting and controlling influence over the cell populations involved in generation of the immune response. DQ is analogous to the I-A region of mice and appears to

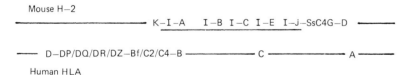

Figure 4.1 Murine (H-2) and human (HLA) histocompatibility system; H-2K and H-2D correspond to HLA-B and -A respectively. Murine H-2I region is divided into several sub-regions 1-A, 1-B, etc. which correspond to HLA-D/DR loci

restrict interaction between antigen presenting cells and T-inducer cells. HLA-DR is the analogue of I-E in the mouse. Clearly, further complexities and expansion of the recognized polymorphisms at these and as yet unidentified loci are to be expected, but there is sufficient evidence to conclude that the biological role of this complex part of the sixth chromosome is regulation of immunological responses.

HLA and MS: population studies

HLA antigen associations with MS have been demonstrated in population studies by comparing the frequency of individual antigens in patients and controls, excluding relatives from each group and comparing individuals of the same ethnic group, since the frequency of most HLA antigens differs between populations. The early studies investigated HLA-A and -B antigens and in many populations these have subsequently been updated by investigating products of the HLA-D region. The existing results can be classified into five groups (*Table 4.2*).

Table 4.2 HLA association in population studies of patients with multiple sclerosis

Country	No. patients studied	Antigen	Frequency (%) Patients	Controls	Relative risk
North Europeans	>1000	A3	32	21	2.9
and	>1000	B7	35	22	4.1
North Americans	>1000	Dw2	53	18	5.5
	>1000	DR2	60	20	5.2
North Europeans	60	DR3	35	12	2.9
Anglo-Saxon Australians	70	Dw2	70		
S. European Australians	14	Dw2	7		
Black Americans	35	A3	52	18	4.9
	35	Dw2	35	0	17
Iranians	35	A11	20	3	8
	35	B7	25	8	3.9
Greeks	81	A3	44	26	2.2
	81	B7	33	13	3.3
Coloured South Africans	24	A3	8	17	0.5
	24	B7	17	21	0.8
	16	DR2	56	33	1.7
Italians	29	DR4	31	12	9.9
	176	DR2	37	23	1.9
Japanese	20	Bw22	40	15	3.8
	11	DR6	55	18	4.8
	29	DR2	55	33	2.5
	29	DR4	52	31	2.3
Orkney Islanders	51	A3	25	30	0.8
	51	B7	35	36	1.0
	51	Dw2	44	40	1.1
	51	DR2	55	50	1.2
Hungarian gypsies	2	DR2	2/2	56	1.8
Spaniards	25	B18	36	18	2.5
Spanish (Canary Islands)	13	B12	70	30	5.2
Israelis	23	A1	43	19	3.3
Jordanian Arabs	32	DR4	88	35	13.1
Asian Indians	27	B12	63	9	18
Parsi Indians	7	B12	86	13	6.8
Non-Parsi Indians	11	B12	73	5	14.2
Asian Indians	26	A9	39	26	1.5
	26	B5	31	15	2.1
	26	B12	19	16	1.2

(For references *see* text).

First, studies of MS patients living in northern Europe involving several hundreds of cases and thousands of controls have shown an association with HLA-A3, -B7, -Dw2 and -DR2 (Batchelor, Compston and McDonald, 1978); the strongest association is with HLA-DR2 and the relative risk (RR) for developing MS in an individual with this antigen is 5.2. The strength of these associations decreases through southern Europe; the HLA-DR2 association is still seen in France (Delasnerie-Laupetre, Suet-Hubert and Marcelli-Barge, 1982) and Hungary (Palffy, 1982), but with some exceptions (*see below*) other populations in this area of Europe have not been investigated. The same associations are seen in migrant populations from northern Europe in North America (Opelz *et al.*, 1977) and South-East Australia (Stewart *et al.*, 1977).

Second, there are asociations with HLA-A3 (RR = 4.9) and Dw2 (RR = 17) in black Americans (Dupont *et al.*, 1977), with B7 (RR = 3.9) in Iranians (Lotfi *et al.*, 1978), and with A3 (RR = 2.23) and B7 (RR = 3.33) in Greeks (Georgaras *et al.*, 1984). There is an increased frequency of DR2 in coloured South Africans (RR = 1.7) (Fewster and Kies, 1984). The situation is uncertain in Italy where an association with HLA-DR4 (RR = 9.9) was initially reported (*see* Batchelor, Compston and McDonald, 1978); subsequently an increased frequency of HLA-DR2 (RR = 1.9) has been described in patients with MS (Tiwari *et al.*, 1980b). The extent to which northern European genes have been introduced into these populations is unknown.

Third, there is no significant association between HLA-A3, B7, Dw2 or DR2 in patients with MS from the Orkney Islands (Poskanzer *et al.*, 1980b), but the frequency of HLA-B7, Dw2 and DR2 in these patients is not significantly different from that found in other North European individuals with MS (Compston, 1981). The lack of an association in Orcadian patients has arisen because the frequency of these antigens in normal Orcadians is significantly higher than in normal controls from northern Europe, the UK or USA. HLA-DR2 is, therefore, very common in the normal population from an area which has the highest prevalence of MS yet to be reported; this finding is consistent with a relationship between these antigens and susceptibility to MS, but the lack of a significant difference in frequency between patients and unaffected individuals, selected as controls in the Orcardian study, remains unexplained. Furthermore, estimates of heritability in patients with MS from the Shetland Isles where HLA typing was not carried out suggests that there is only a slight genetic contribution to the aetiology of MS (Roberts, Roberts and Poskanzer, 1983). Conversely, the prevalence of HLA-DR2 in normal American Indians (Troup *et al.*, 1982) and the prevalence of MS in this population are both low. An association between HLA-DR2 and MS is seen in Hungarians, but in Hungarian gypsies the prevalence of MS appears to be very low ($2/10^5$) despite a high frequency of HLA-DR2 in the normal Hungarian gypsy population (Gyodi *et al.*, 1981; Palffy, 1982). However, it should be pointed out that only two Hungarian gypsies with MS have been identified and both these were HLA-DR2 positive.

Fourth, different HLA associations are found in some non-European populations, adding to the evidence that genetic susceptibility to MS cannot entirely be accounted for by the presence of the HLA-A3, B7, Dw2 and DR2 haplotype. HLA-B18 is increased in Spaniards with MS (RR = 2.5) (*see* Batchelor, Compston and McDonald, 1978) and HLA-B12 in Spanish patients from the Canary Islands (RR = 5.2) (Gantes and Gonzalez, 1983). There are no HLA-DR antigen associations with MS in Israelis (Brautbar *et al.*, 1982); in Jordanian Arabs an antigen closely related to DR4 is increased in patients with MS (RR = 13.1) (Kurdi *et al.*, 1977). An association with HLA-B12 (RR = 18) has been reported in Asian Indians (Wadia, Trikinnay and Krishnaswamy, 1981) and this is found in both Parsi and non-Parsi Indians (Trikinnay, Wadia and Krishnaswamy, 1982). However, a subsequent study of Indian patients from the same city (Bombay) showed no HLA-A or -B antigen associations (Singhal, 1982). An association between MS and the presence of HLA-DR6 was initially reported in Japanese patients (RR = 4.8), but more recent studies demonstrate a higher frequency of DR2 and DR4 in patients with MS than in controls (55% vs 33%: RR = 2.46 for DR2; 52% vs 31%; RR = 2.34 for DR4) although the differences do not reach statistical significance (Naito, Tabira and Kuroiwa, 1982).

Fifth, although the main association in northern Europeans is with HLA-DR2, there is a subsidiary significant association with HLA-DR3. Not only is there a slight increase in the frequency of DR3 overall (de Moerloose *et al.*, 1979), but there is a disturbance in the distribution of this antigen in patients with MS. The frequencies of DR2 and DR3 in the normal population are 21% and 27% respectively; both antigens are detected in 4% and neither in 56% of individuals. The corresponding figures in patients with MS are 60% (DR2), 36% (DR3), 16% (both) and 20% (neither). A higher proportion of patients than controls have DR2 and DR3, there is an increase in the frequency of DR3 in patients without DR2 and fewer MS patients have neither antigen than controls (*Figure 4.2*).

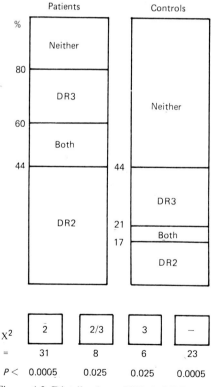

Figure 4.2 Distribution of HLA-DR2 and DR3 in MS patients and controls from northern Europe together with χ^2 and P values for comparisons of all combinations of DR2 and DR3

Any explanation for the HLA associations demonstrated in populations studied in patients with MS must take into account the specifically different associations seen in some non-northern European populations, the lack of an association in Orcadians and the low prevalence of MS in Hungarian gypsies despite a high frequency of DR2 in their normal populations, and the DR2/DR3 pattern seen in northern European patients with MS.

HLA and MS: family studies

Linkage studies in families with multiple cases can also be used to investigate relationships between MS and the HLA system. Chromosomal recombinations during meiosis separate closely placed genes at a frequency dependent on the distance between their respective loci, but recombinations occur with unusual frequency in the MHC. The probability that the distribution of HLA haplotypes in a given pedigree has arisen because of linkage between the HLA system and a disease susceptibility gene or its phenotypic expression (the disease itself) can be calculated for several hypothetical recombination frequencies and is known as the Lod score. The highest Lod score represents the most likely distance between the susceptibility gene and the HLA complex; Lod scores of greater than 3 are taken as proof for linkage. Difficulties arise in applying linkage analysis to diseases such as MS in which susceptibility is probably under polygenic control, environmental factors influence expression of genetic susceptibility, there is no diagnostic test for the disease and age of onset is variable. In addition, the chance that sibling pairs, the commonest relationship between affected individuals, will share one or other HLA haplotype is 75% and it may be necessary to combine evidence from different pedigrees in order to demonstrate higher than expected rates of haplotype sharing and calculate Lod scores.

Compston and Howard (1982) collated published details of HLA typing in 145 multiplex families, not derived from a systematic sample, including 123 with two affected individuals (*Table 4.3*). Observed rates of haplotype sharing were 85/103 (83%) in siblings, 11/11 (100%) in parent/offspring pairs, 4/8 (50%) in cousins and 0/1 (0%) in a pair of first cousins once removed; these are not significantly different from the expected rates of 75%, 100%, 25% and 12.5% respectively. However, in 22 families containing three or more affected individuals, a common haplotype was shared by all cases in 15 (68%) families compared with an expected rate of 35%.

Table 4.3 Multiplex MS families; haplotype sharing between pairs of affected members*

No. cases in family	No. families	No. case pairs	No. pairs with a shared haplotype	
			Observed	Expected
2	123	123	100	90.4
3	20	60	51	42.0
4	2	12	12	6.2
Total	145	195	163*	138.6*

$P<0.00005$ (one tailed)
*Families are taken from the literature: *see* Compston and Howard (1982)

Overall, the observed rate of haplotype sharing between affected individuals (115/145, 79%) was significantly higher than expected (98/145; 67%). However, expected rates of haplotype sharing are lower in families where three or more individuals have the disease, particularly if these are distantly related, than in sibling pairs; if case pairs within all these families are considered, 163/195 (84%) pairs shared one or other haplotype compared with the expected total of 139/195 (70%; $P<0.005$).

Previous analyses of these and other families have led to the conclusion that there is evidence for HLA-linked susceptibility to MS involving a gene situated 5–20 recombination units from the HLA-D locus (Alter *et al.*, 1976; Visscher *et al.*, 1979; Haile *et al.*, 1980; Stewart *et al.*, 1981; Suarez, O'Rourke and van Eerdewegh, 1982). Others have extended this type of analysis to correct for estimated age of disease onset and genetic heterogeneity, concluding that there is tight linkage between susceptibility to MS and the HLA complex in families where HLA-DR2 is associated with MS, whereas there is no evidence for linkage in the remaining families (Tiwari *et al.*, 1980a; Haile *et al.*, 1981; Ho *et al.*, 1982; Kinnunen *et al.*, 1984).

Ebers *et al.* (1982) investigated HLA haplotype sharing in 40 sibling pairs derived from a population sample of 611 patients with MS, including 60 multiplex families. The observed (30/40) and expected (29/40) rates of haplotype sharing were similar. The importance of a population-based sample was stressed by Ebers who compared his findings with those reported by Stewart *et al.* (1981) based on a sample derived from families identified in Australia together with those collected from 10 other published sources in which observed haplotype sharing (87/100; 87%) was higher than expected (75/100; 75%; $P<0.002$). When 35 pairs in whom haplotype assignment was unequivocal were studied alone, corresponding rates were 31/35 (88%) and 26/35 (74%). In multiplex families with affected cousins, in whom chance haplotype sharing is less likely than in siblings, Stewart *et al.* (1981) reported that the observed rate (10/17; 59%) was higher than the expected (4.25/17; 25%).

Based on an analysis of HLA haplotype segregation in multiplex families with sib pair or parent/child combinations, Weitkamp (1981) concluded that more than one gene must be contributing to disease susceptibility and subsequently reported (Weitkamp, 1983) that the frequency of like-sexed sib pairs affected by MS is higher than expected, suggesting an interaction between sex and HLA in determining susceptibility to MS.

Difficulties arise in reconciling the family and population studies. Even in the pooled family studies which are not population-based, evidence for linkage is too weak to maintain the strong associations seen in population studies. The difference would be consistent with significant heterogeneity, for which there is evidence from population studies in northern Europeans and the multiplex MS families of whom some appear tightly linked and others not linked to the HLA system. But if there is significant heterogeneity in patients with MS this is not evident from clinical comparisons between sporadic or familial cases and considerable clinical variations are seen between affected individuals within a single multiplex family (Ebers, 1983).

The attempt to impose patterns of Mendelian inheritance on susceptibility to MS under the hypothesis that there is a functionally distinct MS susceptibility gene in the HLA linkage group ignores the known biological functions of the HLA system which offer a ready explanation for HLA associations with any disease in which there is independent evidence for involvement of genetic, environmental and immunological factors. By analogy with murine immune response genes, the presence of individual HLA-gene products or linked haplotypes influence patterns of immune responsiveness and under appropriate environmental conditions might lower the threshold for establishing an immunological process. In these circumstances population associations with HLA antigens would arise and related individuals sharing HLA haplotypes, exposed to similar environmental conditions, would stand a higher chance of developing the disease than genetically dissimilar relatives, providing some evidence for HLA linkage in multiplex families. However, relatives who share neither HLA haplotype, but have been exposed to the appropriate environmental events, might each develop MS, irrespective of genetic background and the same argument would apply to sporadic cases who lack the HLA antigen associated with MS in their population. Nevertheless, the results of population and family studies add to the evidence from pedigree analysis indicating that genetic factors, and more specifically gene products encoded within the HLA complex, influence susceptibility to MS probably through an effect on regulation of immune response.

MS and HLA-linked immunological abnormalities

In view of the immunological functions of histocompatibility systems, many attempts to identify HLA-linked abnormalities of immune responsiveness, especially to measles, have been made in patients with MS, but this line of investigation has not yet helped in understanding the mechanism of genetic susceptibility to the disease.

There have been several reports of higher serum measles antibody titres in HLA-A3 and -B7 positive individuals with MS compared with patients and/or controls lacking this antigen (Jersild *et al.*, 1973b; Paty *et al.*, 1977); these differences are not always seen in comparisons of individuals with HLA-B7 (Myers *et al.*, 1976) and in other studies, higher measles antibody levels are present only in females with MS (Fewster *et al.*, 1977), in patients with MS irrespective of HLA type (Whitaker *et al.*, 1976), or in individuals with HLA-A3 whether or not they have MS (Arnason *et al.*, 1974). Conversely, in patients with MS studied in the Orkney and Shetland Islands (Poskanzer *et al.*, 1980a) increased measles antibody titres were found in normal controls with HLA-B7 compared with normal individuals lacking these antigens or patients with MS irrespective of HLA type. CSF measles antibody synthesis is increased in Dw2 positive patients with MS compared with patients lacking this antigen (Salmi *et al.*, 1983). Visscher *et al.* (1981) showed that measles antibody titres are significantly lower in siblings sharing neither HLA haplotype than in those who shared one or both haplotypes with the affected individual. Other studies in German (Kuwert and Hoher, 1976), Australian (Stewart *et al.*, 1977), Scandinavian (Ilonen *et al.*, 1977), North American (Eldridge *et al.*, 1978) and Japanese (Saito *et al.*, 1976) individuals have shown no correlations between HLA antigens and measles antibody titre in family studies or in comparisons between unrelated patients and controls.

Neither Visscher *et al.* (1981) nor Poskanzer *et al.* (1980a) found evidence for abnormal immune activity to a wide range of viruses other than measles. HLA-Dw2/DR2 linked reduction in cellular immune response to measles (Walker, Cook and Harrison, 1981) and herpes simplex virus (Paty *et al.*, 1977) have been reported in MS patients compared with other cases and all controls. Lehrich and Arnason (1976) found increased herpes simplex virus 1 and 2 antibody titres in HLA-A3 or -B7 positive individuals, whether or not they had MS, but this increase was not confirmed by Whitaker *et al.* (1976).

However, Stewart *et al.* (1977) found no evidence for altered immune responses to herpes and other viruses in MS patients compared with matched spouse controls and no correlations with HLA type in any of these groups. Interferon (IFN) production in response to viral antigens is reduced in both Dw2 positive patients and controls (Salonen *et al.*, 1982); a more marked difference in IFN synthesis by mitogen-stimulated peripheral blood lymphocytes is seen in comparisons between Dw2 positive patients and controls than in individuals without this antigen (Vervliet *et al.*, 1983).

Wentzel, Roberts and Bates (1984) found no HLA-linked difference in T or B lymphocyte numbers in a study of 96 patients with MS, although in HLA-B8 positive patients there were quantitative differences in lymphocyte sub-populations in samples studied at various stages of the disease.

Compston *et al.* (1986) assessed serum antibodies against 16 viruses and retrospective details of exposure to childhood and more recent infectious illnesses in 177 patients with isolated or recurrent demyelination and 164 controls. Overall, differences in age of infection or antibody titre to rubella, measles, mumps and parainfluenza I viruses were identified, especially in patients with optic neuritis which in most instances could be attributed to the results observed between HLA-DR2 positive cases and controls. Influenza A and B antibody titres were higher in controls compared with cases, irrespective of HLA type. With the exception of increased varicella zoster and adenovirus antibody titres in patients with demyelination who were HLA-DR2 and 3 negative, which did not result in a difference between all cases and controls, no serological or clinical differences were observed between HLA-DR3 positive or HLA-DR2/3 negative cases and controls.

In a similar retrospective survey, Lamoureux *et al.* (1983) reported an increased frequency of HLA-DR3 in 48 cases with a history of recurrent respiratory tract infection in childhood, whereas HLA-Bw42 and DRw8 were increased in 61 cases without this history. Lamoureux, Lapierre and Ducharme (1983) reported that 30% of patients without a history of childhood infection had suffered from MS for more than 15 years compared with 12% in the HLA-DR3 associated group with a history of recurrent childhood infection, suggesting that the presence of HLA-DR3 is associated with a more severe course and shorter survival. But other interpretations of these findings are possible and there have been several attempts to correlate the presence of HLA antigens with severity or progress of MS.

HLA and MS: clinical course

Stendahl-Brodin *et al.* (1979) found a significant association between the presence of Dw2 and development of moderately severe disability within five years of onset; Jersild *et al.* (1973b) had already claimed a higher prognosis coefficient in patients with the equivalent antigen Ld7a. Arnason (1975) found more severe disease in an unspecified number of patients with HLA-A3 or -B7 than in those without these antigens and Bertrams, Hoher and Kuwert (1974) showed that progressive disease with superimposed relapses, which they considered to be more severe than other forms of the disease, was associated with HLA-B7. Olsson, Link and Muller (1976) correlated severe disability, young age of onset and high CSF IgG concentration and Stendahl-Brodin *et al.* (1979) showed an association between the presence of oligoclonal bands or a high IgG index and HLA-Dw2.

These and many other studies have suggested that a form of MS exists, characterized by the presence of Dw2/DR2 or linked alleles, early onset and more severe or rapid disability, sometimes with increased CSF IgG production and abnormal reactivity to a variety of antigens with evidence for milder disease progression in HLA-DR3 positive cases (Ilonen *et al.*, 1977; Engell *et al.*, 1982). Dejaegher *et al.* (1983) found a higher frequency of HLA-DR2 in patients developing MS after the age of 31 years; older age at onset has previously been shown to be associated with increased disease severity (Confavreux, Aimard and Devic, 1982). However, others have found a positive correlation between the presence of HLA-DR3 and disease severity (Madigand *et al.*, 1982; Delasnerie-Laupetre, Suet-Hubert and Marcelli-Barge, 1982) so that the significance of these associations is uncertain. More recently, Meyer Rienecker *et al.* (1982) have correlated less severe disease progression with the presence of HLA-A25/B18.

In their double-blind controlled trial of immunosuppression in the treatment of MS, Mertin *et al.* (1982) found that the presence of HLA-A3 was associated with an increased number of relapses in the control groups, but this difference was no longer seen in immunosuppressed patients. Madigand *et al.* (1982) found that patients with HLA-DR3 were significantly less responsive to azathioprine than HLA-DR2 positive cases. Ebers and Paty (1979), Poser *et al.* (1981) and Wentzel, Roberts and Bates (1984) were unable to confirm these reports of an association between HLA antigens and severity or category of disease.

HLA and MS: complement components

Genes determining alleles of the complement components C2, C4 and Bf map between the HLA-D region and HLA-B locus and are in linkage disequilibrium with certain of their alleles. Complement components and HLA-D region alleles could interact functionally and influence immunological damage against cell membranes; for example some patients with hereditary C2 deficiency, which is associated with HLA-Dw2 (Nerl, Grosse-Wilde and Valet, 1978), develop an autoimmune disease resembling systemic lupus erythematosus.

IgG synthesized in the CNS of patients with MS is complement fixing and capable of activating the complement cascade with the formation of membrane attack complexes. There is no difference in median CSF C2 (Delasnerie-Laupretre, Suet-Hubert and Marcelli-Barge, 1982) or C3 (Jans *et al.*, 1984) concentrations between patients with severe, moderate or mild forms of MS. Jans *et al.* (1984) also reported elevated serum and reduced CSF concentrations of C4 in MS patients compared with controls. C3 and/or C4 activation products and immune complexes were detected more frequently in serum than CSF from MS patients (11/32 vs 0/32 and 17/32 vs 9/31, respectively). These early components can be re-synthesized by infiltrating cells in the CNS and it is difficult to determine from their local concentrations whether complement activation has occurred. Late components are synthesized predominantly in the liver so that their CNS concentration should fall following complement activation.

Using a highly sensitive radio-immunoassay, Morgan, Campbell and Compston (1984) found a significant decrease in CSF concentration of the terminal complement component, C9, in patients with MS compared with individuals under investigation for backache or a variety of other neurological diseases.

There have also been attempts to correlate serum and CSF complement component concentrations with the presence of MHC region alleles. Trouillas *et al.* (1975) described persistent or fluctuating low C3 levels, low total complement haemolytic activity or low factor B levels affecting a total of 30% of patients with MS and subsequently showed (Trouillas *et al.*, 1976) that these complement abnormalities were associated with the presence of HLA-B18, an antigen known to be in linkage disequilibrium with BfF1, whereas complement activity was normal in patients with HLA-B7. Family studies confirmed that these complement abnormalities segregated in association with HLA type (Trouillas and Betuel, 1977) but multiplex families were not studied. Delasnerie-Laupretre, Suet-Hubert and Marcelli-Barge (1982) reported lower CSF C2 levels in HLA-B18 positive individuals and these were further decreased in cases who were both HLA-B18 and DR2 positive. Bertrams *et al.* (1976) also described C2 hypocomplementaemia in HLA-Dw2 positive MS patients. In a study of 13 sibling pairs, all concordant for MS, Schroder *et al.* (1983) found a significant association between MS and the C4 haplotype A4/B2 compared with healthy siblings; since this C4 haplotype is known to be in linkage disequilibrium with the C2 deficiency allele – itself linked to Dw2 – this finding adds to the evidence that complement component concentrations or function are influenced by MHC region gene products in individuals with MS.

Alleles of the Bf system have been investigated in patients with MS. Stewart, Basten and Kirk (1979) found an increased frequency of the BfS alleles (84%) in 162 patients compared with 470 controls (80%) and a corresponding decrease in BfF alleles (14% vs 19% respectively) which they attributed to the known linkage disequilibrium between HLA-DR2 and BfF. But Bertrams (1982) found no disturbance in the distribution of Bf alleles in 200 MS patients compared with 536 normal controls. Fielder *et al.* (1981) compared the frequencies of HLA-DR antigens and alleles of the Bf locus in patients with demyelination; the frequency of HLA-DR2 was significantly increased in patients with optic neuritis (40%), isolated demyelinating lesions affecting other parts of the CNS (52%), and clinically definite MS (55%) compared with normal controls (19%; $0.05 < P0.0005$). The expected results of typing for Bf alleles based on known linkage disequilibrium between DR2 and BfS were not found in each category of patients with demyelination; the decreased frequency of BfF was only present in patients with clinically definite MS (14% vs 36% in controls), whereas the frequency of BfF was increased in patients with optic neuritis (49%) and suspected MS (38%) compared with controls (36%; P not significant). The suggestion that these differences implicate HLA-DR2 as a marker of susceptibility to demyelination in general, whereas alleles of the Bf system confer differences in rate of progression of disease through an effect on complement function, requires confirmation in a prospective study with comparable duration of follow-up in each group of patients.

Attempts to understand genetic susceptibility to MS in terms of HLA linked influences on immune reactivity have not so far been successful, perhaps because, in the absence of a diagnostic test for the disease, correlations have necessarily been made with non-specific immunological abnormalities.

IMMUNOGLOBULIN ALLOTYPES

Apart from the three classes of MHC genes, each of which influences immune response, the polymorphic immunoglobulin genes present on chromosome 14 will also influence immune responsiveness and may interact with MHC gene products. There is some evidence that genetic susceptibility to MS is partly conferred by differences in immunoglobulin structure and function.

Immunoglobulin class is determined by the heavy chains (IgA, D, E, G and M) and there are sub-classes within each of these categories (e.g. IgG1, IgG2, IgG3 and IgG4). Additional alterations in amino acid structure, known as Gm allotypes, are found for each immunoglobulin sub-class and these may confer differences in Ig function. There are four IgG1, one IgG2 and 13 IgG3 Gm allotypes. These can be identified and quantitated in serum using haemagglutination inhibition techniques and their distribution varies between populations. Pandey, Goust and Salier (1981) identified nine Gm markers in patients with MS and controls finding a significant association between MS and the presence of the G1m1, 17; G3m 21 phenotype (RR = 3.6), whereas Propert, Bernard and Simons (1982) reported that the presence of G1m3; G3m5, 13,14 reduces susceptibility to MS. An additional series of Australian MS patients typed for 12 Gm alleles demonstrated a significant increase in frequency of G1m1, 17; G3m21,26 overall, but in this study Gm allotype frequencies were abnormal in only one of the three contributing groups of patients (Stewart and Kirk, 1983).

RESTRICTION FRAGMENT LENGTH POLYMORPHISMS AND MS

The application of recombinant DNA techniques has already led to important advances in understanding several single gene diseases. The HLA complex, originally investigated and described by serological and cellular methods, has now been investigated using restriction enzymes and DNA probes for class 1, 2 and 3 MHC genes or their fragments. It is already clear that this approach to HLA typing in patients with MS and other diseases in which polygenic inheritance is involved might clarify some of the difficulties that arise in interpretation of population and family studies using HLA phenotypes.

HLA-DR2 is associated with increased susceptibility to MS and resistance to insulin-dependent diabetes; DR2 positive individuals who develop diabetes cannot be distinguished serologically or using cellular techniques from DR2 positive patients with MS or normal controls. Using the Eco Ri restriction enzyme to generate a 2.2 kilobase DNA fragment detected with an HLA-DQ (formerly HLA-DC) beta chain probe, Cohen *et al.* (1984) found a strong correlation between the presence of this fragment and serological typing for HLA-DR2 in the normal population but not in HLA-DR2 positive insulin-dependent diabetes. The same genotypic and phenotypic patterns were present in patients with MS as in normal controls. Using a different restriction enzyme (BamHI), a 12 kilobase-pair fragment detected by an HLA-DQ beta chain probe was found to be present in 11/45 normal controls, most of whom were HLA-DR4 positive and in 4/24 HLA-DR2 positive individuals. The same fragment was present in 8/24 MS patients of whom four were HLA-DR2 positive. The combined presence of HLA-DR2 and this 12 kilobase-pair fragment increased the relative risk for developing MS from 4 to 8.8. Four fragments were informative using the EcoRV enzyme and a beta chain HLA-DQ probe; the 7.3 kilobase fragment was present in all DR1, 2 and 6 (equivalent to HLA-DQw1) patients with MS or controls. The 12.8 kilobase fragment was found only in MS patients who were DR2 positive, but was detected in some normal controls with other HLA-DR antigens. The 23.5 kilobase fragment was present in all HLA-DR7 positive MS patients but in only some normal controls with this antigen; the 10 kilobase fragment was found less frequently in HLA-DR3 positive patients with MS than corresponding controls.

These results do not immediately clarify the relationship between MS and the HLA system, but they illustrate the complex typing patterns which can be obtained using serological and recombinant DNA techniques; the extension of these methods may well unravel some of the problems raised by HLA phenotype studies.

SUMMARY

There have been three stages in understanding the genetic basis of MS; first, the epidemiological approach using pedigree analysis in multiplex families established the concept of genetic susceptibility to the disease and indicated that inheritance is more likely to be polygenic than due to a single Mendelian gene. Second, HLA phenotype studies identified a small area on the sixth human chromosome as uniquely important in determining susceptibility to MS but failed to identify the mechanism; these studies confirmed the probable involvement of polygenic inheritance and provided evidence for genetic heterogeneity. Third, the HLA studies have prepared the way for genotypic analysis using recombinant DNA technology, concentrating in the first instance on the major histocompatibility complex and loci determining immunoglobulin chains on the 14th chromosome.

References

ALTER, M., HARSHE, M., ANDERSON, V. E., EMME, L. and YUNIS, E. J. (1976) Genetic associations of multiple sclerosis and HL-A determinants. *Neurology*, **26**, 31–36

ARNASON, B. G. W. (1975) Histocompatibility testing in multiple sclerosis. In *Multiple Sclerosis Research*, edited by A. N. Davison, J. H. Humphrey, A. L. Liversedge, W. I. McDonald and J. S. Porterfield, pp. 80–84. London: HMSO

ARNASON, B. G. W., FULLER, T. C., LEHRICH, J. R. and WRAY, G. H. (1974) Histocompatibility types and measles antibodies in multiple sclerosis and optic neuritis. *Journal of the Neurological Sciences*, **22**, 419–428

BATCHELOR, J. R., COMPSTON, D. A. S. and McDONALD, W. I. (1978) HLA and multiple sclerosis. In *The HLA System. British Medical Bulletin*, **34**, 279–284

BEEBE, G. W., KURTZKE, J. F., KURLAND, L. T., AUTH, T. L. and NAGLER, B. (1967) Studies in the natural history of multiple sclerosis. III. Epidemiological analysis of the army experience in World War II. *Neurology*, **17**, 1–7

BERTRAMS, J. (1982) Factor B alleles and multiple sclerosis. *Lancet*, **1**, 288

BERTRAMS, J., HOHER, P. G. and KUWERT, E. K. (1974) HL-A antigens in multiple sclerosis. *Lancet*, **1**, 1287

BERTRAMS, J., OPSERKUCH, W., GROSSE-WILDE, H., LUBOLDT, W., SCHUPPIEN, W. and KUWERT, E. (1976) C2 hypocomplementemia in multiple sclerosis. *Lancet*, **2**, 1358–1359

BODMER, J. and BODMER, W. (1984) Histocompatibility. *Immunology Today*, **5**, 251–254

BRAUTBAR, C., AMAR, A., COHEN, N. *et al.* (1982) HLA-D typing in multiple sclerosis: Israelis tested with European homozygous typing cells. *Tissue Antigens*, **19**, 189–197

COHEN, D., COHEN, O., MARCADET, A. *et al.* (1984) Class II HLA-DC B chain DNA restriction fragments differentiate among HLA-DR2 individuals in insulin-dependent diabetes and multiple sclerosis. *Proceedings of the National Academy of Sciences, USA*, **81**, 1774–1778

COMPSTON, D. A. S. (1981) Multiple sclerosis in the Orkneys. *Lancet*, **2**, 98

COMPSTON, D. A. S. and HOWARD, S. V. (1982) HLA typing in multiple sclerosis. *Lancet*, **2**, 661

COMPSTON, D. A. S., VAKARELIS, B. N., McDONALD, W. I., BATCHELOR, J. R. and MIMS, C. A. (1986) Viral infection in patients with multiple sclerosis and HLA-DR matched controls. *Brain* (in press)

CONFAVREUX, C., AIMARD, G. and DEVIC, M. (1980) Course and prognosis of multiple sclerosis assessed by the computerised data processing of 349 patients. *Brain*, **103**, 281–300

DAVENPORT, C. B. (1922) Multiple sclerosis from the standpoint of geographic distribution and race. *Archives of Neurology and Psychiatry*, **8**, 51–58

DEJAEGHER, L., DE BRUYERE, M., KETELAER, P. and CARTON, H. (1983) HLA antigens and progression of multiple sclerosis: part II. *Journal of Neurology*, **229**, 167–174

DELASNIERE-LAUPETRE, N., SUET-HUBERT, C. and MARCELLI-BARGE, A. (1982) Cerebrospinal fluid C2 and HLA system in multiple sclerosis. *Tissue Antigens*, **19**, 79–84

DE MOERLOOSE, PH., JEANNET, M., MARTINS DE SILVA, B., WERNER-FAVRE, CH., ROHR, J. and GAUTHIER, G. (1979) Increased frequency of HLA-DRw2 and DRw3 in multiple sclerosis. *Tissue Antigens*, **13**, 357–360

DUPONT, B., LISAK, R. P., JERSILD, C. *et al.* (1977) HLA antigens in black American patients with multiple sclerosis. *Transplantation Proceedings*, **9** (Suppl. I), 181–185

EBERS, G. C. (1983) Genetic factors in multiple sclerosis. *Neurological Clinics*, **1**, 645–654

EBERS, G. C., BULMAN, D. E., SADOVNICK, A. D. *et al.* (1984) A population based twin study in multiple sclerosis. *American Journal of Human Genetics*, **36** (Suppl.), 495

EBERS, G. C., COUSIN, H. K., FEASBY, T. E. and PATY, D. W. (1981) Optic neuritis in familial MS. *Neurology*, **31**, 1138–1142

EBERS, G. C. and PATY, D. W. (1979) The major histocompatibility complex: the immune system and multiple sclerosis. *Clinics of Neurology and Neurosurgery*, **81-2**, 69–86

EBERS, G. C., PATY, D. W., STILLER, C. R., NELSON, R. F., SELAND, T. P. and LARSEN, B. (1982) HLA typing in multiple sclerosis sibling pairs. *Lancet*, **1**, 88–90

ELDRIDGE, R., MCFARLAND, H., SEVER, J., SADOWSKY, D. and KREBS, H. (1978) Familial multiple sclerosis: clinical, histocompatibility and viral serological studies. *Annals of Neurology*, **3**, 72–80

ENGELL, T., RAUS, N. E., THOMSEN, M. and PLATZ, P. (1982) HLA and heterogeneity of multiple sclerosis. *Neurology*, **32**, 1043–1046

FEWSTER, M. E. and KIES, B. (1984) HLA antigens in multiple sclerosis in coloured South Africans. *Journal of the Neurological Sciences*, **66**, 179–181

FEWSTER, M. E., MYERS, L. W., ELLISON, G. W. and WALFORD, R. L. (1977) Histocompatibility types and measles antibodies in multiple sclerosis. *Journal of the Neurological Sciences*, **34**, 287–296

FIELDER, A. H. L., BATCHELOR, J. R., VAKARELIS, B. N., COMPSTON, D. A. S. and MCDONALD, W. I. (1981) Optic neuritis and multiple sclerosis; do factor B alleles influence progression of disease? *Lancet*, **2**, 1246–1248

GANTES, M. and GONZALEZ, T. (1983) HLA-B12 antigen and multiple sclerosis in a Spanish population (Canary Islands). *Tissue Antigens*, **22**, 172–173

GEORGARAS, A., CONSTANTOPOULOS, C., LYGIDACIS, C. and ZERVAS, J. (1984) HAL antigens and multiple sclerosis in Greeks. *Journal of Neurology, Neurosurgery and Psychiatry*, **47**, 751–752

GILBERT, J. J. and SADLER, M. (1983) Unsuspected multiple sclerosis. *Archives of Neurology*, **40**, 533–536

GYODI, E., TAUSZIK, T., PETRENYI, G. Y. *et al.* (1981) The HLA antigen distribution in the gipsy population in Hungary. *Tissue Antigens*, **18**, 1–12

HAILE, R. W., HODGE, S. E., VISSCHER, B. R. *et al.* (1980) Genetic susceptibility to multiple sclerosis: a linkage analysis with age-of-onset corrections. *Clinical Genetics*, **18**, 160–167

HAILE, R. W., ISELIUS, L., HODGE, S. E., MORTON, N. E. and DETELS, R. (1981) Segregation and linkage analysis of 40 multiplex multiple sclerosis families. *Human Heredity*, **31**, 252–258

HO, H-Z., TIWARI, J. L., HAILE, R. W., TERASAKI, P. I. and MORTON, N. E. (1982) HLA linked and unlinked determinants of multiple sclerosis. *Immunogenetics*, **15**, 509–517

ILONEN, J., HERVA, E., REUNANEN, M. *et al.* (1977) HLA antigens and antibody responses to measles and rubella viruses in multiple sclerosis. *Acta Neurologica Scandinavica*, **55**, 299–309

JAMES, W. H. (1984) Multiple sclerosis and birth order. *Journal of Epidemiological and Community Health*, **38**, 21–22

JANS, H., HELTBERG, A., ZEEBERG, I. *et al.* (1984) Immune complexes and the complement factor C4 and C3 in cerebrospinal fluid and serum from patients with chronic progressive multiple sclerosis. *Acta Neurologica Scandinavica*, **69**, 34–38

JERSILD, C., AMMITZBOLL, T., CLAUSEN, J. and FOG, T. (1973a) Association between HL-A antigens and measles antibody in multiple sclerosis. *Lancet*, **1**, 151–152

JERSILD, C., HANSEN, G. S., SVEJGAARD, A., FOG, T., THOMSEN, M. and DUPONT, B. (1973b) Histocompatibility determinants in multiple sclerosis with special reference to clinical course. *Lancet*, **2**, 1221–1224

KINNUNEN, E., KOSKIMIES, S., LAGERSTEDT, A. and WILKSTROM, J. (1984) Histocompatibility antigens in familial multiple sclerosis in a high-risk area of the disease. *Journal of the Neurological Sciences*, **65**, 147–155

KURDI, A., AYESH, I., ABDALLAT, A. *et al.* (1977) Different B-lymphocyte alloantigens associated with multiple sclerosis in Arabs and North Europeans. *Lancet*, **1**, 1123–1125

KUWERT, E. K. and HOHER, P. G. (1976) Lack of association between HLA system and antibodies to whole virus and virus sub-units of members of the paromyxovirus group in MS patients and controls. In *HLA and Disease*, Paris: Inserm (abstract), p.70

LAMOUREUX, G., DUQUETTE, P., LAPIERRE, Y., COSGROVE, B., BOURRET, G. and LABRIE, L. (1983) HLA antigen-linked genetic controls in multiple sclerosis patients resistant and susceptible to infection. *Journal of Neurology*, **230**, 91–104

LAMOUREUX, G., LAPIERRE, Y. and DUCHARME, G. (1983) Past infectious events and disease evolution in multiple sclerosis. *Journal of Neurology*, **230**, 81–90

LEHRICH, J. R. and ARNASON, B. G. W. (1976) Histocompatibility types and viral antibodies. *Archives of Neurology*, **33**, 404–405

LOTFI, J., NIBKIN, B., DERAKSHAN, J., AGHAI, Z. and ALA, F. (1978) Histocompatibility antigens (HLA) in multiple sclerosis in Iran. *Journal of Neurology, Neurosurgery and Psychiatry*, **41**, 699–701

MACKAY, R. F. and HIRANO, A. (1967) Forms of benign multiple sclerosis. *Archives of Neurology*, **17**, 588–600

MADIGAND, M., OGER, J. J-F., FAUCHET, R., SABOURARD, O. and GENETET, B. (1982) HLA profiles in multiple sclerosis suggest two forms of the disease and existence of protective haplotypes. *Journal of the Neurological Sciences*, **53**, 519–529

MERTIN, J., RUDGE, P., KREMER, M. *et al.* (1982) Double blind controlled trial of immunosuppression in the treatment of multiple sclerosis: final report. *Lancet*, **2**, 351–354

MEYER-RIENECKER, H. J., WEGENER, S., HITZSCHKE, B. and RICHTER, K. V. (1982) Multiple sclerosis – relation between HLA haplotype A25, B18 and disease progression. *Acta Neurologica Scandinavica*, **66**, 709–712

MORGAN, B. P., CAMPBELL, A. K. and COMPSTON, D. A. S. (1984) Terminal component of complement (C9) in cerebrospinal fluid of patients with multiple sclerosis. *Lancet*, **2**, 251–254

MYERS, L. W., ELLISON, G. W., FEWSTER, M. E., TERASAKI, P. I. and OPELZ, G. (1976) HLA and the immune response to measles in multiple sclerosis. *Neurology*, **26**, 54–55

NAITO, S., TABIRA, T. and KUROIWA, Y. (1982) HLA studies of multiple sclerosis in Japan. In *Multiple Sclerosis East and West*, edited by Y. Kuroiwa and L. T. Kurland, pp. 215–222. Basel: Karger

NERL, C., GROSSE-WILDE, H. and VALET, G. (1978) Association of low C2 and C4 serum levels with the HLA-Dw2 allele in healthy individuals. *Journal of Experimental Medicine*, **148**, 704–713

OLSSON, J. E., LINK, H. and MULLER, R. (1976) Immunoglobulin abnormalities in multiple sclerosis. Relation to clinical parameters disability, duration, age of onset. *Journal of the Neurological Sciences*, **27**, 233–245

OPELZ, G., TERASAKI, P. I., MYERS, L. *et al.* (1977) The association of HLA antigens A3, B7 and Dw2 with 330 multiple sclerosis patients in the United States. *Tissue Antigens*, **9**, 54–58

PALFFY, G. Y. (1982) MS in Hungary, including the gipsy population. In *Multiple Sclerosis East and West*, edited by Y. Kuroiwa and L. T. Kurland, pp. 149–158. Basel: Karger

PANDEY, J. R., GOUST, J-M. and SALIER, J-P. (1981) Immunoglobulin G heavy chain (Gm) allotypes in multiple sclerosis. *Journal of Clinical Investigation*, **67**, 1797–1800

PATY, D. W., DOSSETOR, J. B., STILLER, C. R. *et al.* (1977) HLA in multiple sclerosis – relationship to measles antibody mitogen responsiveness and clinical course. *Journal of the Neurological Sciences*, **32**, 371–379

POSER, S., RITTER, G., BAUER, H. J., GROSSE-WILDE, H., KUWERT, E. K. and RAUN, N. E. (1981) HLA antigens and the prognosis of multiple sclerosis. *Journal of Neurology*, **225**, 219–221

POSKANZER, D. C., SEVER, J. L., TERASAKI, P. I., PRENNEY, L. B., SHERIDAN, J. L. and PARK, M. S. (1980a) Multiple sclerosis in the Orkney and Shetland Islands. V. The effect on viral titres of histocompatibility determinants. *Journal of Epidemiological and Community Health*, **34**, 265–270

POSKANZER, D. C., TERASAKI, P. I., PRENNEY, L. B., SHERIDAN, J. L. and PARK, M. S. (1980b) Multiple sclerosis in the Orkney and Shetland Islands. III. Histocompatibility determinants. *Journal of Epidemiological and Community Health*, **34**, 253–257

PROPERT, D. N., BERNARD, C. C. A. and SIMONS, M. J. (1982) Gm allotypes and multiple sclerosis. *Journal of Immunogenetics*, **9**, 359–361

ROBERTS, D. F. and BATES, D. (1982) The genetic contribution to multiple sclerosis. *Journal of the Neurological Sciences*, **54**, 287–293

ROBERTS, D. F., ROBERTS, M. J. and POSKANZER, D. C. (1983) Genetic analysis of multiple sclerosis in Shetland. *Journal of Epidemiological and Community Health*, **37**, 281–285

SADOVNICK, A. D. and McLEOD, P. M. J. (1981) The familial nature of multiple sclerosis: empiric recurrence risks for first, second and third degree relatives of patients. *Neurology*, **31**, 1039–1041

SAITO, S., NAITO, S., KAWANAMI, S. and KUROIWA, Y. (1976) HLA studies on multiple sclerosis in Japan. *Neurology*, **26** (6 part 2) 49

SALONEN, R., KONEN, J., REUNANEN, M. and SALMI, A. (1982) Defective production of interferon associated with HLA-Dw2 antigen in static multiple sclerosis. *Journal of the Neurological Sciences*, **55**, 197–206

SALMI, A., REUNANEN, M., KONEN, J. and PANELIUS, M. (1983) Intrathecal antibody synthesis to virus antigens in multiple sclerosis. *Clinical and Experimental Immunology*, **52**, 241–249

SCHRODER, R., ZANDER, H., ANDREAS, A. and MAUFF, G. (1983) Multiple sclerosis: immunogenetic analyses of sib-pair double case families. II. Studies on the association of multiple sclerosis with C2, C4, Bf, C3, C6 and GLO polymorphisms. *Immunology*, **164**, 160–170

SINGHAL, B. S. (1982) Clinical profile and HLA-studies in Indian multiple sclerosis patients from the Bombay region. In *Multiple Sclerosis East and West*, edited by Y. Kuroiwa and L. T. Kurland, pp. 123–134. Basel: Karger

STENDAHL-BRODIN, L., LINK, H., MOLLER, E. and NORRBY, E. (1979) Genetic basis of multiple sclerosis, HLA antigens, disease progression and oligoclonal IgG in CSF. *Acta Neurologica Scandinavica*, **59**, 297–308

STEWART, G. J., BASTEN, A., GUINAN, J., BASHIR, H., CAMERON, J. and McLEOD, J. G. (1977) HLA-Dw2 viral immunity and family studies in multiple sclerosis. *Journal of the Neurological Sciences*, **32**, 153–167

STEWART, G. J., BASTEN, A. and KIRK, R. L. (1979) Strong linkage disequilibrium between HLA-Dw2 and BfS in multiple sclerosis and in the normal population. *Tissue Antigens*, **14**, 86–97

STEWART, G. J. and KIRK, R. L. (1983) The genetics of multiple sclerosis: the HLA system and other genetic markers. In *Multiple Sclerosis*, edited by J. F. Hallpike, C. W. M. Adams and W. W. Tourtellotte, pp. 97–128. London: Chapman and Hall

STEWART, G. J., McLEOD, J. G., BASTEN, A. and BASHIR, H. V. (1981) HLA family studies and multiple sclerosis a common gene, dominantly inherited. *Human Immunology*, **3**, 13–29

SUAREZ, B., O'ROURKE, D. and VAN EERDEWEGH, P. (1982) Power of the affected-sib pair method to detect disease susceptibility loci of small effect: an application to multiple sclerosis. *American Journal of Medical Genetics*, **12**, 309–326

SUTHERLAND, J. M. (1956) Observations on the prevalence of MS in Northern Scotland. *Brain*, **79**, 635–654

TIWARI, J. L., HODGE, S. E., TERASAKI, P. I. and SPENCE, M. A. (1980a) HLA and the inheritance of multiple sclerosis: linkage analysis of 72 pedigrees. *American Journal of Human Genetics*, **32**, 103–111

TIWARI, J. L., MORTON, N. E., LALOUEL, J. M. *et al.* (1980b) Multiple sclerosis. In *Histocompatibility Testing 1980*, UCLA Tissue Typing Laboratory, Los Angeles, pp. 687–692

TRIKINNAY, V. S., WADIA, N. H. and KRISHNASWAMY, P. R. (1982) Multiple sclerosis and HLA-B12 in Parsi and non-Parsi Indians. A clarification. *Tissue Antigens*, **19**, 155–157

TROUILLAS, P., AIMARD, G., BERTHOUX, F. and DEVIC, M. (1975) MS with hypocomplementaemia. *Lancet*, **2**, 932

TROUILLAS, P., BERTHOUX, F., BETUEL, H., BOUISSON, D., AIMARD, G. and DEVIC, M. (1976) Hypocomplementaemic MS. Heterozygous C2 deficiency linked to HLA A10, B18. *Lancet*, **2**, 1023

TROUILLAS, P. and BETUEL, H. (1977) Hypocomplementaemic and normocomplementaemic multiple sclerosis. *Journal of the Neurological Sciences*, **32**, 425–435

TROUP, G. M., SCHANFIELD, M. S., SINGARAJU, C. H. *et al.* (1982) Study of HLA alloantigens of the Navajo Indians of N. America. II HLA-A, B, C, DR and other genetic markers. *Tissue Antigens*, **20**, 339–351

VERVLIET, G., CLAEYS, H., VAN HAVER, H. *et al.* (1983) Interferon production and natural killer (NK) activity in leukocyte cultures from multiple sclerosis patients. *Journal of the Neurological Sciences*, **60**, 137–150

VISSCHER, B. R., DETELS, R., DUDLEY, J. *et al.* (1979) Genetic susceptibility to multiple sclerosis. *Neurology*, **29**, 1354–1360

VISSCHER, B. R., SULLIVAN, C. B., DETELS, R. *et al.* (1981) Measles antibody titres in multiple sclerosis patients and HLA matched and unmatched siblings. *Neurology*, **31**, 1142–1145

WADIA, N. H., TRIKINNAD, V. S. and KRISHNASWAMY, P. R. (1981) HLA antigens in multiple sclerosis amongst Indians. *Journal of Neurology, Neurosurgery and Psychiatry*, **44**, 849–851

WALKER, J. E., COOK, J. D. and HARRISON, P. (1981) HLA and immune responses to viral antigens in patients with multiple sclerosis (MS): (abstract). *Neurology*, **31**, 146–147

WEITKAMP, L. R. (1981) HLA and disease: predictions for HLA haplotype sharing in families. *American Journal of Human Genetics*, **33**, 776–784

WEITKAMP, L. R. (1983) Multiple sclerosis susceptibility: interaction between sex and HLA. *Archives of Neurology*, **40**, 399–401

WENTZEL, J., ROBERTS, D. F. and BATES, D. (1984) Multiple sclerosis HLA and lymphocyte surface markers. *Acta Neurologica Scandinavica*, **69**, 65–73

WHITAKER, J. N., HERRMANN, K. L., ROGENTINE, N., STEIN, S. F. and KOLLINS, L. L. (1976) Immunogenetic analysis and serum viral antibody titres in multiple sclerosis. *Archives of Neurology*, **33**, 399–403

WILLIAMS, A., ELDRIDGE, R., McFARLAND, H., HOUFF, S., KREBS, H. and McFARLIN, D. (1980) Multiple sclerosis in twins. *Neurology*, **30**, 1139–1147

XU, X. and McFARLIN, D. (1984) Oligoclonal bands in CSF: twins with MS. *Neurology*, **34**, 769–774

5
Immunological abnormalities
Robert P. Lisak

INTRODUCTION

As described elsewhere in this volume, the presence of mononuclear inflammatory cells within the central nervous system (CNS) of patients with multiple sclerosis (MS) has led to the hypothesis that immunopathological mechanisms are important in the pathogenesis and aetiology of MS. Indeed, there seems little question that MS is an immunopathologically mediated disease. Some researchers have suggested that such reactions are directed towards self antigens (autoantigens) within the CNS, a true autoimmune disease. Others have postulated that the reactions are directed toward viral antigens within the CNS. Still another hypothesis is that the CNS vasculature is the site for a potentially non-organ specific reaction, such as immune complex deposition which, for unknown reasons, is somehow restricted to that vasculature. The presence of a putative immunopathological reaction or a persistent CNS viral infection (two of the most widely held hypotheses for the cause of MS) would also suggest the possibility of abnormalities of normal immunoregulatory mechanisms. As reviewed below, the evidence for any of these hypotheses is indirect and frequently controversial. It also seems certain that there are abnormalities of immunoregulation in patients with MS, but as detailed later it is not clear which of these are primary and which are important in development of the disease.

IMMUNOPATHOLOGICAL REACTIONS

There are several ways in which the immune system can damage rather than protect the host. These immunological mechanisms are termed immunopathological reactions. The basic reactions themselves, i.e. the production of antibodies, formation of immune complexes, development of cell-mediated immunity, are not abnormal. Indeed, such immune reactions are necessary for preservation of the host. What makes immunopathological reactions pathological is that they are misdirected, excessive, self-perpetuating, or inappropriate.

There have been several classifications proposed, the most widely used being that of Coombs and Gell (1968) (*Table 5.1*). As we have learned more about the

74

Table 5.1 Immunopathological reactions (modified from Coombs and Gell, 1968)

Type I	Reaginic
Type II	Antibody reaction to self (auto-) antigen Directly cytolytic or toxic Alteration of cell membranes and surface receptors (a) Increased sequestration of cells (b) Block of receptor binding of ligand (c) Down-regulation of receptor (d) Stimulation of receptor function
Type III	Immune complex deposition
Type IV	Cell-mediated reactions T-cell-mediated (a) Delayed hypersensitivity (b) Cytotoxic Antibody dependent cell-mediated cytotoxicity (ADCC) Natural killer cells (NK)

immune system, it has become clear that one can readily subdivide type II (antibody to self antigens) and type IV (cell-mediated reactivity) reactions, leading to other modified classifications (Sell, 1975). In order to understand better the discussion of immunopathological mechanisms in relation to multiple sclerosis (MS), a brief overview is provided.

Reaginic immunity (*Table 5.1*; type I) involves the reaction of antibodies, frequently of the IgE isotype (class) and an antigen (generally exogenous), which then initiate release and activation of vasoactive substances. These substances can have local and/or systemic effects. Histamine and leukotrienes are examples of such mediators and hay fever and other inhalation allergies, certain types of asthma, and generalized anaphylaxis are examples of such reaginic reactions.

Antibody to self antigens (*Table 5.1*; type II) are true autoimmune reactions. The original view was that the reaction between an autoantibody and autoantigen lead to activation of mediators, principally the complement pathway, which then lead to cell damage, lysis and/or infiltration of inflammatory cells. Antibody to basement membrane, platelets, red cells and haptenes bound to tissue are examples of such reactions. One of the reactions mediated by antibodies to the acetylcholine receptor in patients with myasthenia gravis is a complement-mediated reaction (reviewed in Lisak, Levinson and Zweiman, 1985). It has also become clear that autoantibodies can modify cells and lead to tissue destruction via increased sequestration and phagocytosis.

As we have found antibodies to self antigens with receptor functions, it has become clear that such autoantibodies can cause disease without initiating actual tissue destruction. Thus, antibodies can directly block interaction of a ligand such as acetylcholine with its receptor or cause specific down-regulation of a receptor by cross-linking antigenic determinants (epitopes) on adjacent receptor molecules which results in a decrease in available receptor (reviewed in Lisak, Levinson and Zweiman, 1985). Antibodies can also cause an increase in thyroid function because of interaction of an autoantibody (long-acting thyroid stimulator) and a receptor on thyroid cells (Volpe, 1981).

It is now clear that antibodies to a particular target organ, tissue, cell or even to the same autoantigen may induce immunopathological changes in more than one manner (Lisak, Levinson and Zweiman, 1985). In addition, antibodies may induce cellular reactions (*see below*) in which the antibody determines the specificity but the actual cytotoxicity is mediated by the cells.

The deposition of circulating immune complexes (consisting of antigen and antibody) in vessels of the body or on circulating blood elements, with subsequent activation of complement pathways, can lead to tissue damage or cell sequestration and subsequent accelerated destruction (*Table 5.1*; type III reaction). Serum sickness, lupus nephritis, periarteritis nodosa, certain drug-induced thrombocytopenias are among just a few examples of this type of reaction.

Cell-mediated damage (*Table 5.1*; type IV) comprises the remaining immunopathological reactions. Several types of reactions involving different subpopulations of inflammatory cells are now known to be involved. The classical reaction was the delayed type hypersensitivity reaction, similar to the tuberculin skin test reaction but directed at an autoantigen. We now know that these lesions are initiated by antigen specific T cells of the helper/inducer phenotype (T4 in man) and that type II antigens (DR, DC or DQ) of the major histocompatibility complex (MHC) are important in these reactions. The release of lymphokines (soluble peptides) from lymphocytes is important in amplifying these reactions, in part by involving other cells such as monocyte-macrophages. Other T-cell mediated reactions are mediated by antigen-specific cytotoxic T cells (T8 in man) that can cause cytotoxic reactions only if the target cell bears type I (HLA-A or B) MHC antigens.

At least two other reactions seem to be encompassed within cell-mediated reactions. One, already mentioned, is antibody dependent cell-mediated cytotoxicity (ADCC). In these reactions, antibody reacts with specific antigen. Antigen binding by immunoglobulin depends upon the so called Fab portion of the molecule which leaves the Fc portion free. The Fc portion can then interact with inflammatory cells (killer cells or K cells) that have specific receptors for the Fc portion of immunoglobulin. These cells, which themselves are not specific for the antigen, then initiate the tissue damage. If complement interacts with the Fc portion of the immunoglobulin then the complement can interact with receptors for complement on inflammatory cells and these cells also mediate tissue damage.

The other mechanism is termed natural killer cell (NK) cell reaction and seems to involve cells identical to or of the same lineage as K cells. This reaction is not antigen specific and the factors that determine target cell susceptibility are not well understood. It is known that these cells seem to be stimulated by lymphokines such as γ-interferon and interleukin-2 (IL-2). It is thought that the normal NK cells are important in early reactions to tumour and viral infections.

Reaginic reactions

There is little to suggest that an autoantibody of the IgE class (isotype) directed against a CNS constituent is involved in the pathogenesis of MS. There have been fragmentary reports of such anti-CNS IgE antibodies (Campbell, 1971), but there have not been any published large series which systematically examine this possible immunopathological mechanism. It should be pointed out, however, that mast cells, which are important in reaginic reactions, are present within the CNS

(Rosenblum, 1973) and prostaglandins, important mediators and modulators of inflammation, are also demonstrable in the nervous system (Dore-Duffy, Ho and Longo, 1985). On the other hand, the pathological lesions in MS are not typical of reagin type reactions.

Antibody-mediated reactions to CNS constituents

The search for an autoimmune immunopathological reaction to a constituent of myelin and/or oligodendrocytes has been a major focus of MS research for many years. The logic behind such research is supported by several observations, including: (1) an increase in cerebrospinal fluid (CSF) immunoglobulin (principally IgG, but sometimes IgM and IgA as well) (Mingioli *et al.*, 1978) and/or a restricted (oligoclonal) pattern of immunoglobulin (Lowenthal, Vansande and Karcher, 1960; Laterre *et al.*, 1970; Ebers, 1984) are the most common and least controversial immunological abnormalities in patients with MS; (2) using several formulae (Lefvert and Link, 1985; Tourtellotte *et al.*, 1985; Whitaker, 1985) and occasionally direct measurement (Cutler, Watters and Hammerstad, 1970), it has been shown that there is an increased rate of immunoglobulin synthesis within the CNS in patients with MS; (3) immunoglobulin is found in plaques in the CNS of patients with MS (Tourtellotte and Parker, 1967; Mehta *et al.*, 1982) and immunoglobulin positive cells are found in lesions as well (Esiri, 1977; Mussini, Hauw and Escourolle, 1977); (4) the serum of animals with experimental allergic encephalomyelitis (EAE) induced in laboratory animals by sensitization with whole CNS tissue or unfractionated myelin contains antibodies to myelin components (principally to galactocerebroside GalC, an important glycolipid) which have demyelinating (Bornstein and Appel, 1961; Dubois-Dalq, Niedieck and Bayse, 1970), myelination inhibition (Bornstein and Raine, 1970; Fry *et al.*, 1974) and oligodendrocyte toxic effects *in vitro* (Bornstein and Appel, 1961; Hirayama *et al.*, 1983); (5) antibodies to constituents of other tissues have been shown to be important in other putative. and proven autoimmune diseases of man; and (6) early studies in patients with MS (*see below*) were compatible with the possibility of an antibody-mediated pathogenic mechanism.

There have been countless studies using a wide array of assays to detect antibodies to CNS constituents in the serum and CSF of patients with MS (reviewed in Lisak *et al.*, 1968; Lisak, 1980; Lisak *et al.*, 1984). These have included the relatively insensitive precipitin reactions and more sensitive assays such as indirect immunofluorescence, immunoperoxidase, enzyme linked immunoabsorbent assays (ELISA), radioimmunoassays of several types, complement-mediated lysis or *in vitro* demyelination, and even extremely sensitive assays such as lysis of or changes in spin resonance of antigen-containing liposomes. Substrates for these assays have included frozen CNS tissues (Edgington and D'Alessio, 1970; Lisak *et al.*, 1975), crude extracts of CNS or myelin (reviewed in Lisak *et al.*, 1968, 1984), myelinated organotypic cultures (Bornstein and Appel, 1965; Seil, 1977), cultures of CNS cells or cultures enriched for oligodendrocytes (Abramsky *et al.*, 1977; Kennedy and Lisak, 1979; Traugott, Snyder and Raine, 1979; Steck and Regli, 1980; Hirayama, Lisak and Silberberg, 1986), as well as chemically purified components of CNS myelin. Included in this last category are myelin basic protein (MBP) (Lisak *et al.*, 1968; Lennon and Mackay, 1972; Panitch, Hoffer and Johnson, 1980), myelin proteolipid (Trotter, 1983), gangliosides (Arnon *et al.*, 1980; Endo *et al.*, 1984) and GalC (Ruutianen, Reunenen and Frey, 1982; Rostami *et al.*, 1983). MBP and GalC have been clearly shown to be autoantigens in experimental animals (reviewed in Lisak, 1984; Kies, 1985). For example, antibodies to GalC have been shown to mediate demyelination (Dubois-Dalq, Niedielle and Bayse, 1970; Fry *et al.*, 1974) and oligodendrocyte toxicity *in vitro* (Hirayama *et al.*, 1983) and *in vivo* (Sergott *et al.*, 1984). Myelin associated glycoprotein (MAG) is likely to be an important autoantigen in certain patients with progressive demyelinative neuropathies (Latov, 1984; Steck and Murray, 1985). MAG has not as yet been systematically or widely studied as an autoantigen in MS but mouse monoclonal antibodies to MAG have been shown to induce demyelination in the guinea pig optic nerve after intraneural injection (Sergott *et al.*, 1985a).

In reviewing these studies there have been several roadblocks in unequivocally demonstrating disease specific antibodies in the serum or CSF of patients with MS which would be necessary to imply an antibody-mediated immune disease. Non-specific binding of human immunoglobulin to myelin and oligodendrocytes perhaps mediated in part by the Fc portion of immunoglobulin (not the antigen binding portion of immunoglobulin), or the presence of antibodies to myelin or oligodendrocytes in the serum of controls and normals, has confounded analysis (Allerand and Yahr, 1964; Aarli *et al.*, 1975). Another problem is the observation that serum from normal subjects can be shown to mediate demyelination *in vitro* (reviewed in Seil, 1977) and *in vivo* (Sergott *et al.*, 1985b) perhaps because of activation of the alternate pathway (Silberberg, Manning and Schreiber, 1984) or classical pathways (Vanguri *et al.*, 1982) of complement. Moreover, it has been demonstrated that sera of patients that cause active *in vitro* demyelination do not seem to have immunoglobulin that binds to the surface of viable intact myelin or oligodendrocytes cultured *in vitro* (Johnson and Bornstein, 1978). This would suggest that the serum demyelinating factor is not an antibody.

It is possible that there is an increase in the amount of antibodies to an important CNS constituent in the serum and/or CSF of patients with MS when compared with controls or normal subjects, but because of technical considerations this has proved difficult to demonstrate unequivocally. If such antibodies were present in a higher titre in appropriate patients they might indeed be important in disease pathogenesis, even if present in lesser amounts in controls. It is also possible that antibodies present in both patients with MS and control subjects, or other circulating substances (immune complexes, activated complement, other non-immunoglobulin acute phase reactants, proteinases) could be important in demyelination if they came into contact with myelin and/or oligodendrocytes because of changes in the blood–brain barrier (known to occur in acute exacerbations of MS) brought about by some of the other immunological mechanisms described elsewhere.

Immune complex deposition

There is increasing evidence that deposition of immune complexes (antigen–antibody) is responsible for a wide variety of lesions in many putative immunopathological diseases of man, including serum sickness, lupus nephritis, primary vasculitides, certain drug-induced thrombocytopenias, etc. The presence of aggregated immunoglobulins (immune complexes or cryoglobulins) in the vessels of different organs can initiate damage through activation of the complement cascade and associated changes in clotting factors. In addition, these complexes can serve as stimuli for cell migration (chemotaxis) and can damage vascular structures including the endothelium. Such damaged vessels would allow the passage of potentially tissue damaging circulating materials including serum enzymes (proteinases) as well as inflammatory cells. It is, therefore, reasonable to consider the possibility that deposition of immune complexes in vessels within the CNS might be important in the pathogenesis of MS (reviewed in Reik, 1980).

Several groups have now reported the presence of immune complexes in the serum and CSF of patients with MS (Tachovsky *et al.*, 1976; Goust *et al.*, 1978; Coyle *et al.*, 1980). Abnormalities in serum and CSF complement pathway profiles have been reported (Delasnerie-Laupretre, 1984; Morgan, Campbell and Compston, 1984). Such abnormalities could represent activation of complement pathways by deposition of immune complexes in the CNS. However, it is also possible that such changes could represent activation induced by binding to CNS constituents of antibodies directed against CNS components, or non-specific activation.

The mere presence of immune complexes in the serum and/or CSF does not necessarily imply deposition of these complexes and resultant CNS tissue damage. Indeed, the pathological changes in the CNS of patients with MS do not resemble the more classic immune complex deposition lesions. It is conceivable that complexes could cause alterations in the vascular endothelium and contribute to cell-mediated lesions (Nightingale and Hurley, 1978; Reik, 1980) or allow potentially cytotoxic or demyelinating factors which themselves are not specific for MS to cross the blood–brain barrier and contribute to demyelination (Hirayama, Lisak and Silberberg, 1986).

Persistent circulating immune complexes may also be important in the pathogenesis of MS by interfering with normal immunoregulatory mechanisms. However, it is also possible that immune complexes persist in the serum and CSF as a result of defective immunoregulation.

There is interest in circulating immune complexes from the point of view of identifying the antigen complexed with the immunoglobulin. Even if the complexes simply are a result of immunological damage (i.e. an epiphenomenon), it would be of interest to identify a single antigen, either a viral or CNS antigen, in the immune complexes of patients with MS. There have been very few studies addressing this question. To date, a single viral or CNS antigen has not been identified in MS patients nor a different single antigen in different individual patients with MS (Coyle and Procyk-Dougherty, 1984).

Thus, while circulating immune complexes have been identified in the serum and CSF of patients with MS, the role, if any, in the aetiology and/or pathogenesis of MS for immune complexes is not clear.

T-Cell mediated reactions to CNS components

Many studies have been directed at the possible role of cell-mediated immune reactions (especially T cell) to constituents of myelin as an important pathogenic mechanism in the inflammation and demyelination seen in patients with MS. The striking similarities between lesions of MS and both acute and recurrent-chronic progressive experimental allergic encephalomyelitis (EAE) have served as a major stimulus for such investigative efforts.

Acute EAE can be actively induced in most species by sensitization of animals with whole CNS, myelin, a purified component of myelin (MBP), or certain amino acid sequences of MBP (reviewed in Kies, 1985). There is some controversy as to whether the entire spectrum of clinical and pathological disease (Paterson, 1984) can be induced by sensitization with this protein or the active peptides in all species, but in most, inflammation and some demyelination can be demonstrated. Passive transfer of acute EAE has been accomplished with mononuclear inflammatory cells from sensitized animals (reviewed in Hinrichs, 1984), but attempts to transfer EAE with serum, especially from animals sensitized with MBP, have · not been reproducibly successful. Results of experiments manipulating the immune system of animals have suggested that the disease is T-cell dependent and initiated and that B cells and antibodies are of lesser or perhaps no importance (Blaw, Cooper and Good, 1967; Gonatas and Howard, 1974). T cells have been identified as early inflammatory cells in the EAE lesion (Traugott *et al.*, 1981) and in the mouse and rat the T-cell subset associated with helper/inducer function and delayed type hypersensitivity has been described as initiating EAE lesions (Sriram *et al.*, 1982; Hickey *et al.*, 1983). Macrophages are also important but cytotoxic/suppressor T cells seem to accumulate later (Hickey and Gonatas, 1984) as the animal recovers from the acute attack. This sequence has similarities to certain MS lesions as described by some (Traugott and Raine, 1984; Traugott, 1985) although not all (Booss *et al.*, 1983; Weiner *et al.*, 1984) groups of investigators.

Recently, acute EAE has been passively transferred with MBP specific T-cell lines of helper/inducer type obtained from the lymphoid system (Ben-Nun, Wekerle and Cohen, 1981; reviewed in Wekerle and Fierz, 1985). Burns *et al.* (1984) have also recovered MBP reactive T cells from the spinal cords of rats with EAE and have demonstrated that these T cells, also of the helper/inducer phenotype, are capable of passive transfer of EAE as well.

The essentially uniphasic nature of acute EAE and the relatively limited demyelination led some to feel that EAE was not a satisfactory experimental model of MS, although it should be noted that very early lesions of MS are rarely, if ever, studied and significant demyelination can be seen in acute EAE in non-human primates (Behan *et al.*, 1973). More recently, the development of chronic and relapsing EAE in several species (reviewed in Raine and Traugott, 1984; Lublin, 1985) has once again re-emphasized EAE as an important model for MS and focused attention on those immunological mechanisms involved in EAE as potentially important in MS. Although early studies in the guinea pig suggested that recurrent EAE could only be induced by sensitization with whole CNS, recent studies in the mouse, using both active induction and passive transfer, have supported the view that MBP reactive T cells are fundamental in the pathogenesis of chronic and recurrent EAE. Indeed, it is not clear whether a second antigen or another immune mechanism, such as antibody mediated damage, is involved.

Since T-cell immunity to MBP seemed to be of importance in EAE, there have been scores of studies of reactivity of peripheral blood cells in patients with MS searching for reactivity to CNS constituents, especially MBP. These studies have employed many different *in vitro* techniques. As reviewed by Lisak *et al.* (1984), it is not clear whether MS-specific enhanced reactivity to MBP can be reproducibly demonstrated using peripheral blood cells. Moreover, Burns has demonstrated that MBP-specific T-cell lines and clones can be recovered from the blood of normal subjects (Burns *et al.*, 1983). This may explain the low levels of MBP induced in cell reactivity *in vitro* reported by some investigators in control subjects. Therefore, the mere presence of MBP autoreactive T cells in a patient need not imply a pathogenic role for such cells. It will probably require frequency analysis to demonstrate potentially pathological specific increases in peripheral blood T-cell reactivity to MBP. There are no studies using modern T-cell cloning techniques to look for T cells in MS patients and controls that are specific for potentially encephalitogenic peptides (sequences) of MBP. In addition, we do not know which amino acid sequences of MBP are encephalitogenic in man.

Peripheral blood cells of patients with MS have been reported to be cytotoxic to and to cause demyelination of CNS organ cultures obtained from rodents (Berg and Kallen, 1964). Such studies have been cited as evidence of a cytotoxic T-cell reaction to the CNS in patients with MS. However, we now know that such reactions are not likely to occur across histocompatibility barriers. Therefore, these reactions may have been ADCC reactions or local antibody synthesis. However, soluble antigen could be released in these cultures and antigen presentation by cells within the blood cell population or by glial cells such as astrocytes, under the influence of lymphokines such as interferon, could allow for a true T-cell mediated reaction. It has been demonstrated that astrocytes can be induced to present antigen to MBP specific T-cell lines in the context of major histocompatibility complex (MHC; HLA in man) type II antigens (Ia or DR) (Fontana, Fierz and Wekerle, 1984). It is of considerable interest that MHC type II antigens have been recently described on astrocytes as well as macrophages, but not oligodendrocytes, in MS lesions (Traugott, Scheinberg and Raine, 1985). Once a reaction commences within the CNS it is conceivable that the MHC type II positive astrocytes could be important in the maintenance of the immunological reaction. In addition, lymphokines and monokines (including interleukin-1 (IL-1) and prostaglandins), could have the capacity to cause demyelination and/or CNS symptoms without demyelination (Fontana and Fierz, 1985). Interleukins and other mediators produced by inflammatory cells could also serve to stimulate proliferation of astrocytes, which is a prominent finding in MS lesions.

Some of the difficulties in the study of cell-mediated immunological reactions in MS using peripheral blood may be due to the dilution of antigen specific cells among a large circulating population. In addition, it is possible that the more reactive cells are within the CNS and CSF (Norohna, Richman and Arnason, 1980) as has been suggested in EAE. Using techniques developed to study the relatively few cells found in the CSF of patients with MS even during acute exacerbations, it was possible to demonstrate that CSF lymphocytes of patients with active MS had greater reactivity to MBP than CSF of patients with clinically stable MS or other neurological disorders (Lisak and Zweiman, 1977). Perhaps more important was the demonstration that the CSF lymphocytes were more reactive to MBP than peripheral blood mononuclear cells from the same patient. The paucity of available cells made it impossible to test the cells of the same subjects with other antigens. Therefore, antigen specific disease specific hypersensitivity to MBP was not demonstrated. Increased reactivity to MBP by CSF lymphocytes of MS patients has been reported by others (Czlonkowska *et al.*, 1982) and also to measles (Reunanen *et al.*, 1980).

It is now clear that T cells that react specifically with tetanus toxoid (Burns, Zweiman and Lisak, 1984), an antigen that it not a likely pathogenic agent in MS, can be recovered from the CSF of patients with MS. Therefore, future studies of CSF lymphocytes in patients with MS and control subjects will require: (1) frequency analysis; (2) testing of different amino acid sequences from MBP; (3) testing of CNS and non-CNS antigens including non-suspect antigens; and/or (4) demonstration of prior *in vivo* activation of cells reactive to one particular antigen.

Only such studies would strongly support the pathogenic role for CNS autoantigen-reactive T cells (Lisak *et al.*, 1984).

Another explanation for the failure to demonstrate increased reactivity to a myelin or oligodendrocyte component is that the tests are performed using antigens such as MBP or cells (oligodendrocytes, myelinated tissue culture) obtained from the CNS of normal human or experimental animals. There have been attempts to demonstrate MS specific antigens in the CNS of patients with MS. To date, there is no compelling evidence for such an antigen nor for a specific reaction (cellular or humoral) to MS origin CNS components (Lisak *et al.*, 1984).

Other cell-mediated reactions

There have been many studies that address natural-killer (NK) and antibody dependent cell-mediated cytotoxicity (ADCC; killer cell (K)) function in patients with MS (*see below*). These have been primarily designed to investigate NK- and K-cell functions as indicators of general abnormal immunoregulatory activity rather than examining the possibility that such cells cause lesions within the CNS with myelin, myelin components or oligodendrocytes as the target of the cell-mediated reaction. Although glial tumours have been employed as *in vitro* targets for NK reactions, there are no published studies using cultured adult human oligodendrocytes as targets.

ADCC reactions to CNS antigens have not been extensively investigated. MBP has been coated on to the surface of erythrocytes, the red blood cells serving as the indicator cells of cytotoxicity (Frick and Stickl, 1980, 1982; Eggers *et al.*, 1981). While MS serum is reported to mediate increased ADCC reactions to these cells, the biological relevance is not clear since: (1) MBP is not an external component of oligodendrocytes or myelin; and (2) in some studies there are significant technical questions raised by the assay as performed. Convincing studies employing cultured oligodendrocytes or CNS myelinated cultures, MS serum or CSF and effector cell populations from patients with MS and controls are not available.

Monocyte-macrophages are prominent in the inflammatory lesion in MS. It had long been assumed that these cells were simply serving a non-specific phagocytic function. As we have learned more about the functions of macrophages, it has become clear that their presence in MS lesions may be important in other ways. They may be present as part of a delayed type hypersensitivity reaction and contribute to propagation of the lesion as well as demyelination and cytotoxicity, perhaps by secretion of various monokines (IL-1, prostaglandins, leukotrienes) (Fontana and Grob, 1985; Dore-Duffy, Ho and Longo, 1985; Zweiman and Lisak, 1986). They also may be important in immune phagocytosis through the interaction of antibodies (immunoglobulins) to myelin and the macrophage receptors for the Fc portion of immunoglobulin (antibodies) and/or complement (Prineas *et al.*, 1984).

VIROLOGICAL RELATED IMMUNOLOGICAL ABNORMALITIES

General considerations

A considerable amount of investigative activity is centred around the possibility of a viral aetiology of MS. The evidence for this hypothesis is indirect and is based on several pieces of evidence. Among these are: (1) epidemiological, including the Faroe islands experience which has characteristics of a point source epidemic; (2) the clear-cut demonstration of naturally occurring persistent viral infections in man (herpes simplex and varicella-zoster) and animals, in which latency within the nervous system has been clearly demonstrated; (3) the demonstration that there are transmissible disorders of the CNS of man and other animals in which the characteristics of the 'infective' agent differs from that of known conventional viruses or other known infectious agents (Jacob-Creutzfeld disease, Kuru, scrapie); (4) claims of isolation of viral agents or demonstration of fingerprints of such agents employing immunohistological techniques, electron microscopy or, more recently, genetic probes (Haase *et al.*, 1984); and (5) immunological studies (to be reviewed below) which suggest an altered immune response to one or more viruses in patients with MS. Discussion of the epidemiological considerations is found elsewhere in this volume (*see* Chapter 3) and detailed consideration of latent viral diseases of man and other animals, 'prion'-mediated disorders and the lack of specificity and reproducibility of the demonstration of viruses in the CNS or other organs of patients with MS is beyond the scope of this chapter (*see* Johnson, 1982, and ter Meulen *et al.*, 1984).

Humoral immunity

The strongest immunological evidence for a role for viruses in the aetiology of MS rests on serological data. Several groups have demonstrated that patients with MS have significantly, albeit modestly, elevated titres to measles virus in their serum (Fraser, 1977; Haire, 1977). This evidence, along with the long-standing description of post-infectious acute disseminated encephalomyelitis following measles, was the major impetus for the search for measles or a related virus (canine distemper) as a possible persistent infectious agent in MS brain. Further interest in measles virus resulted from the demonstration of elevated titres in the CSF, generally higher in the CSF than the serum on a milligram of immunoglobulin basis (Norrby, Line and Olsson, 1974; Norrby, 1978). This suggests that the CSF antimeasles antibody was being synthesized within the nervous system. Analogies were made to subacute sclerosing panencephalitis (SSPE). However, more recent studies have cast considerable doubt on the specificity of the heightened humoral immune response to measles or any other as yet unidentified virus in MS.

Elevated serum and CSF titres can be demonstrated to other viruses including mumps, herpes simplex, varicella-zoster, rubella and vaccinia (Haire, 1977; Nordal, Vandvick and Norrby, 1978). One might argue that a different virus is involved in different patients, but elevated titres to several viruses are frequently found in the same patient and indirect evidence for intra-CNS synthesis of antibodies to several viruses can also be found in the same patient. As noted earlier in this chapter and elsewhere in this volume (Chapter 6), the IgG in the CSF and within plaques is most often found in a restricted spectrotype pattern (oliogoclonal bands). Employing absorption with antigen or immunofixation techniques, it has also become clear that very little of the IgG (the major oligoclonal bands or the polyclonal IgG) can be accounted for by antibody to viruses, although the antiviral antibodies in CSF themselves show a restricted spectrotypic pattern (Nordal, Vandvick and Norrby, 1978). In SSPE and other known infections the vast majority of the CSF IgG is antibody to the infectious agent (Vandvick *et al.*, 1976; Porter, Sinnamon and Gilles, 1977). Another argument against the oligoclonal bands necessarily representing evidence for CNS infection is the demonstration of oligoclonal IgG in the CSF and CNS of animals with acute EAE (Rostami *et al.*, 1982), recovering from acute EAE (Whitacre *et al.*, 1981), and with chronic-recurrent EAE (Mehta, Lassman and Wisnewski, 1981). Thus, oligoclonal bands may simply represent the consequences of subacute and chronic CNS inflammation.

Since there is an increase in antibodies to several viruses in the serum of patients with MS and intra-CNS synthesis of antibodies to several viruses (and bacteria as well) but no hard evidence for specific infection of the CNS in patients, we need to examine the possible explanations.

The increase in antibodies to several viruses could represent the result of a modest decrease in normal broad-based regulatory immunological control mechanisms. It has been reported that family members have a higher serum titre to several viruses than do friends of patients with MS, although not as high as the patients themselves (Brody *et al.*, 1972).

The reason for increased intra-CNS synthesis of antibodies to several viruses is not known. It has been suggested that during exacerbations, or perhaps at other times, B cells and T cells enter the CNS. For unknown reasons these lymphocytes persist, perhaps proliferate and secrete immunoglobulins (antibodies) despite the absence of specific antigen. Why B cells, or T cells for that matter, should persist in the absence of specific antigen is not clear. A relative lack of normal suppressor mechanisms within the CNS could be important. Material within the CNS such as proteases (Bever and Whitaker, 1985), myelin constituents or immunoglobulin itself (Berman and Weigle, 1977) could have direct or indirect stimulatory effects on B cells. T cells reacting to antigen within the CNS of patients with MS, or perhaps activated elsewhere and migrating through a defective blood–brain barrier, could secrete lymphokines which could then non-specifically stimulate all the B cells that happen to be within the CNS. However, it seems clear that initial B-cell activation is not mediated by lymphokines (Fauci, 1982; Howard and Paul, 1983; Calvert *et al.*, 1984). Therefore, an anti-immunoglobulin such as an anti-idiotype (antibodies directed against the antigen binding portion of other antibodies), or other stimulatory factors would have to be involved if there is no specific antigen within the CNS to initiate B-cell activation.

Cell-mediated immunity

Over the years there has also been interest in cell-mediated immune responses to different viruses in patients with MS. There have been several approaches. One hypothesis is that there are reduced levels of cell-mediated reactivity, for unknown reasons, which then allow for persistent infection (Utermohlen and Zabriskie, 1973). In this scheme, the persistent virus or viral antigen serves as a source of continuous antigenic stimulation which contributes to the elevated levels of antibodies to the virus in the serum and CSF. The proof of reduced cell-mediated immunity was based on several *in vitro* assays, some of which may have been measuring other than T-cell reactivity (Nordal *et al.*, 1976). It is not clear how decreased reactivity to several viruses in the same patient could be compatible with a single persistent pathogenic virus. There is no evidence that fluctuations in *in vitro* reactivity to viruses correlate with clinical changes in patients (Lisak *et al.*, 1978). *In vivo* assays (skin tests) have also been employed but a review of these studies fails to provide conclusive proof of significant reduction of reactivity to one or more viruses.

Two other possibilities are that patients have increased levels of cell-mediated immunity to one or more viruses as a result of persistent infection or an excessive response because of abnormal immunoregulation. Such an increased response could be pathogenic under certain circumstances. If a virus persisted within the nervous system and the patient had normal T-cell reactivity to that virus, damage could be inadvertently directed at cells containing that virus (Wisniewski, 1977). However, in order for a cytotoxic T cell to proceed against a virus resident in a cell, that cell must have type I MHC antigens on its surface (Zinkernagel and Doherty, 1974). There is no evidence that unstimulated oligodendrocytes are MHC type I antigen positive. It has been suggested that certain lymphokines can induce specific MHC antigens on the surface of oligodendrocytes (Wong *et al.*, 1984; Suzumura, Lisak and Silberberg, 1986). Therefore, an inflammatory response within the CNS might result in lymphokine release which could then alter the oligodendrocyte so that it could be involved as a target of a cytotoxic T-cell response. While there have been several studies recently describing type II MHC antigens on astrocytes and vascular endothelial cells in lesions of patients with MS (Traugott, 1985; Traugott, Scheinberg and Raine, 1985), there is little information about the presence or absence of type I antigens on oligodendrocytes in MS lesions. If the virus was resident in astrocytes (which might be induced to bear MHC antigens), lymphocytes or macrophage-monocytes within the CNS, T-cell cytotoxic reactions could proceed. It is also possible that NK-cell or K-cell reactions directed at a virus with the CNS could be the explanation for the cellular infiltration seen in the MS lesion.

It has long been suggested that a viral infection might induce an autoimmune disease by: (1) altering a CNS antigen (Steck *et al.*, 1976); (2) sensitizing the host to that antigen (Tschannen, Steck and Schafer, 1979). There is experimental evidence for this in animals but none in man. Another possible interaction of viruses and autoimmunity in MS is the possibility that reactivity to a viral or bacterial antigen with homology to a CNS antigen could induce a cytotoxic response to the self-antigen. There is increasing experimental evidence for such potential cross-reactivity with MBP (Finne, Leinonen and Mahela, 1983; Waksman, 1984; Fujinani and Oldstone, 1985; Jahnke, Fischer and Alvord, 1985).

Animal models

There has been renewed interest in animal models of viral induced demyelination. Most of the acute experimental viral infections of laboratory animals do not produce a primary inflammatory demyelinating disease of the CNS with relative sparing of neurons and axons. However, demyelinating lesions have recently been produced by experimental manipulation or by allowing animals to recover from acute encephalitis or poliomyelitis (Weiner, 1973; Dal Canto and Lipton, 1975; Nagashima *et al.*, 1978; ter Meulen *et al.*, 1984). The subsequent development of lesions that resemble those of EAE has been reported. At this stage the CNS has little, if any, viral material detectable by conventional immunological or virological methods. It has been suggested that this late pathogenic lesion in some models results from either a cell-mediated reaction to a persistent viral antigen or the induction of an autoimmune disease within the CNS. While these hypotheses are quite attractive, until quite recently there has been no direct proof to support either of these two alternatives. However, Watanabe, Wege and ter Meulen (1983) have been able to transfer EAE, employing cells of animals that have developed a late demyelinative lesion following intracerebral inoculation with a coronavirus. Cell-mediated immunity to myelin basic protein seems to be involved. As yet, passive transfer with antigen specific T-cell lines or clones, either from spleen, lymph nodes, blood or CNS (*see* earlier discussion) has not been reported in this fascinating model.

ABNORMALITIES OF IMMUNOREGULATION

As pointed out earlier, immunopathological reactions can be thought of as typical immune reactions that are excessive, inappropriate, or misdirected. If MS is a disease that is mediated by one or more immunopathological reactions, then it seems likely that there must be a breakdown or failure in the control or regulation of one or more aspects of the immune system. If MS is caused by a persistent infection with a virus or an abnormal immune response triggered by a virus, it would seem most likely to be a common virus. If this is true, then one must assume that there is a reason for viral persistence with tissue damage or for the triggering of an aberrant or unusual response by the immune system. For these reasons there are many investigations of immunoregulation in patients with MS.

Normal regulation of the immune response involves incompletely understood interactions of several subpopulations of cells as well as products of these cells. There are both antigen and antibody specific as well as non-specific suppressive and enhancing interactions (Bona and Pernis, 1984; Tada, 1984). In addition to interactions between cells of the immune system there are interactions with other organ systems including the nervous system (reviewed by Besedovsky, del Ray and Sorkin, 1984; Martin, 1984; Tecoma and Huey, 1985).

Over the past few years there has been a flurry of studies examining blood and, more recently, CSF cells of patients with MS for evidence of impaired immunoregulation. These have included both quantitative studies of lymphocyte subsets and functional studies. Until recently, most functional studies and many quantitative studies have employed blood cells which may only give an indirect or perhaps even an erroneous impression of regulatory mechanisms at play in the CNS. The major shortcoming of studies of abnormal immunoregulation is that the nature of the antigen of importance is not known in MS, as opposed to the situation in myasthenia gravis. In that disorder, studies of both non-specific and specific defects in immunoregulation are possible since the acetylcholine receptor has been clearly identified as the important autoantigen (Lisak, Levinson and Zweiman, 1985; Levinson *et al.*, 1985). A second major problem in MS is that we do not know which are the important immunopathogenic mechanisms, again differing from myasthenia gravis (Lisak, Levinson and Zweiman, 1985; Ashizawa and Appel, 1985). Investigators, therefore, have studied regulation of T-cell, B-cell, K-cell and NK-cell function, but not to specific CNS antigens. While useful data have come from these studies, it is difficult to put these in perspective.

Quantitative studies

There have been many studies of levels of subsets of lymphocytes using several assays to determine if there is a numerical imbalance of helper and suppressor T cells as well as total lymphocytes, total T cells and B cells. Most of the recent studies have employed one of several series of monoclonal antibodies which identify subpopulations of lymphocytes with different putative *in vitro* and *in vivo* functions. The earliest of these studies seemed to indicate a decrease in levels of blood suppressor/cytotoxic T cells, often to very low levels, which were seen either in acute exacerbations or progressive disease (Bach *et al.*, 1980; Reinherz *et al.*, 1980). Since that time there have been many studies, some of which have supported this association, others showing only modest decreases in suppressor T cells and a resultant increase in the helper/suppressor ratio, and others which fail to show consistent changes (Compston, 1983; Kastrukoff and Paty, 1984; Rice *et al.*, 1984). Despite several panel discussions and supplements to journals dealing with this point, it is unlikely that a consensus will be reached (Panel discussion, 1984). Some of the difficulties may relate to technical questions (which monoclonal antibodies are employed, visual assessment of immunofluorescence versus the use of cell sorters, etc.), others to the simple fact that there are clearly subsets within the lymphocyte subsets (oversimplification of the problem). The major problem probably arises from the great difficulty in assessing what is going on within the CNS even with the most careful clinical observations.

The explanation for the observed decrease in suppressor/cytotoxic cells in the blood of patients with MS, when observed, is also not clear. It seems unlikely to represent cell lysis and it has been suggested that the decrease in the blood may represent migration of these T8$^+$ (suppressor/cytotoxic) cells into the CNS. Most studies of the CSF cell subpopulations do not support that compartment as the site of homing of suppressor/cytotoxic T cells (Cashman *et al.*, 1982; Hauser *et al.*, 1983). Several groups have examined lesions in the CNS of patients with MS and at least one group believes that the chronic active plaques and perhaps active lesions could be the site of the rapidly shifting suppressor/cytotoxic cells (Weiner *et al.*, 1984; Panel discussion, 1984). Not all groups find a predominance of suppressor/cytotoxic T cells in MS lesions (Traugott and Raine, 1984; Traugott, 1985). Moreover, it is impossible to quantitate truly the number of any inflammatory cell subset throughout the neuraxis. In addition, different lesions in the same patient are likely to be of different chronological ages. Acute lesions of classic relapsing-remitting MS have not been studied with current immuno-histological techniques and reagents.

It has been suggested that suppressor cells are not lost from the blood but rather the antigens on these cell surfaces cannot be detected because of *in vivo* down-regulation by circulating antilymphocyte antibodies (Antel *et al.*, 1982; Reder *et al.*, 1984). Sera of MS patients frequently contain antilymphocyte antibodies (Schocket *et al.*, 1977; Lisak, Mercado and Zweiman, 1979). Down-regulation of specific lymphocyte antigens by mouse monoclonal antibodies to lymphocytes can be demonstrated *in vitro*, as can apparent reappearance *in vitro*. It is clear that the T-cell antigens detected with some of the monoclonal antibodies have important functions in T cells (Huddlestone and Oldstone, 1982; Achito and Reinherz, 1985). There is, however, no evidence that the blood of patients with MS contains antilymphocyte antibodies directed against any of the known epitopes detected by currently employed monoclonal antibodies.

Because most of the available monoclonal antibodies to human mononuclear cells have been directed at markers of T-cell subsets, most of the quantitative studies of blood and CSF lymphocytes (as well as *in situ* studies of lesions themselves) have been concerned with T-cell subsets. As a new generation of monoclonal antibodies to B-cell differentiation antigens (B1, B2, PC-1, PCA-1, Leu 12) and monocyte markers becomes available, we will probably see similar studies of blood, inflammatory cells in CSF and the CNS. As studies evolve, we will have to compare the results of quantitative measurement with these to functional B-cell assays of the same populations in an attempt to determine if there is any biological importance to the quantitative findings.

Functional studies

While assessing the numbers of frequencies of subpopulations of lymphocytes may prove useful, one must show that there are functional consequences of such changes. Indeed, it is abnormal function of cells involved in immune regulation that would lead to autoimmunity or persistent infection.

Antel, Arnason and Medof (1979) first demonstrated that there was a decrease in the capacity of blood lymphocytes to generate concanavalin-A suppressor activity using an assay that measures T-cell suppression of mitogen (non-specific) induced T-cell proliferation. This has been confirmed (Gonzalez, Dau and Spitler, 1978), although there is no direct correlation with the levels of suppressor cells as assessed by monoclonal antibodies to the T8 antigen (Bach, 1985). In addition, there is some evidence that suppressor cells are activated in certain phases of the disease (Huddlestone and Oldstone, 1982). It seems likely that T cells are directly or indirectly involved in the pathogenesis of MS. However, this is not certain and, therefore, whether changes in suppressor cell control of T-cell reactivity (non-specific or to an as yet unidentified auto- or viral antigen) are important in the pathogenesis of MS is not clear.

Other workers have described an increase *in vitro* in blood B-cell activity (Levitt, Griffin and Egan, 1980; Kelley *et al.*, 1981; Goust, Hogan and Arnaud, 1982), although there is some controversy as to whether the defect is the result of reduced suppression by T cells, excess help by T cells, inherently increased B-cell activity or some combination of these factors. These functional studies cannot be readily attributed to frequency (numbers) of suppressor or helper cell populations, at least using the first generation of monoclonal antilymphocyte antibodies (Antel *et al.*, 1984). In addition, the role of monocytes and their products, such as prostaglandins, on B-cell and T-cell responses is not clear (Dore-Duffy, Ho and Longo, 1985). Moreover, since serum immunoglobulin levels in patients with MS are normal or minimally elevated (Wilkerson *et al.*, 1977) and spectrotype restriction is not prominently observed in serum immunoglobulins, it is not clear what one is to make of these data related to blood T-cell/B-cell interactions. They may be important if these cells either enter the CNS or at least reflect intra-CNS and intra-CSF cellular interactions.

Recently it has been shown that CSF lymphocytes may exhibit vigorous *in vitro* B-cell activity (Levinson *et al.*, 1983). It is not clear whether this represents decreased suppressor activity by T cells, monocytes or NK-cells or inherent increased B-cell activity. It is also possible that material within the CNS or CSF may serve as a polyclonal (or oligoclonal) stimulator for B cells (*see above*).

Several groups have described a decrease in *in vitro* NK-cell activity in the blood of patients with MS, as well as a decrease in interferon production. However, the demonstration of decreased NK-cell activity and interferon production has not been universally confirmed (reviewed in Neighbor, 1984). Merrill has described a decrease in NK activity which seems to correlate with increased macrophage production of prostaglandin E (PGE) (Merrill, Myers and Ellison, 1984), which is seen in patients with active disease as originally described by Dore-Duffy and co-workers (reviewed in Dore-Duffy, Ho and Longo, 1985). The relative sensitivity of lymphocytes of patients with MS to the *in vitro* and *in vivo* regulatory effects of the various interferons is not well worked out and there is controversy in this area as well.

Merrill and colleagues have also reported decreased NK activity *in vitro* by CSF lymphocytes as well as reduced interferon-positive cells when compared to patients with other neurological diseases (Merrill, Myers and Ellison, 1984). While they have also described elevated CSF levels of PGE and a correlation between PGE production and decreased interferon, there was no effect of indomethacin (an inhibitor of prostaglandin synthesis) on CSF NK-cell activity (Merrill *et al.*, 1983). It has also been reported that there is an increase in blood cell ADCC activity in MS patients (Merrill *et al.*, 1982).

There is now considerable evidence that patients with MS differ from normal subjects in regard to cellular immunoregulatory mechanisms and in the *in vitro* production of and response to several immunomodulating substances. Both quantitative and functional abnormalities have been reported, but their relation to disease activity and pathogenesis is not clear. It is now clear that lesions within the CNS itself can have effects on the regulatory status of the immune system, inducing changes in immunoregulation and immune reactivity. It is also known that lymphocytes may interact with neuropeptides. Moreover, groups of investigators differ on experimental details and even as to whether certain of these abnormalities can be consistently demonstrated in patients with MS. Until a target antigen is identified and it becomes clear which immunopathogenic reactions are important, studies of immunoregulation such as have been reviewed above will need to be interpreted with great caution.

SUMMARY

There can be little doubt that MS is an inflammatory disorder of the CNS accompanied by several immunological abnormalities. The inflammatory response seems to be important in the initiation of the demyelination and is accompanied, associated with or perhaps caused by abnormalities in the immune system. These abnormalities are detectable within the systemic immune system and in the nervous system, including the CSF. Indeed, the very presence of a significant number of inflammatory cells in the nervous system is abnormal since such cells are not a normal component of the nervous system, at least not in readily detectable numbers. It is likely that inflammatory cells pass through some portions of the nervous system in small numbers (Stohl and Gonatas, 1978).

There has been an outpouring of studies (reviewed above) examining many different aspects of immunological responses of patients with MS. While there seems to be agreement that the immune system is not normal, the reader and reviewer are likely to come away frustrated and often confused by the frequently contradictory studies. Several review articles appear each year and despite often heroic attempts at understanding the reasons for the conflicting data and the development of imaginative and elegant schemes to synthesize a clear cut story for the aetiology and pathogenesis of MS, the final answer is not close at hand. For those who are not intimately involved in research in MS or experimental models or involved in the care of such patients, as well as for many of those who are, the reasons for this difficulty may not be readily apparent.

The reasons are many but can be considered in four general inter-related areas; the extreme complexity of the immune and nervous systems, the long duration of the disease, the difficulty in assessing the activity of the disease, and the necessary reliance on *in vitro* tests frequently employing sera and cells from the blood rather than CNS or CSF derived material.

In recent years we have learned a great deal about the inter-relationships between different subsets of cells of the immune system and their products in health and disease in experimental animals using both *in vitro* and *in vivo* assays. Such progress has rapidly been applied to human immunobiology and immunopathology. However, these very studies of experimental animals and man reveal how much more there is to learn and understand. Thus, we frequently see unfortunate oversimplification. It has also become clear that there are inter-relationships between the CNS and the immune systems under normal circumstances as well as the demonstration that abnormalities of the CNS may affect normal immunological function. Thus, both the immune system and the CNS may be modified directly or indirectly by drugs and therapies not previously thought to have an effect on either system. This can contribute to problems in correlation with disease activity (*see below*) and may affect several *in vitro* assays of immunological function.

As reviewed in Chapter 3, epidemiological evidence suggests that there may be a 5–30 year latency between exposure to an important, albeit unknown, environmental factor and the first symptoms of MS. In addition, it is not uncommon for immunological and virological studies to be performed on CNS material obtained 30 years after the onset of disease and many years after obvious clinically active disease.

Early studies of immunological abnormalities in patients with MS frequently failed to take into consideration the type of disease (relapsing-remitting, relapsing-progressive, progressive from the outset), disease activity (acute exacerbation, recovery from exacerbation, slow progression, rapid progression), age, sex and medications. Although there are still unfortunate exceptions, it is unusual to see such reports today. In addition, studies which examine abnormal reactivity in which disease specific antigenic reactivity is a vital part of the hypothesis now generally include appropriate neurological and immunological disease control subjects. Despite attention to these issues, clinical differences probably contribute to much of the disparity in immunological studies. Based on pathological studies and more recently on neuroimaging (*see* Chapter 2) with computerized assisted tomography and magnetic resonance imaging as well as evoked responses (*see* Chapter 7), it is clear that lesions may occur in the absence of clinical manifestations. It is also clear that an acute exacerbation of apparently circumscribed type may actually be associated with many more active lesions of varying size which are not associated with any discernable symptomatology. We do not know if an acute exacerbation represents a new lesion or is simply due to a lesion which has reached sufficient size to cause new symptoms (*see* Chapter 7). We do not know if inflammation and demyelination are continuous in stable, progressive, or relapsing-exacerbating disease. We do not even know if all exacerbations represent demyelination or just oedema or symptoms produced in part by products of activated lymphocytes, monocytes or glial cells (Fontana and Grob, 1985). In addition, fatigue, fever, etc. may produce new symptoms by affecting a known or clinically silent existing lesion, despite strict clinical criteria used by many workers to try to distinguish acute exacerbations from fluctuating clinical manifestations of other causes.

The vast majority of immunological studies of patients with MS employ *in vitro* assays to assess humoral and cell-mediated responses. *In vitro* assays have several advantages including providing objective quantitative measurements, allowing dissection of complex immunological phenomena, and safe testing of reactivity to potential autoantigens. They have drawbacks as well. Among these are assumptions that a particular technique has a certain correlation with an *in vivo* function. For certain techniques there is a need for considerable volumes of blood or other body fluids. Over the years, as more has been learned about the immune system, it has become clear that we have at times been either incorrect or at least simplistic in our interpretations of the meaning of certain *in vitro* tests. The problem of available number of cells and/or volume of fluid is a major limiting factor in MS research. As indicated, one would like to know about the reactivity of CSF and CNS cells and immunoglobulin as well as kinetics of cell migration and trafficking, immunoglobulin synthesis, etc. Even with miniaturization of techniques, it is not always feasible to perform such studies, because of technical and ethical considerations. This had led to some reliance on experimental models but even here there are technical limitations in studying cells and antibodies within the CNS and CSF.

Despite these limitations in our ability to interpret easily complex immunological and neurological phenomena, our new knowledge and understanding and the availability of new technology in immunology, neurobiology, virology, molecular biology, clinical electrophysiology and imaging of the nervous system, should allow significant progress in our understanding of the immune system in the aetiology and pathogenesis of MS. This should then lead to rational, effective and safe treatment and/or prevention of the disorder.

References

AARLI, J. A., APARICIO, S. R., LUMSDEN, C. E. and TONDER, O. (1975) Binding of normal human IgG to myelin sheaths, glia and neurons. *Immunology*, **28**, 171–185

ABRAMSKY, O., LISAK, R. P., SILBERBERG, D. H. and PLEASURE, D. E. (1977) Antibodies to oligodendroglia in patients with multiple sclerosis. *New England Journal of Medicine*, **297**, 1207–1211

ACUTO, O. and REINHERZ, E. L. (1985) The human T-cell receptor. *New England Journal of Medicine*, **312**, 1100–1111

ALLERAND, D. and YAHR, M. D. (1964) Gammaglobulin affinity for normal human tissue of the central nervous system. *Science*, **144**, 1141–1142

ANTEL, J. P., ARNASON, B. G. W. and MEDOF, M. E. (1979) Suppressor cell function in multiple sclerosis – correlation with clinical disease activity. *Annals of Neurology*, **5**, 338–342

ANTEL, J. P., OGER, J., JACKEVICIUS, S., KUO, H. H. and ARNASON, B. G. W. (1982) Modulation of T lymphocyte differentiation antigens: potential relevance for multiple sclerosis. *Proceedings of the National Academy of Science, USA*, **79**, 3330–3334

ANTEL, J. P., ROSENKOETTER, M., REDER, A., OGER, J. J.-F. and ARNASON, B. G. W. (1984) Correlation of *in vitro* IgG secretion with T suppressor cell number and function in multiple sclerosis. *Neurology*, **34**, 1155–1160

ARNON, R., CRISP, E., KELLY, R., ELLISON, G. W., MYERS, L. W. and TOURTELLOTTE, W. W. (1980) Antiganglioside antibodies in multiple sclerosis. *Journal of Neurological Sciences*, **46**, 179–186

ASHIZAWA, T. and APPEL, S. H. (1985) Immunopathologic events at the endplate in myasthenia gravis. In *Immunoneurology, Volume II, Springer Seminars in Immunopathology*, edited by A. J. Steck and R. P. Lisak, **8**, 177–196

BACH, M. A. (1985) Immunoregulatory T-cells in multiple sclerosis: markers and functions. In *Immunoneurology, Volume I, Springer Seminars in Immunopathology*, edited by A. J. Steck and R. P. Lisak, **8**, 45–56

BACH, M. A., PHAN-DINH, F., TOURNIER, E. *et al.* (1980) Deficit in suppressor T-cells in active multiple sclerosis. *Lancet*, **2**, 1221–1224

BEHAN, P. O., KIES, M. W., LISAK, R. P., SHEREMATA, W. and LAMARCHE, J. B. (1973) Immunologic mechanisms in experimental encephalomyelitis in nonhuman primates. *Archives of Neurology*, **29**, 4–9

BEN-NUN, A., WEKERLE, H. and COHEN, I. R. (1981) The rapid isolation of clonable antigen-specific T lymphocyte lines capable of mediating autoimmune encephalomyelitis. *European Journal of Immunology*, **11**, 195–199

BERG, O. and KALLEN, B. (1964) Effect of mononuclear blood cells from multiple sclerosis patients on neuroglia in tissue culture. *Journal of Neuropathology and Experimental Neurology*, **23**, 550–559

BERMAN, M. A. and WEIGLE, W. O. (1977) B lymphocyte activation by the Fc region of IgG. *Journal of Experimental Medicine*, **146**, 241–256

BESEDOVSKY, H., DEL RAY, A. and SORKIN, E. (1984) Immunoregulation by neuroendocrine mechanisms. In *Neuroimmunology*, edited by P. O. Behan and F. Spreafico, pp. 445–450. New York: Raven Press

BEVER, C. T. and WHITAKER, J. N. (1985) Proteinases in inflammatory demyelinating disease. In *Immunoneurology, Volume II, Springer Seminars in Immunopathology*, edited by A. J. Steck and R. P. Lisak, **8**, 235–250

BLAW, M. E., COOPER, M. D. and GOOD, R. A. (1967) Experimental allergic encephalomyelitis in agammaglobulinemic chickens. *Science*, **158**, 1198–1200

BONA, C. A. and PERNIS, B. (1984) Idiotypic networks. In *Fundamental Immunology*, edited by W. E. Paul, pp. 577–592. New York: Raven Press

BOOSS, J., ESIRI, M. M., TOURTELLOTTE, W. W. and MASON, D. Y. (1983) Immunohistological analysis of T lymphocyte subsets in the central nervous system in chronic progressive multiple sclerosis. *Journal of Neurological Sciences*, **62**, 219–232

BORNSTEIN, M. B. and APPEL, S. H. (1961) The application of tissue culture to the study of experimental 'allergic' encephalomyelitis. I. Patterns of demyelination. *Journal of Neuropathology and Experimental Neurology*, **20**, 141–157

BORNSTEIN, M. B. and APPEL, S. H. (1965) Tissue culture studies of demyelination. *Annals of the New York Academy of Science*, **122**, 280–286

BORNSTEIN, M. B. and RAINE, C. S. (1970) Experimental allergic encephalomyelitis: antiserum inhibition of myelination *in vitro*. *Laboratory Investigation*, **23**, 536–542

BRODY, J. A., SEVER, J. L., EDGAR, A. and McNEW, J. (1972) Measles antibody titers of multiple sclerosis patients and their siblings. *Neurology*, **22**, 492–499

BURNS, J. B., ROSENZWEIG, A., ZWEIMAN, B. and LISAK, R. P. (1983) Isolation of myelin basic protein-reactive T-cell lines from normal human blood. *Cellular Immunology*, **81**, 435–440

BURNS, J., ROSENZWEIG, A., ZWEIMAN, B., MOSKOVITZ, A. and LISAK, R. P. (1984) Recovery of myelin basic protein reactive T-cells from spinal cords of Lewis rats with autoimmune encephalomyelitis. *Journal of Immunology*, **132**, 2690–2692

BURNS, J., ZWEIMAN, B. and LISAK, R. P. (1984) Tetanus toxoid reactive T lymphocytes in the cerebrospinal fluid of multiple sclerosis patients. *Immunological Communication*, **13**, 361–369

CALVERT, J. E., MARUYAMA, S., TEDDER, T. F., WEBB, C. F. and COOPER, M. D. (1984) Cellular events in the differentiation of antibody secreting cells. *Seminars in Hematology*, **21**, 226–243

CAMPBELL, B. (1971) Discussion of Kibler, R. F., Paty, D. W. and Sher, V. Immunology of multiple sclerosis. In *Immunological Disorders of the Nervous System, Research Publication Association of Nervous and Mental Diseases*, edited by L. P. Rowland, pp. 109–110. Baltimore: Williams and Wilkins

CASHMAN, N., MARTIN, C., EIZENBAUM, J.-F., DEGOS, J.-D. and BACH, M.-A. (1982) Monoclonal antibody-defined immunoregulatory cells in multiple sclerosis cerebrospinal fluid. *Journal of Clinical Investigation*, **70**, 387–392

COMPSTON, A. (1983) Lymphocyte subpopulations in patients with multiple sclerosis. *Journal of Neurology, Neurosurgery and Psychiatry*, **46**, 106–114

COOMBS, R. R. A. and GELL, P. G. H. (1968) Classification of allergic reactions responsible for clinical hypersensitivity and disease. In *Clinical Aspects of Immunity*, edited by P. G. H. Gell and R. R. A. Coombs, pp. 575–596. Philadelphia: F. A. Davis

COYLE, P. K., BROOKS, B. R., HIRSCH, R. *et al.* (1980) Cerebrospinal fluid lymphocyte populations and immune complexes in active multiple sclerosis. *Lancet*, **2**, 229–231

COYLE, P. K. and PROCYK-DOUGHERTY, Z. (1984) Multiple sclerosis immune complexes: an analysis of component antigens and antibodies. *Annals of Neurology*, **16**, 600–667

CUTLER, R. W. P., WATTERS, G. V. and HAMMERSTAD, J. P. (1970) The origin and turnover rates of cerebrospinal fluid albumin and gammaglobulin in man. *Journal of Neurological Sciences*, **10**, 259–268

CZLONKOWSKA, A., POLTARAK, M., CENDROWSKI, W. and KARLAK, J. (1982) Sensitization of cerebrospinal fluid and peripheral blood lymphocytes to myelin basic protein in multiple sclerosis. *Acta Neurologica Scandinavica*, **66**, 121–129

DAL CANTO, M. C. and LIPTON, H. L. (1975) Primary demyelination in Theiler's virus infection. *Laboratory Investigation*, **33**, 626–637

DELASNERIE-LAUPRETRE, N., PREVOT, D., MARTIN-MONDIERE, C., EIZENBAUM, J.-F., DEGOS, J.-D. and SOBEL, A. T. (1981) Serum and cerebrospinal fluid C2 in multiple sclerosis. *Journal of Laboratory and Clinical Immunology*, **6**, 23–25

DORE-DUFFY, P., HO, S.-Y. and LONGO, M. (1985) The role of prostaglandins in altered leukocyte function in multiple sclerosis. In *Immunoneurology, Volume II, Springer Seminars in Immunopathology*, edited by A. J. Steck and R. P. Lisak, **8**, 305–319

DUBOIS-DALQ, M., NIEDIECK, B. and BAYSE, M. (1970) Action of anticerebroside sera on myelinating tissue cultures. *Pathology European*, **5**, 331–347

EBERS, G. C. (1984) Oligoclonal banding in MS. *Annals of the New York Academy of Science*, **436**, 206–212

EDGINGTON, T. S. and D'ALESSIO, D. J. (1970) The assessment by immunofluorescence methods of humoral antimyelin antibodies in man. *Journal of Immunology*, **105**, 248–255

EGGERS, A. E., TARNUN, L., PLANK, C. R. and GAMBOA, E. T. (1981) Hyperreactivity to myelin basic protein in multiple sclerosis. *Journal of Neurological Sciences*, **52**, 385–390

ENDO, T., STEWART, S. S., KUNDU, S. K., OSOVITZ, S. and MARCUS, D. M. (1984) Antibodies to glycosphingolipids in patients with multiple sclerosis. *Annals of the New York Academy of Science*, **436**, 213–220

ESIRI, M. (1977) Immunoglobulin-containing cells in multiple sclerosis lesions. *Lancet*, **2**, 478–480

FAUCI, A. S. (1982) Human B lymphocyte function: cell triggering and immunoregulation. *Journal of Infectious Diseases*, **145**, 602–612

FINNE, J., LEINONEN, M. and MAHELA, P. H. (1983) Antigenic similarities between brain components and bacteria causing meningitis. Implications for vaccine development and pathogenesis. *Lancet*, **2**, 355–357

FONTANA, A., FIERZ, W. and WEKERLE, H. (1984) Astrocytes present myelin basic protein to encephalitogenic T-cell lines. *Nature*, **307**, 273–276

FONTANA, A. and FIERZ, W. (1985) The endothelium-astrocyte immune control system of the brain. In *Immunoneurology, Volume I, Springer Seminars in Immunopathology*, edited by A. J. Steck and R. P. Lisak, **8**, 57–70

FONTANA, A. and GROB, P. J. (1985) Lymphokines and the brain. In *Lymphokines, Springer Seminars in Immunopathology*, edited by A. L. De Weck, **7**, 375–378

FRASER, K. B. (1977) Multiple sclerosis: a virus disease? *British Medical Bulletin*, **33**, 34–39

FRICK, E. and STICKL, H. (1980) Antibody dependent lymphocyte cytotoxicity against basic protein of myelin in multiple sclerosis. *Journal of Neurological Sciences*, **46**, 187–197

FRICK, E. and STICKL, H. (1982) Specificity of antibody-dependent lymphocyte cytotoxicity against cerebral tissue constituents in multiple sclerosis. *Acta Neurologica Scandinavica*, **65**, 30–37

FRY, J. M., WEISSBARTH, S., LEHRER, G. M. and BORNSTEIN, M. B. (1974) Cerebroside antibody inhibits sulfatide synthesis and myelination and demyelinates in cord tissue cultures. *Science*, **183**, 540–542

FUJINAMI, R. S. and OLDSTONE, M. B. A. (1985) Virus induced autoimmunity through molecular mimicry. *Federation Proceedings*, **44**, 1921

GONATAS, N. K. and HOWARD, J. C. (1974) Inhibition of experimental allergic encephalomyelitis in rats severely depleted of T-cells. *Science*, **185**, 839

GONZALEZ, R. L., DAU, P. C. and SPITLER, L. E. (1978) Altered regulation of mitogen responsiveness by suppressor cells in multiple sclerosis. *Clinical and Experimental Immunology*, **36**, 78–84

GOUST, J. M., CHENAIS, F., CARNES, J. E., HAMES, C. G., FUDENBERG, H. H. and HOGAN, E. L. (1978) Abnormal T-cell subpopulations and circulating immune complexes in the Guillain-Barré syndrome and multiple sclerosis. *Neurology*, **28**, 421–425

GOUST, J.-M., HOGAN, E. L. and ARNAUD, P. (1982) Abnormal regulation of IgG production in multiple sclerosis. *Neurology*, **32**, 228–234

HAASE, A. T., STOWRING, L., VENTURA, P. *et al.* (1984) Detection by hybridization of viral infection of the human central nervous system. *Annals of the New York Academy of Science*, **436**, 10;3–108

HAIRE, M. (1977) Significance of virus antibodies in multiple sclerosis. *British Medical Bulletin*, **33**, 40–44

HAUSER, S. L., REINHERZ, E. L., HOBAN, C. J., SCHLOSSMAN, S. F. and WEINER, H. L. (1983) CSF cells in multiple sclerosis: monoclonal antibody analysis and relationship to peripheral blood T-cell subsets. *Neurology*, **33**, 575–579

HICKEY, W. F. and GONATAS, N. K. (1984) Suppressor T lymphocytes in the spinal cord of Lewis rats recovered from acute experimental allergic encephalomyelitis. *Cellular Immunology*, **85**, 284–288

HICKEY, W. F., GONATAS, N. K., KIMURA, H. and WILSON, D. B. (1983) Identification and quantitation of T lymphocyte subsets found in the spinal cord of the Lewis rat during acute experimental allergic encephalomyelitis. *Journal of Immunology*, **131**, 2805–2809

HINRICHS, D. J. (1984) Requirements for and regulation of adoptively transferred paralytic EAE. In *Immunoregulatory Processes in Experimental Allergic Encephalomyelitis and Multiple Sclerosis*, edited by A. A. Vandenbark and J. C. M. Raus, pp. 63–98. Amsterdam: Elsevier

HIRAYAMA, M., SILBERBERG, D. H., LISAK, R. P. and PLEASURE, D. (1983) Long-term culture of oligodendrocytes isolated from rat corpus callosum by Percoll density gradient. Lysis by polyclonal antigalactocerebroside serum. *Journal of Neuropathology and Experimental Neurology*, **42**, 16–28

HIRAYAMA, M., LISAK, R. P. and SILBERBERG, D. H. (1986) Serum-mediated oligodendrocyte cytotoxicity in multiple sclerosis patients and controls. *Neurology*, (in press)

HOWARD, M. and PAUL, W. E. (1983) Regulation of B-cell growth and differentiation by soluble factors. *Annual Review of Immunology*, **1**, 307–333

HUDDLESTONE, J. R. and OLDSTONE, M. B. A. (1982) Suppressor T-cells are activated *in vivo* in patients with multiple sclerosis coinciding with remission from acute attack. *Journal of Immunology*, **129**, 915–917

JAHNKE, U., FISCHER, E. H. and ALVORD, E. C. JR (1985) Sequence homology between certain viral proteins related to encephalomyelitis and neuritis. *Science*, **229**, 282–284

JOHNSON, A. B. and BORNSTEIN, M. B. (1978) Myelin-binding antibodies *in vitro*: immunoperoxidase studies with experimental allergic encephalomyelitis, anti-galactocerebroside and multiple sclerosis sera. *Brain Research*, **159**, 173–182

JOHNSON, R. T. (1982) *Viral Infections of the Nervous System*. Chapter 10, pp. 263–270. New York: Raven Press

KASTRUKOFF, L. F. and PATY, D. W. (1984) A serial study of peripheral blood T lymphocyte subsets in relapsing-remitting multiple sclerosis (MS). *Annals of Neurology*, **15**, 250–256

KELLEY, R. E., ELLISON, G. W., MYERS, L. W., GOYMERAC, V., LARRICK, S. B. and KELLY, C. C. (1981) Abnormal regulation of *in vitro* IgG production in multiple sclerosis. *Annals of Neurology*, **9**, 267–272

KENNEDY, P. G. E. and LISAK, R. P. (1979) A search for antibodies to glial cells in the serum and cerebrospinal fluid of patients with multiple sclerosis and Guillain-Barré syndrome. *Journal of Neurological Sciences*, **44**, 125–133

KIES, M. W. (1985) Species-specificity and localization of encephalitogenic sites in myelin basic protein. In *Immunoneurology, Volume II, Springer Seminars in Immunopathology*, edited by A. J. Steck and R. P. Lisak, **8**, 295–304

LATERRE, E. C., COLLEWOERT, A., HERMANS, J. F. and SFAELLO, Z. (1970) Electrophoretic morphology of gammaglobulins in cerebrospinal fluid of multiple sclerosis and other diseases of the nervous system. *Neurology*, **20**, 982–990

LATOV, N. (1984) Immunological abnormalities associated with chronic peripheral neuropathies: plasma cell dyscrasia and neuropathy. In *Neuroimmunology*, edited by P. O. Behan and F. Spreafico, pp. 261–274. New York: Raven Press

LEFVERT, A. K. and LINK, H. (1985) IgG production within the central nervous system: a critical review of proposed formulae. *Annals of Neurology*, **17**, 13–20

LENNON, V. and MACKAY, I. R. (1972) Binding of ^{125}I basic protein by serum and cerebrospinal fluid. *Clinical and Experimental Immunology*, **11**, 595–603

LEVINSON, A. I., SANDBERG-WOLLHEIM, M., LISAK, R. P. et al. (1983) Analysis of B-cell activation of cerebrospinal fluid lymphocytes in multiple sclerosis. *Neurology*, **33**, 1305–1310

LEVINSON, A. I., LISAK, R. P., ZWEIMAN, B. and KORNSTEIN, J. J. (1985) Phenotypic and functional analysis of lymphocytes in myasthenia gravis. In *Immunoneurology, Volume II, Springer Seminars in Immunopathology*, edited by A. J. Steck and R. P. Lisak, **8**, 209–234

LEVITT, D., GRIFFIN, N. B. and EGAN, M. L. (1980) Mitogen-induced plasma cell differentiation in patients with multiple sclerosis. *Journal of Immunology*, **124**, 2117–2121

LISAK, R. P. (1980) Multiple sclerosis: evidence for immunopathogenesis. *Neurology*, **30**, 99–105

LISAK, R. P. (1984) Antibodies to galactocerebroside: probes for the study of antibody-determined neurologic damage. In *Neuroimmunology*, edited by P. O. Behan and F. Spreafico, pp. 167–177. New York: Raven Press

LISAK, R. P., HEINZE, R. G., FALK, G. A. and KIES, M. W. (1968) Search for anti-encephalitogen antibody in human demyelinative diseases. *Neurology*, **18**, 122–128

LISAK, R. P., LEVINSON, A. I. and ZWEIMAN, B. (1985) Autoimmune aspects of myasthenia gravis. In *Concepts in Immunopathology*, edited by J. M. Cruse and R. E. Lewis Jr, pp. 65–101. Basel: Karger

LISAK, R. P., MERCADO, F. and ZWEIMAN, B. (1979) Cold reactive antilymphocyte antibodies in neurological diseases. *Journal of Neurology, Neurosurgery and Psychiatry*, **42**, 1054–1057

LISAK, R. P. and ZWEIMAN, B. (1977) *In vitro* cell-mediated immunity of cerebrospinal fluid lymphocytes to myelin basic protein in primary demyelinating disease. *New England Journal of Medicine*, **297**, 850–853

LISAK, R. P., ZWEIMAN, B., BURNS, J. B., ROSTAMI, A. and SILBERBERG, D. H. (1984) Immune response to myelin antigens in multiple sclerosis. *Annals of the New York Academy of Science*, **436**, 221–230

LISAK, R. P., ZWEIMAN, B. and NORMAN, M. E. (1975) Antimyelin antibodies in neurologic diseases: immunofluorescent demonstration. *Archives of Neurology*, **32**, 163–167

LISAK, R. P., ZWEIMAN, B., WATERS, D., KAPROWSKI, H. and PLEASURE D. E. (1978) Cell-mediated immunity to measles, myelin basic protein and central nervous system extract in multiple sclerosis. A longitudinal study employing direct buffy coat migration assays. *Neurology*, **28**, 798–803

LOWENTHAL, A., VANSANDE, M. and KARCHER, D. (1960) The differential diagnosis of neurological disease by fractionating electrophoretically the CSF-globulins. *Journal of Neurochemistry*, **6**, 51–60

LUBLIN, F. D. (1985) Relapsing experimental allergic encephalomyelitis – an autoimmune model of multiple sclerosis. In *Immunoneurology, Volume II, Springer Seminars in Immunopathology*, edited by A. J. Steck and R. P. Lisak, **8**, 197–208

MARTIN, J. B. (1984) Neuroendocrine regulation of the immune response. In *Neuroimmunology*, edited by P. O. Behan and F. Spreafico, pp. 433–443. New York: Raven Press

MASSANARI, R. M., PATERSON, P. Y. and LIPTON, H. L. (1979) Potentiation of experimental allergic encephalomyelitis in hamsters with persistent encephalitis due to measles virus. *Journal of Infectious Diseases*, **139**, 297–303

MEHTA, P. D., LASSMANN, H. and WISNIEWSKI, H. M. (1981) Immunologic studies of chronic relapsing EAE in guinea pigs: similarities to multiple sclerosis. *Journal of Immunology*, **127**, 334–338

MEHTA, P. D., MILLER, J. A. and TOURTELLOTTE, W. W. (1982) Oligoclonal IgG bands in plaques from multiple sclerosis brains. *Neurology*, **32**, 372–376

MERRILL, J. E., GERNER, R. H., MYERS, L. W. and ELLISON, G. W. (1983) Regulation of NK cell cytotoxicity by prostaglandin E in the blood and CSF of patients with MS and other neurological diseases. *Journal of Neuroimmunology*, **4**, 223–227

MERRILL, J. E., MYERS, L. W. and ELLISON, G. W. (1984) Cytotoxic cells in peripheral blood and cerebrospinal fluid of multiple sclerosis patients. *Annals of the New York Academy of Science*, **436**, 192–205

MERRILL, J. E., WAHLIN, B., SIDEN, A. and PERLMANN, P. (1982) Elevated direct and IgM enhanced ADCC activity in multiple sclerosis patients. *Journal of Immunology*, **128**, 1728–1735

MINGIOLI, E. S., STROBER, W., TOURTELLOTTE, W. W., WHITAKER, J. N. and MCFARLIN, D. E. (1978) Quantitation of IgG, IgA and IgM in the CSF by radioimmunoassay. *Neurology*, **28**, 991–995

MORGAN, B. P., CAMPBELL, A. K. and COMPSTON, D. A. S. (1984) Terminal component of complement (C9) in cerebrospinal fluid of patients with multiple sclerosis. *Lancet*, **2**, 251–255

MUSSINI, J.-M., HAUW, J.-J. and ESCOURELLE, R. (1977) Immunofluorescent studies if intra-cytoplasmic immunoglobulin binding lymphoid cells (CILC) in the central nervous system: report of 32 cases including 19 with multiple sclerosis. *Acta Neuropathology (Berlin)*, **40**, 227–232

NAGASHIMA, K., WEGE, H., MEYERMANN, R. and TER MEULEN, T. (1978) Coronavirus induced subacute, demyelinating encephalomyelitis in rats: a morphological analysis. *Acta Neuropathology (Berlin)*, **44**, 63–70

NEIGHBOR, P. A. (1984) Studies of interferon production and natural killing by lymphocytes from multiple sclerosis patients. *Annals of the New York Academy of Science*, **436**, 181–191

NIGHTINGALE, G. and HURLEY, J. V. (1978) Relationship between lymphocyte migration and vascular endothelium in chronic inflammation. *Pathology*, **10**, 27–44

NORDAL, H. J., FROLAND, S. S., VANDVICK, B. and NORRBY, E. (1976) Measles virus-induced migration inhibition of human leukocytes *in vitro*: an expression of cell-mediated immunity? *Scandinavian Journal of Immunology*, **5**, 969–977

NORDAL, H. J., VANDVICK, B. and NORRBY, E. (1978) Multiple sclerosis: local synthesis of electrophoretically restricted measles, rubella, mumps and herpes simplex virus antibodies in the central nervous system. *Scandinavian Journal of Immunology*, **7**, 473–479

NOROHNA, A. B. C., RICHMAN, D. P. and ARNASON, B. G. W. (1980) Detection of *in vivo* stimulated cerebrospinal fluid lymphocytes by flow cytometry in patients with multiple sclerosis. *New England Journal of Medicine*, **303**, 713–717

NORRBY, E. (1978) Viral antibodies in multiple sclerosis. *Progress in Medical Virology*, **24**, 1–39

NORRBY, E., LINK, H. and OLSSON, J. E. (1974) Measles virus antibodies in multiple sclerosis, comparison of antibody titres in cerebrospinal fluid and serum. *Archives of Neurology*, **30**, 285–292

Panel Discussion on Diagnostic Values of Blood T-Cell Levels in Multiple Sclerosis (1984) *Annals of the New York Academy of Science*, **436**, 247–293

PANITCH, H. S., HOFFER, C. L. J. and JOHNSON, K. P. (1980) CSF antibody to myelin basic protein. Measurements in patients with multiple sclerosis and subacute sclerosing panencephalitis. *Archives of Neurology*, **37**, 206–209

PATERSON, P. Y. (1984) Contribution of humoral and cellular processes to lesion formation in experimental allergic encephalomyelitis. In *Immunoregulatory Processes in Experimental Allergic Encephalomyelitis and Multiple Sclerosis*, edited by A. A. Vandenbark and J. C. M. Raus, pp. 127–150. Amsterdam: Elsevier

PORTER, K. G., SINNAMON, D. G. and GILLES, R. R. (1977) *Cryptococcus neoformans*-specific oligoclonal immunoglobulins in cerebrospinal fluid in cryptococcal meningitis. *Lancet*, **1**, 1262

PRINEAS, J. W., KWON, E. E., CHO, E.-S. and SHARER, L. R. (1984) Continual breakdown and regeneration of myelin in progressive multiple sclerosis plaques. *Annals of the New York Academy of Science*, **436**, 11–32

RAINE, C. S. and TRAUGOTT, U. (1984) Immunopathology of the lesion in multiple sclerosis and chronic relapsing experimental allergic encephalomyelitis. In *Immunoregulatory Processes in Experimental Allergic Encephalomyelitis and Multiple Sclerosis*, edited by A. A. Vandenbark and J. C. M. Raus, pp. 151–212. Amsterdam: Elsevier

REDER, A. T., ANTEL, J. P., OGER, J., McFARLAND, T. A., ROSENKOETTER, M. and ARNASON, B. G. W. (1984) Low T8 antigen density on lymphocytes in active multiple sclerosis. *Annals of Neurology*, **16**, 242–249

REIK, L., JR (1980) Disseminated vasculomyelinopathy: an immune complex disease. *Annals of Neurology*, **7**, 291–296

REINHERZ, E. L., WEINER, H. L., HAUSER, S. L., COHEN, J. A., DISTASO, J. A. and SCHLOSSMAN, S. F. (1980) Loss of suppressor T-cells in active multiple sclerosis. Analysis with monoclonal antibodies. *New England Journal of Medicine*, **303**, 125–129

REUNANEN, M., SAHUI, A., ILONEN, J. and HERVA, E. (1980) Proliferation of multiple sclerosis cerebrospinal fluid lymphocytes after stimulation with measles virus antigen. *Acta Neurologica Scandinavica*, **62**, 293–299

RICE, G. P. A., FINNEY, D. F., BRAHEMY, S. L., KNOBLER, R. L., SIPE, J. C. and OLDSTONE, M. B. A. (1984) Disease activity markers in multiple sclerosis. Another look at suppressor cells defined by monoclonal antibodies OKT4, OKT5 and OKT8. *Journal of Neuroimmunology*, **6**, 75–84

ROSENBLUM, W. I. (1973) A possible role for mast cells in the production of the pial vasospasm. *Brain Research*, **49**, 75–83

ROSTAMI, A., ECCLESTON, P. A., SILBERBERG, D. H., MANNING, M. C., BURNS, J. B. and LISAK, R. P. (1983) Absence of antibodies to galactocerebroside in the sera and cerebrospinal fluid of human demyelinating disorders. *Neurology*, **33** (Suppl. 2), 130

ROSTAMI, A., LISAK, R. P., BLANCHARD, N., GUERRERO, F., ZWEIMAN, B. and PLEASURE, D. E. (1982) Oligoclonal IgG in the cerebrospinal fluid of guinea pigs with acute experimental allergic encephalomyelitis. *Journal of Neurological Sciences*, **53**, 433–441

RUUTIANEN, J., REUNANEN, M. and FREY, H. (1982) Galactocerebroside antibodies in multiple sclerosis. *Acta Neurologica Scandinavica*, **65** (Suppl. 90), 260–261

SCHOCKET, A., WEINER, H. L., WALKER, J., McINTOSH, K. and KOHLER, P. F. (1977) Lymphocytotoxic antibodies in patients with multiple sclerosis. *Clinical Immunology and Immunopathology*, **7**, 15–23

SEIL, F. J. (1977) Tissue culture studies of demyelinating disease. A critical review. *Annals of Neurology*, **2**, 345–355

SELL, S. (1975) *Immunology, Immunopathology and Immunity*, 2nd edn, pp. 126–130; 276–282. Hagerstown, MD: Harper and Row

SERGOTT, R. C., BROWN, M. J., LISAK, R. P., MILLER, S. L. and McGARRY, R. (1985a) Monoclonal antibody to myelin associated glycoprotein (MAG) produces cell-associated demyelination *in vivo. Neurology*, **35** (Suppl.1), 295

SERGOTT, R. C., BROWN, M. J., LISAK, R. P. and SILBERBERG, D. H. (1985b) Optic nerve demyelination induced by human serum: patients with multiple sclerosis or optic neuritis and normal subjects. *Neurology*, **35**, 1438–1442

SERGOTT, R. C., BROWN, M. J., SILBERBERG, D. H. and LISAK, R. P. (1984) Antigalactocerebroside serum demyelinates optic nerve *in vivo. Journal of Neurological Sciences*, **64**, 297–303

SILBERBERG, D. H., MANNING, M. C. and SCHREIBER, A. D. (1984) Tissue culture demyelination by normal human serum. *Annals of Neurology*, **15**, 575–580

SRIRAM, S., SOLOMON, D., ROUSE, R. V. and STEINMAN, L. (1982) Identification of T-cell subsets and B lymphocytes in mouse brain experimental allergic encephalomyelitis lesions. *Journal of Immunology*, **129**, 1649–1651

STECK, A. J. and MURRAY, N. (1985) Monoclonal antibodies to myelin associated glycoprotein reveal antigenic structures and suggest pathogenic mechanisms. In *Immunoneurology, Volume I, Springer Seminars in Immunopathology*, **8**, 29–44

STECK, A. and REGLI, F. (1980) Oligodendrocyte binding antibodies in multiple sclerosis: ^{125}I protein A studies. *Neurology*, **30**, 540–542

STECK, A. J., SIEGRIST, P., HERSCHKOWITZ, N. and SCHAEFER, R. (1976) Phosphorylation of myelin basic protein by vaccinia virus cores. *Nature*, **263**, 436–438

STOHL, W. and GONATAS, N. K. (1978) Chronic permeability of the central nervous system to mononuclear cells in experimental allergic encephalomyelitis in the Lewis rat. *Journal of Immunology*, **120**, 844–850

SUZUMURA, A., LISAK, R. P. and SILBERBERG, D. H. (1986) The expression of MHC antigens on oligodendrocytes: induction of polymorphic H-2 expression by lymphokines. *Journal of Neuroimmunology* (in press)

TACHOVSKY, T. G., LISAK, R. P., KOPROWSKI, H., THEOFILOPOULUS, A. N. and DIXON, F. J. (1976) Circulating immune complexes in multiple sclerosis and other neurological diseases. *Lancet*, **2**, 997–999

TADA, T. (1984) Help, suppression, and specific factors. In *Fundamental Immunology*, edited by W. E. Paul, pp. 481–517. New York: Raven Press

TECOMA, E. S. and HUEY, L. Y. (1985) Minireview. Psychic distress and the immune response. *Life Sciences*, **36**, 1799–1812

ter MEULEN, V., CARTER, M. J., WEGE, H. and WATANABE, R. (1984) Mechanisms and consequences of virus persistence in the human nervous system. *Annals of the New York Academy of Sciences*, **436**, 86–96

TOURTELLOTTE, W. W. and PARKER, J. A. (1967) Multiple sclerosis: brain immunoglobulin-G and albumin. *Nature*, **214**, 683–686

TOURTELLOTTE, W. W., STAUGAITUS, S. M., WALSH, M. J. *et al.* (1985) The basis of intra-blood–brain-barrier IgG synthesis. *Annals of Neurology*, **17**, 21–27

TRAUGOTT, U. (1985) Characterization and distribution of lymphocyte subpopulations in multiple sclerosis plaques versus autoimmune demyelinating lesions. In *Immunoneurology, Volume I, Springer Seminars in Immunopathology*, edited by A. J. Steck and R. P. Lisak, **8**, 71–96

TRAUGOTT, U. and RAINE, C. S. (1984) Further lymphocyte characterization in the central nervous system in multiple sclerosis. *Annals of the New York Academy of Science*, **436**, 163–178

TRAUGOTT, U., SCHEINBERG, L. C. and RAINE, C. S. (1985) On the presence of Ia-positive endothelial cells and astrocytes in multiple sclerosis lesions and its relevance to antigen presentation. *Journal of Neuroimmunology*, **8**, 1–14

TRAUGOTT, U., SHEVACH, E., CHIBA, J., STONE, S. H. and RAINE, C. S. (1981) Autoimmune encephalomyelitis: simultaneous identification of T and B-cells in the target organ. *Science*, **214**, 1251–1253

TRAUGOTT, U., SNYDER, D. S. and RAINE, C. S. (1979) Oligodendrocyte staining by multiple sclerosis serum is nonspecific. *Annals of Neurology*, **6**, 13–20

TROTTER, J. L. (1983) Studies on the role of myelin proteolipid protein in chronic progressive experimental encephalomyelitis and multiple sclerosis. *Annals of Neurology*, **14**, 115

TSCHANNEN, R., STECK, A. J. and SCHAFER, R. (1979) Mechanisms in the pathogenesis of post-infectious vaccinia encephalomyelitis in the mouse. *Neuroscience Letters*, **15**, 295–300

UTERMOHLEN, V. and ZABRISKIE, J. B. (1973) Suppressed cellular immunity to measles antigen in multiple sclerosis patients. *Lancet*, **2**, 1147–1148

VANDVICK, B., NORRBY, E., NORDAL, H. J. and DEGRE, M. (1976) Oligoclonal measles virus-specific IgG antibodies isolated from cerebrospinal fluids, brain extracts, and sera from patients with subacute sclerosing panencephalitis and multiple sclerosis. *Scandinavian Journal of Immunology*, **5**, 979–992

VANGURI, P., KOSKI, C. L., SILVERMAN, B. and SHIN, M. L. (1982) Complement activation by isolated myelin. Activation of the classical pathway in the absence of myelin-specific antibody. *Proceedings of the National Academy of Science, USA*, **79**, 3290–3291

VOLPE, R. (1984) Autoimmune thyroid disease. *Hospital Practice*, **19**, 141–151, 155–158

WAKSMAN, B. H. (1984) The pathogenic significance of cross reactions in autoimmune disease of the nervous system. *Immunology Today*, **5**, 346–348

WATANABE, R., WEGE, H. and TER MEULEN, V. (1983) Adoptive transfer of EAE-like lesions from rats with coronavirus-induced demyelinating encephalomyelitis. *Nature*, **305**, 150–153

WEINER, H. L., BHAN, A. K., BURKS, J. *et al.* (1984) Immunohistochemical analysis of the cellular infiltrate in multiple sclerotic lesions. *Neurology*, **34** (Suppl. 1), 112

WEINER, L. P. (1973) Pathogenesis of demyelination induced by a mouse hepatitis virus (JHM virus). *Archives of Neurology*, **28**, 298–303

WEKERLE, H. and FIERZ, W. (1985) T-cell approach to demyelinating diseases. In *Immunoneurology, Volume I, Springer Seminars in Immunopathology*, edited by A. J. Steck and R. P. Lisak, **8**, 97–110

WHITACRE, C. C., MATTSON, D. H., PATERSON, P. Y., ROSS, R. P., PETERSON, D. J. and ARNASON, B. G. W. (1981) Cerebrospinal fluid and serum oligoclonal IgG bands in rabbits with experimental allergic encephalomyelitis. *Neurochemistry Research*, **6**, 87–96

WHITAKER, J. N. (1985) Quantitation of the synthesis of immunoglobulin G within the central nervous system. *Annals of Neurology*, **17**, 11–12

WISNEWSKI, H. M. (1977) Immunopathology of demyelination. *British Medical Bulletin*, **33**, 54–59

WILKERSON, L. P., LISAK, R. P., ZWEIMAN, B. and SILBERBERG, D. H. (1977) Antimyelin antibody in multiple sclerosis: no change during immunosuppression. *Journal of Neurology, Neurosurgery and Psychiatry*, **40**, 872–875

WONG, G. H. W., CLARK-LEWIS, I., HARRIS, A. W. and SCHRADER, J. W. (1984) Effect of cloned interferon on expression of H-2 and Ia antigens of cell lines of hemopoietic, lymphoid, epithelial fibroblastic and neuronal origin. *European Journal of Immunology*, **14**, 52–56

ZINKERNAGEL, R. M. and DOHERTY, P. C. (1974) Restriction of an *in vitro* T-cell-mediated cytotoxicity in lymnphocyte choriomeningitis within a syngeneic or semiallogeneic system. *Nature*, **248**, 701–702

ZWEIMAN, B. and LISAK, R. P. (1986) Cell-mediated immunity in neurologic diseases. *Human Pathology* (in press)

6
Pathogenesis of demyelination
Donald H. Silberberg

INTRODUCTION

Multiple sclerosis (MS) is defined by the striking pathological alterations which it produces. The importance of the histological picture is twofold: first, as there is no specific diagnostic test for MS, the accuracy of the clinical diagnosis rests on the discovery of characteristic histopathology; second, any attempts to explain the process of MS must be consistent with what is observed microscopically. It is entirely possible that more than one route may lead to the complex series of changes in the central nervous system that we know as MS. However, the relatively uniform age distribution throughout the world and the many other features that individuals with MS share with one another speak strongly for a unifying hypothesis. Before considering the possible mechanisms which might lead to these changes, one must have in mind the neuropathology of MS.

NEUROPATHOLOGY

Clinical inferences

It is likely that the events which lead to neurological dysfunction occur quickly, over the course of hours to days. However, the brain, optic nerve and spinal cord rarely are subject to the pathologist's examination until months to many years after the event. With important exceptions, the neuropathologist must try to reconstruct events from a late, static picture. Pathological examination almost always reveals many more areas of demyelination than could be suspected on the basis of the clinical history and examination of the patient. Similarly, examination of the patient with computerized tomographic (CT) or nuclear magnetic resonance imaging very often reveals many more lesions than were expected clinically (*see* Chapter 2). Additionally, it is relevant to note that asymptomatic plaques are discovered at post-mortem with sufficient frequency to make it likely that the MS process takes place in many people who remain clinically well (*see Figure 7.7*).

Increased numbers of lymphocytes and other monoclonal cells are found in the cerebrospinal fluid during disease activity. A related clinical point, which is not often mentioned, is the frequency with which individuals with MS describe headache just before or during the evolution of new symptoms. Since the chief pain-sensitive intracranial structures are the meninges and blood vessels, this would be consistent with Lumsden's (1970) suggestion, and later observations by others, that lymphocytic infiltration of the meninges and Virchow-Robin spaces may be among the earliest events.

Despite the difficulties involved in correlating the histological picture with the timing of the actual evolution of a given lesion, several approaches have been used to try to delineate the crucial early changes. The approaches include: (1) observations of smaller lesions in patients dying of complications of acutely progressing MS, in whom it can be assumed that activity is still present and evolving in those lesions; (2) studies of very well-fixed tissue obtained shortly after death, which permit a search for the least perturbation in slightly demyelinated lesions. This has permitted attempts to reconstruct the probable sequence of events. Potential criticisms of hypotheses based on these observations include the likelihood that some of the changes described at the plaque edge are a secondary reaction to the pathogenic process taking place deeper within the lesion (or elsewhere). Similarly, the early appearance of invading cells from outside the central nervous system may be a reaction to submicroscopic alterations in the myelin-oligodendrocyte unit. Nevertheless, the construction of a scaffold helps to clarify thinking about the process.

The probable sequence of events

The early lesion

As mentioned above, lymphocytic infiltration of meninges, the Virchow-Robin spaces, and then individual perivenous spaces may be the earliest event (*Figure 6.1*). Lesions appear first along the course of small veins (Dawson, 1916; Adams, 1975); often several parallel veins in a particular small area show focal infiltration

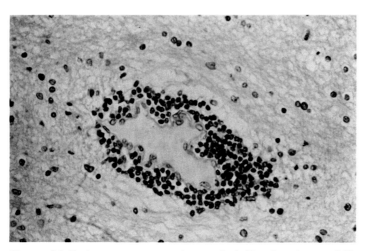

Figure 6.1 Perivenous mononuclear cell infiltration in an MS plaque stained with haematoxylin and eosin

by lymphocytes, plasma cells, and macrophages, and early demyelination (Raine, Powers and Suzuki, 1974; Adams, 1975, 1977). Macrophages, some of which show capping with surface immunoglobulin G, ingest fragments of myelin of normal appearance, which often maintains its periodicity within the cell. These intracellular fragments of myelin still contain the protein most characteristic of myelin, myelin basic protein, and myelin-associated glycoprotein (Prineas *et al.*, 1984b). At first, the outer lamellae of myelin peel off and are ingested; ultimately the axon is left bare of myelin. While the axon may develop spheroids indicating damage, this is relatively uncommon, hence the nosology of MS as a demyelinating disease, sparing the axon.

Although the perivenular process is spotty, small lesions eventually coalesce to form the familiar 1–2 cm lesions. Lesion progression also occurs at the outer margin. This area becomes hypercellular, crowded with hypertrophied astrocytes, macrophages, lymphocytes and plasma cells. Some of the oligodendrocytes within demyelinated areas may represent survivors (Raine, Scheinberg and Waltz, 1981) while others present may represent newly appearing cells as attempts at remyelination begin.

The cerebrospinal fluid contains lymphocytes, plasma cells, polymorphonuclear lymphocytes, monocytes, eosinophils, lipid-laden macrophages, fibroblasts, and extracellular as well as intracellular myelin fragments (Herndon and Kasckow, 1978). This suggests the possibility that some of the myelin destruction occurs extracellularly, although the free fragments may have been released from degenerating or lysed macrophages.

Interstitial oedema is often a prominent feature of the more acute lesions. It is most easily seen around veins, but extends into the damaged areas. The histological appearance correlates well with the enlargement and radiolucency which is often seen in recent-onset lesions by CT imaging.

Blood–brain barrier

The CT brain scan has also permitted visualization of the impairment of the blood–brain barrier (BBB) during life. Over 50% of the individuals who are studied shortly following the onset of an acute attack show 'enhancement', leakage of intravenously injected iodine compounds, which are radiopaque (Ebers *et al.*, 1984). This leakage through the BBB disappears spontaneously over the course of a few weeks to months. Interestingly, contrast-enhancement can be transiently reversed by the administration of corticosteroids (Troiano *et al.*, 1984). Additional evidence for impairment of the BBB is the appearance of haptoglobin polymers in the cerebrospinal fluid in MS, an occurrence which is very uncommon among normal subjects (Takeoka *et al.*, 1983). As noted below (in retinal vessels, p. 103) focal alterations in the permeability of retinal venules, which are in most respects identical to intracranial vessels, occur as well (McDonald, 1983).

Alteration of the BBB may be of crucial importance, in that this could be the step which permits entry of immunocompetent cells, antibody, or other effectors which lead to myelin destruction. However, it is important to note that a break in the BBB occurs as part of many infections and other inflammatory brain lesions, so it is equally possible that it represents an epi- or secondary phenomenon. Nevertheless, its existence may add to a cascade of events which might otherwise be more benign or self-limited.

Progression

The white matter beyond the immediate zone of demyelination shows a number of abnormalities. Hypertrophied, fibrillary, often binucleate astrocytes are numerous. The number of lymphocytes and plasma cells increases. As the disorder progresses, the brain seems to acquire a more or less permanent population of plasma cells, presumably the source of the oligoclonal IgG found in the cerebrospinal fluid (Prineas and Wright, 1978). IgG can be demonstrated readily, particularly at plaque borders, using immunofluorescence or peroxidase techniques.

The use of monoclonal antibodies to phenotypic lymphocyte antigens and to the Ia antigen associated with macrophages, and with activated lymphocytes and astrocytes, has permitted more detailed studies in relation to lesion progression. In the presumably more acute lesions the several demonstrable varieties of T lymphocytes and macrophages are found in large numbers throughout the lesion, but are not found in adjacent normal white matter. In the more chronic but still active lesions, lymphocytes are more numerous at the plaque edge, and extend into the white matter of normal appearance. In this instance, macrophages are more dense in the lesion centre (Traugott, Reinherz and Raine, 1983; Traugott, 1985).

Old lesions

Old plaques become more sharply demarcated, both grossly and microscopically (*see Figure 6.2*). Less cellular activity is visible at the plaque margin, and the perivascular cuffing may be less prominent. Individual plaques generally measure

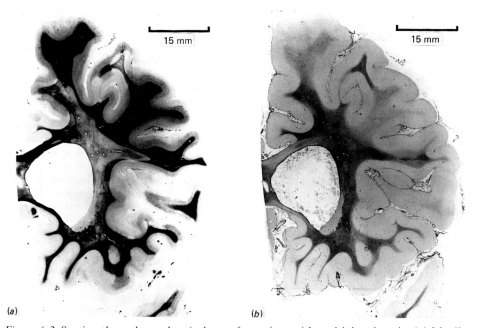

(a)   (b)

Figure 6.2 Section through one hemisphere of a patient with multiple sclerosis. (*a*) Myelin preparation. Note the extensive periventricular demyelination (Heidenhain's stain). (*b*) Section near (*a*) stained for fibrillary astrocytic processes. Note the intense gliosis especially in the obviously demyelinated regions (Holzer stain). (By courtesy of Dr Robin Barnard)

less than 2 cm, but often coalesce to produce large areas of abnormality. Many are located near a ventricular surface (*Figure 6.2*), in the centrum semiovale, optic nerves, cervical cord and brainstem. The reasons for these localizations remain obscure. Both the optic nerves, which are almost always affected, and the cervical spinal cord are subject to motion during life; perhaps mechanical stresses lead to changes in blood vessel permeability, as suggested by Oppenheimer (1978). Plaques occur in grey matter and appear to outnumber those in white matter by 4:1 (Lumsden, 1970). These changes lead to gross atrophy in the more severely affected patients, an observation often made via CT and magnetic resonance imaging, as well as at autopsy.

Within the plaque bare axons are invested by astrocytic processes, leading to the firm texture which led to the name sclerosis. Interestingly, membrane specializations develop between the demyelinated axon and the astrocyte process (Raine, 1978), as if an attempt at interaction takes place. Whether or not this has any functional significance is not known.

The shadow plaque

Areas of partial demyelination, termed shadow plaques, have been used as evidence that some remyelination occurs in patients with MS. Electron microscopy reveals that these areas contain many axons with thinner than normal myelin sheaths and shorter internodes (Suzuki *et al.*, 1969; Prineas and Connell, 1979) which are similar to findings in remyelinating areas following experimental demyelination in several animal models. Thus, shadow plaques may represent both partial demyelination and remyelination. Demyelination may also be seen at the edge of chronic plaques (Prineas and Connell, 1979). Additional evidence for remyelination in MS is the observation by many that Schwann cells invade and produce peripheral-type myelin, particularly in locations which permit ready access to Schwann cells (Ghatak *et al.*, 1973; Ogata and Feigin, 1975). It is noteworthy that these areas of peripheral-type myelin remain intact in the midst of an otherwise actively demyelinating lesion, underscoring the specificity of the MS process (Itoyama *et al.*, 1983).

Retinal vessels

The many clinical descriptions of ophthalmoscopically visible perivenous sheathing in the optic fundus has its histopathological counterpart. Fog (1965) and Arnold *et al.*, (1984) described retinal perivenous accumulation of inflammatory cells in the retinas of patients dying of complications of MS. These perivascular cuffs are very similar to those seen around veins within the CNS. However, since the human retina does not usually contain myelinated axons, the presence of these cells may have pathogenetic significance. Additionally, alterations in the blood–retina barrier can be demonstrated with fluorescein angiography in MS. This allows direct visualization of focal leakage of dye (McDonald, 1983). In most aspects which have been studied, the retinal blood vessels are identical to similar-sized intracranial vessels. Thus an inflammatory response surrounding retinal veins and changes in retinal vessel permeability in MS may indicate that a similar process is occurring around intracranial and intraspinous veins, independent of the presence or absence of oligodendrocytes or myelin at those sites. This would support the possibility that the first point of attack is at or near the blood vessel, and that demyelination occurs as a secondary event.

Peripheral nervous system

Multiple sclerosis has been regarded as a disorder which involves the central nervous system exclusively, except for those instances in which poor nutrition or pressure neuropathies develop. However, reports are accumulating of peripheral nervous system (PNS) abnormalities in ambulatory patients with MS who have no other reason for PNS involvement. Patients with MS have developed an inflammatory demyelinative polyneuropathy (Lassman, Budka and Schnaberth, 1981). Morphological abnormalities, including a 50% or greater reduction in myelin thickness at many internodes (Pollock, Calder and Allpress, 1977), Schwann cell abnormalities (Argyrakis, 1980) and hypertrophic neuropathy (Schoene *et al.*, 1977), have been reported. Electrophysiological studies have shown slowing of motor conduction as demonstrated by collision technique (Hopf, 1963), prolonged refractoriness of sensory axons (Hopf and Eysholdt, 1978) and altered supernormality, a regular part of the recovery cycle of nerve (Eisen, Paty and Horich, 1982).

Since CNS and PNS myelin, and oligodendrocytes and Schwann cells share many features, it should not be surprising to discover subclinical PNS involvement in MS. However, this is not consistent with the observations that Schwann cell-produced myelin within MS plaques appears to be resistant to the demyelination which affects neighbouring oligodendrocyte-produced myelin. It is not clear how often PNS alterations occur in MS. Clearly, further work is needed.

CHEMICAL ALTERATIONS

No convincing evidence indicates that the myelin of those who develop MS is abnormal in any way prior to the beginning of the inflammatory-demyelinating process. Descriptions of the biochemical abnormalities in the white matter distant from plaques have probably not taken into account the very subtle earliest stages of demyelination, which include the presence of enlarged astrocytes and stripping of outer myelin lamellae by phagocytes.

As myelin degenerates, three types of chemical changes which are specifically related to the myelin occur. First, the water content of the myelin, as seen by electron microscopy, and the demyelinating area as a whole, increases. Much or most of the oedema is extracellular. Second, the absolute amounts of the normal constituents such as myelin basic protein, myelin-associated glycoprotein, galactocerebroside, plasmalogen and cholesterol decrease. Third, myelin constituents which are not normally found such as cholesterol esters, neutral fat, and unsaturated lipids, appear. These changes are not specific for MS.

Increased levels of lipolytic and proteolytic enzymes in the plaque and peri-plaque areas have been well documented (*see* review by Allen, 1983). The source of these potentially destructive enzymes is chiefly the lysosomes of invading inflammatory cells, and of astrocytes and microglia. Oligodendrocytes lack lysosomes and thus are an unlikely source. In addition, as myelin degenerates, a number of potentially lytic enzymes are released (Sato *et al.*, 1984). These changes are not seen before observable astrocytic proliferation and hypertrophy occur, and again must be considered unlikely candidates for initial lesion pathogenesis. However, it is entirely possible that one or more of these enzymes plays a role in lesion development, extension, or continuation, as part of a cascade of events which has been initiated by another mechanism. Alternatively, one or more released cell products may enhance an immune attack, such as through activation of a component of the complement system (Vanguri *et al.*, 1982; Cyong *et al.*, 1982).

THE VIROLOGY OF MULTIPLE SCLEROSIS

The epidemiology of multiple sclerosis strongly suggests that one or more infectious agents are involved in its pathogenesis, as discussed by Nathanson *et al.* (*see* Chapter 3). Nevertheless, attempts to support this probability with a reproducible isolation of viral material, identification of virus by electron microscopy, or discovery of a specific immunological response to one or more viruses have not been successful to date.

Viral isolations

On the basis of direct isolation, a number of agents have been identified as aetiological candidates. These include mycoplasma (Chevassut, 1930), protozoa (Bequignon, 1956), spirochaetes (Ichelson, 1957), and viruses including rabies (Bychkova, 1964), herpes simplex type 2 (Gudnadottir *et al.*, 1964), parainfluenza type I (Meulen *et al.*, 1972), coronavirus (Burks *et al.*, 1980), an unidentified fusion agent from bone marrow (Mitchell *et al.*, 1978), and an agent related antigenically to the virus isolated from subacute myelo-optic neuropathy (Melnick *et al.*, 1982). Unfortunately, none of these isolations has been confirmed by subsequent study. It is worth noting that the agents responsible for kuru, and for Creutzfeldt-Jakob disease, both spongiform encephalopathies of man, have not been visualized directly and have been recovered only by direct transmission to primates and then to other species. Similar efforts employing tissues from patients with MS have not transmitted diseases, except for one instance in which intracerebral inoculation in a baby chimpanzee led to cytopathic changes which were attributed to cytomegalic inclusion body virus, a probable contaminant (Rorke *et al.*, 1979).

More recently, two common viruses have been demonstrated in human brain tissue by sensitive techniques of molecular virology. *In situ* hybridization revealed persistent measles virus genome in six out of 12 brains from patients with multiple sclerosis, and in one out of seven normal controls (Haase *et al.*, 1981). Similarly, the Southern blot technique of nucleic acid hybridization was used to demonstrate the herpes simplex genome in four out of five patients with MS and three out of six normal subjects (Fraser *et al.*, 1981). These techniques recognize the viral genome, which was found in both white and grey matter. To date, neither measles nor herpes simplex antigen have been recognized in MS brain. However, it has been recognized since Adams' and Imagawa's work (1962) that levels of serum and cerebrospinal fluid antibodies to measles are elevated in MS (*see* Lisak, Chapter 5).

This correlates more with whether or not an individual has the HLA-A3 or B7 haplotypes than with the presence or absence of MS (Visscher, Sullivan and Detels, 1981). The HLA haplotype may in turn be related to the way in which an individual handles invading viruses.

Immunological evidence of viral pathogenesis

Antibody titres

It has become clear that patients with MS have higher cerebrospinal fluid levels of IgG class antibodies to measles, mumps, rubella, herpes simplex, parainfluenza and influenza viruses than do normal individuals or patients with other neurological diseases (Nordal and Froland, 1978; Arnadottir *et al.*, 1979; Salmi *et al.*, 1983). These antiviral antibodies are produced intrathecally, and the levels produced do not alter with changes in clinical activity of individual patients. Further, each individual patient has an individual pattern of intrathecal antibody titres. To complicate the picture further, it appears that the pattern of oligoclonal IgG which can be recovered from individual plaques from a given patient differ within the same patient (Mattson, Roos and Arnason, 1980). This finding needs verification by other protein separation techniques, since it leads to the conclusion that, although the CSF IgG oligoclonal pattern remains relatively constant throughout a patient's course, that pattern may be a blend of heterogeneous IgG molecular species, each of which emanates from one or more specific plaques. The possible relationship of intrathecal antiviral antibodies to an aetiological agent is further compromised by the fact that IgG which is demonstrably directed towards a virus component makes up only a small portion of the total CSF IgG. The specificity of most of the IgG remains unknown.

That intrathecal synthesis of viral antibodies should occur in MS does not itself indicate an abnormality. Intrathecal antibody synthesis specific for a particular infecting virus, such as mumps or measles is a characteristic part of the host response following primary infection with these agents. What is atypical in MS is the persistent production of more than one antiviral antibody, long after the acute infection presumed to have initiated the plasma cell response has cleared. Salmi *et al.* (1983) have suggested that: 'The intrathecal virus antibody synthesis in MS patients may be best characterized as normal immunoglobulin synthesis by a restricted number of plasma cells in a wrong compartment of the body.' Thus the presence of intrathecal viral antibodies may be more indicative of an abnormality in the blood–brain barrier, or of the immune system, or perhaps signals the presence of something which stimulates continuing IgG synthesis.

Complexes

Immune complexes are found in both blood (Tachovsky *et al.*, 1976) and spinal fluid of many patients with MS. An analysis of CSF complexes revealed that six out of six patients with MS in exacerbation had detectable complexes; three included herpes simplex type I antigen; three had complexed myelin basic protein. Two of the six also had complexed brain glycolipids. Of six patients with other neurological diseases, only one, who had herpes simplex encephalitis, complexed a viral antigen (herpes simplex type 1) (HSV-1)) and one with hypoxic encephalopathy complexed brain glycolipids. A corresponding study of the patients' sera indicated that the complexes arose from within the nervous system (Coyle, 1985). The fact that complexes included only HSV-1 antigen among the several viral antigens tested suggests either that the burden of latent HSV-1 is related to the MS exacerbations, or that this occurs because persistent HSV-1 is commonly present within the CNS and thus available to form complexes when antibody is synthesized. Clearly, more studies are needed to follow this interesting lead. The nature of the remitting and exacerbating behaviour of HSV-1 in man adds to the interest in a possible association with this virus.

PATHOGENIC MECHANISMS

Based on the morphological and viral immune data, and using experimental models to illustrate parallel situations, it is possible to construct pathogenic hypotheses. Any proposed sequence of events must also be consistent with the epidemiology and the clinical course.

As discussed elsewhere in this volume (Chapter 4), the evidence suggests that genetic susceptibility is an important factor in determining whether or not MS will develop. However, genetic capability alone is not sufficient for the development of the disorder. Exogenous factors, as discussed by Nathanson *et al.*(*see* Chapter 3), seem to determine whether or not MS will develop in a genetically susceptible individual. The most reasonable candidate for an exogenous factor is one or more infectious agents, so that any postulated aetiology and pathogenesis would include a role for an infectious process. In addition, the heterogeneous clinical course of identical twins with MS (Williams *et al.*, 1980) suggests that non-genetic factors determine the pace of the illness in affected individuals.

Among the possible pathogenic mechanisms are these.

(1) VIRUS PRODUCES DIRECT ALTERATION IN CELL FUNCTION
Potential targets include:
(a) The oligodendrocyte-myelin unit. There is little reason to consider the oligodendrocyte, and the myelin which it synthesizes, separately. The oligodendrocyte and myelin share most or all of the same antigens, and both are affected morphologically. One oligodendrocyte sends processes to the internodes of many neighbouring axons, so that impairment of one oligodendrocyte is capable of demyelinating a volume of tissue of approximately $1\,mm^3$.
(b) Vascular endothelium. Impairment of function of the vessel's endothelium could lead to the blood–brain barrier leakage which seems to be an early step in lesion development. It has been shown in several experimental systems that exposure to human serum is capable of inducing demyelination. Serum from patients with MS and other disorders (reviewed by Seil, 1977) and from normal individuals (Silberberg, Manning and Schreiber, 1984) can demyelinate myelinated organ cultures of rodent brain and spinal cord. It appears that this is mediated by a non-immunoglobulin molecule, and involves complement activation. Similarly, both MS and normal sera induce demyelination when injected directly into the guinea pig optic nerve (Sergott *et al.*, 1984). The pattern of demyelination produced (*Figure 6.3*) resembles the 'tubular' or 'vesicular' pattern of myelin disruption described by Kirk (1979) in an acute case of MS.

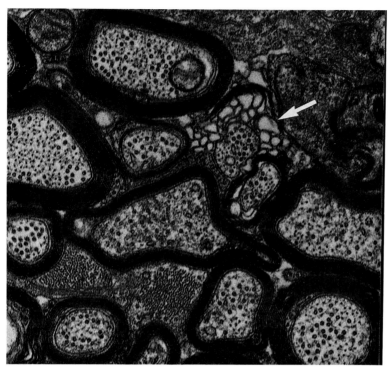

Figure 6.3 Fascicular demyelination of a single axon induced by injection of 15 μl from a patient with active MS, and 20% pooled guinea pig serum. (Original magnification 50 400)

Similarly, disruption of the blood–brain barrier might lead to entry into the CNS of immunocompetent lymphocytes which do not ordinarily have access, and thus to an immune attack.

The presence of virus components in cells might lead to functional alterations well before morphologically visible structural alterations occur. In the case of the oligodendrocyte, this might lead to degeneration of the myelin before changes are visible in the soma. The infiltration by cells of haematogenous origin might then follow and persist in response to a continuing antigenic stimulus provided by persistent virus.

(2) VIRUS-INDUCED, IMMUNE-MEDIATED
Viral infection may expose otherwise hidden antigens to the body's immune system, leading to an inappropriate immune sensitivity directed against the oligodendrocyte-myelin unit, or vascular endothelium.

The proximity of viral antigen to cell membrane can lead to damage to the host cell by the immune attack on the virus.

If the virus and cell have an antigen recognition site in common, the immune response could lead to cell damage.

Viral infection may lead to formation of antibody to the idiotype on the antiviral antibodies which might then react with virus receptors on the surface of normal, uninfected cells.

Infection of the immune system itself may lead to disorders of immunoregulation.

Remyelination

Central nervous system remyelination occurs regularly following demyelination produced in most, but not all experimental systems (Blakemore, Crang and Evans, 1983). The myelin sheath of the remyelinated axons is thinner, and the internodes are shorter than in the primary myelinated tissue. These features permit recognition of remyelination within the plaque areas in MS (Suzuki *et al.*, 1969; Prineas and Connell, 1979; Prineas *et al.*, 1984a). As noted previously in this chapter, remyelination by Schwann cells occurs in areas which are accessible to Schwann cells, such as the root entry zone in the spinal cord. Plaques may contain mixtures of axons showing varying degrees of demyelination, alongside what appear to be remyelinating axons.

The factors which determine whether any remyelination will take place in MS are totally unknown. Experience with tissue culture systems shows that the presence of low levels of antibodies, which in higher concentrations are capable of causing demyelination, can totally and reversibly prevent remyelination. Thus, low concentrations of anti-galactocerebroside antibody will prevent remyelination of antiserum-demyelinated mouse cerebellum cultures (Dorfman, Fry and Silberberg, 1979). If some of the immunoglobulin G present in MS plaques is directed against myelin or oligodendrocyte surface antigens, a similar mechanism could prevent remyelination. Similarly, the functional capacity of partially remyelinated axons in MS is unknown. The question of the extent to which remyelination contributes to the recovery of function which follows most exacerbations is discussed in Chapter 7.

Hopefully, the increasing knowledge of oligodendrocyte biology which is the result of successful isolation of oligodendrocytes, with subsequent maintenance and study in tissue culture systems, will permit a more complete understanding of the factors which influence remyelination. This has the potential for leading to a therapeutic approach independent of our understanding of the aetiology and pathogenesis of multiple sclerosis.

References

ADAMS, C. W. M. (1975) The onset and progression of the lesion in multiple sclerosis. *Journal of Neurological Science*, **25**, 165–182

ADAMS, C. W. M. (1977) Pathology of multiple sclerosis: progression of the lesion. *British Medical Bulletin*, **33**, 15–20

ADAMS, J. M. and IMAGAWA, D. T. (1962) Measles antibodies and multiple sclerosis. *Proceedings of the Society for Experimental Biology and Medicine*, **111**, 562–566

ALLEN, I. V. (1983) Hydrolytic enzymes in multiple sclerosis. In *Progress in Neuropathology, Vol. 5*, edited by H. M. Zimmerman, pp. 1–17. New York: Raven Press

ARGYRAKIS, A. (1980) Ultrastructural changes in peripheral nerves in multiple sclerosis and subacute sclerosing panencephalitis. In *Progress in Multiple Sclerosis Research*, edited by H. J. Bauer, S. Poser and G. Ritter, pp. 360–364. Berlin: Springer-Verlag

ARNADOTTIR, T., REUNANEN, M., MEURMAN, O., SALMI, A., PANELIUS, M. and HALSNEN, P. (1979) Measles and rubella virus antibodies in patients with multiple sclerosis. A longitudinal study of serum and CSF specimens by radioimmunoassay. *Archives of Neurology*, **36**, 261–265

ARNOLD, A. C., PEPOSE, J. S., HEPLER, R. S. and FOOS, R. Y. (1984) Retinal periphlebitis and retinitis in multiple sclerosis: I pathologic characteristic. *Ophthalmology*, **91**, 255–262

BEQUIGNON, R. (1956) De l'etiologie de la sclerose en plaques. *CR Academy of Science (D) (Paris)*, **242**, 1380–1382

BLAKEMORE, W. F., CRANG, A. J. and EVANS, R. J. (1983) The effect of chemical injury on oligodendrocytes. In *Viruses and Demyelinating Diseases*, edited by C. A. Mims, M. L. Cuzner and R. E. Kelly, pp. 167–190. London: Academic Press

BURKS, J. S., DEVALD, B. L., JANKOVSKY, L. D. and GERDES, J. C. (1980) Two coronaviruses isolated from central nervous system tissue of two multiple sclerosis patients. *Science*, **209**, 933–934

BYCHKOVA, E. N. (1964) Viruses isolated from patients with encephalomyelitis and multiple sclerosis. Communication I: pathogenic and antigenic properties. *Voprosy Virusologii*, **9**, 173–176

CHEVASSUT, K. (1930) The aetiology of disseminated sclerosis. *Lancet*, **1**, 552–560

COYLE, P. K. (1985) CSF immune complexes in multiple sclerosis. *Neurology*, **35**, 429–432

CYONG, J-C., WHITKIN, S. S., RIEGER, B., BARBARESE, E., GOOD, R. A. and DAY, N. K. (1982) Antibody-independent complement activation by myelin via the classical complement pathway. *Journal of Experimental Medicine*, **155**, 587–598

DAWSON, J. W. (1916) The histology of disseminated sclerosis. Part II histological study. *Edinburgh Medical Journal, NS*, **17**, 311–344

DORFMAN, S. H., FRY, J. M. and SILBERBERG, D. H. (1979) Antiserum induced myelination inhibition *in vitro* independent of the cytolytic effects of the complement system. *Brain Research*, **177**, 105–114

EBERS, G. C., VINUELA, F. V., FEASBY, T. and BASS, B. (1984) Multifocal CT enhancement in MS. *Neurology*, **34**, 341–346

EISEN, A., PATY, D. and HORICH, M. (1982) Altered supernormality in multiple sclerosis peripheral nerve. *Muscle and Nerve*, **5**, 411

FOG, T. (1965) The topography of plaques in multiple sclerosis with special reference to cerebral plaques. *Acta Neurologica Scandinavica*, **15**, 154–156

FRASER, N. W., LAWRENCE, W. C., WROBLESKA, Z., GILDEN, D. H. and KOPROWSKI, H. (1981) Herpes simplex type I DNA in human brain tissue. *Proceedings of the National Academy of Science, USA*, **78**, 6461–6465

GHATAK, N. R., HIRANO, A., DORON, Y. and ZIMMERMAN, H. M. (1973) Remyelination in multiple sclerosis with peripheral-type myelin. *Archives of Neurology*, **29**, 262–267

GUDNADOTTIR, M., HELGADOTTIR, H., BJARNASON, O. and JONSDOTTIR, K. (1964) Virus isolated from the brain of a patient with multiple sclerosis. *Experimental Neurology*, **9**, 85–95

HAASE, A. T., VENTRUA, P., GIBBS, C. J. JR and TOURTELLOTTE, W. W. (1981) Measles virus nucleotide sequences: detection by hybridization *in situ*. *Science*, **212**, 672–674

HERNDON, R. N. and KASCKOW, J. (1978) Electron microscopic studies of cerebrospinal fluid sediment in demyelinating disease. *Annals of Neurology*, **4**, 513–515

HOPF, H. C. (1963) Electromyographic study on so-called mononeuritis. *Archives of Neurology*, **9**, 307–312

HOPF, H. C. and EYSHOLDT, M. (1978) Impaired refractory periods of peripheral sensory nerves in multiple sclerosis. *Annals of Neurology*, **4**, 449–501

ICHELSON, R. R. (1957) Cultivation of spirochaetes from spinal fluids with multiple sclerosis cases and negative controls. *Proceedings of the Society for Experimental Biology and Medicine*, **95**, 57–58

ITOYAMA, T., WEBSTER, H. F., RICHARDSON, E. P. and TRAPP, B. D. (1983) Schwann cell remyelination of demyelinated axons in spinal cord multiple sclerosis lesions. *Annals of Neurology*, **14**, 339–346

KIRK, J. (1979) The fine structure of the CNS in multiple sclerosis. II. Vesicular demyelination in an acute case. *Neuropathology and Applied Neurobiology*, **5**, 289–294

LASSMANN, H., BUDKA, H. and SCHNABERTH, G. (1981) Inflammatory demyelinating polyradiculitis in a patient with multiple sclerosis. *Archives of Neurology*, **38**, 99–102

LUMSDEN, C. E. (1970) Multiple sclerosis and other demyelinating diseases. *Handbook of Clinical Neurology*, edited by P. J. Vinken and G. W. Bruyn, **Vol. 9**, pp. 217–309. New York: American Elsevier Publishing Co

MATTSON, D. H., ROOS, R. P. and ARNASON, B. G. W. (1980) Isoelectric focusing of IgG eluted from multiple sclerosis and subacute sclerosing panencephalitis brains. *Nature*, **287**, 335–337

McDONALD, W. I. (1983) The significance of optic neuritis. *Transactions of the Ophthalmological Societies of the United Kingdom*, **103**, 230–246

MELNICK, J. L., SEIDEL, E., INOUE, Y. K. and NISHIBE, Y. (1982) Isolation of virus from the spinal fluid of three patients with multiple sclerosis and one with amyotrophic lateral sclerosis. *Lancet*, **1**, 830–833

MEULEN TER, V., KOPROWSKI, H., IWASAKI, Y., KACKELLY, M. and MUELLER, D. (1972) Fusion of cultured multiple-sclerosis brain cells with indicator cells: presence of nucleocapsids and virion with isolation of parainfluenza-type virus. *Lancet*, **1**, 1–5

MITCHELL, D. N., PORTERFIELD, J. S., MICHELETTI, R. *et al.* (1978) Isolation of an infectious agent from bone-marrows of patients with multiple sclerosis. *Lancet*, **2**, 387–391

NORDAL, H. J. and FROLAND, S. S. (1978) Lymphocyte populations and cellular immune reactions *in vitro* in patients with multiple sclerosis. *Clinical Immunology and Immunopathology*, **9**, 87–96

OGATA, J. and FEIGIN, I. (1975) Schwann cells and regenerated peripheral myelin in multiple sclerosis: an ultrastructural study. *Neurology*, **25**, 255–262

OPPENHEIMER, D. R. (1978) The cervical cord in multiple sclerosis. *Neuropathology and Applied Neurobiology*, **4**, 151–162

POLLOCK, M., CALDER, C. and ALLPRESS, S. (1977) Peripheral nerve abnormality in multiple sclerosis. *Annals of Neurology*, **2**, 41–48

PRINEAS, J. W. and CONNELL, F. (1979) Remyelination in multiple sclerosis. *Annals of Neurology*, **5**, 22–31

PRINEAS, J. W., KWON, E. E., CHO, E.-S. and SCHARER, L. R. (1984a) Continual breakdown and regeneration of myelin in progressive multiple sclerosis plaques. In *Multiple Sclerosis: Experimental and Clinical Aspects*, edited by L. Scheinberg and C. S. Raine. *Annals of the New York Academy of Sciences*, **436**, 11–32

PRINEAS, J. W., KWON, E. E., STERNBERGER, N. H. and LENNON, V. A. (1984b) The distribution of myelin-associated glycoprotein and myelin basic protein in actively demyelinating multiple sclerosis lesions. *Journal of Neuroimmunology*, **6**, 251–264

PRINEAS, J. W. and WRIGHT, R. G. (1978) Macrophages, lymphocytes, and plasma cells in the perivascular compartment in chronic multiple sclerosis. *Laboratory Investigation*, **38**, 409–421

RAINE, C. S. (1978) Membrane specializations between demyelinated axons and astroglia in chronic EAE lesions and multiple sclerosis plaques. *Nature*, **275**, 326–327

RAINE, C. S., POWERS, J. M. and SUZUKI, K. (1974) Acute multiple sclerosis. *Archives of Neurology*, **30**, 39–46

RAINE, C. S., SCHEINBERG, L. and WALTZ, J. M. (1981) Multiple sclerosis: oligodendrocyte survival and proliferation in an active established lesion. *Laboratory Investigation*, **45**, 534–546

RORKE, L. B., IWASAKI, Y., KOPROWSKI, H. *et al.* (1979) Acute demyelinating disease in a chimpanzee three years after inoculation of brain cells from a patient with MS. *Annals of Neurology*, **5**, 89–94

SALMI, A., REUNANEN, M., ILONEN, J. and PANELIUS, M. (1983) Intrathecal antibody synthesis to virus antigens in multiple sclerosis. *Clinical Experimental Immunology*, **52**, 241

SATO, S., QUARLES, R. H., BRADY, R. O. and TOURTELLOTTE, W. W. (1984) Elevated neutral protease activity in myelin from brains of patients with multiple sclerosis. *Annals of Neurology*, **15**, 264–267

SCHOENE, W. C., CARPENTER, S., BEHAN, P. O. and GESCHWIND, N. (1977) 'Onion bulb' formations in the central and peripheral nervous system in association with multiple sclerosis and hypertrophic polyneuropathy. *Brain*, **100**, 755–773

SEIL, F. J. (1977) Tissue culture studies of demyelinating disease: a critical review. *Annals of Neurology*, **2**, 345–355

SERGOTT, R. C., BROWN, M. J., SILBERBERG, D. H. and LISAK, R. P. (1984) Antigalactocerebroside serum demyelinates optic nerve *in vivo. Journal of Neurological Sciences*, **64**, 297–303

SILBERBERG, D. H., MANNING, M. C. and SCHREIBER, A. D. (1984) Tissue culture demyelination by normal human serum. *Annals of Neurology*, **15**, 575–580

SUZUKI, K., ANDREWS, J., WALTZ, J. and TERRY, R. (1969) Ultrastructural studies of multiple sclerosis. *Laboratory Investigation*, **20**, 444–454

TACHOVSKY, T. G., LISAK, R. P., KOPROWSKI, H., THEOFILOPOULOS, A. N. and DIXON, F. J. (1976) Circulating immune complexes in multiple sclerosis and other neurological diseases. *Lancet*, **2**, 997–999

TAKEOKA, T., SHINOHARA, Y., FURUMI, K. and MORI, K. (1983) Impairment of blood-cerebrospinal fluid barrier in multiple sclerosis. *Journal of Neurochemistry*, **41**, 1102–1108

TRAUGOTT, U. (1985) Characterization and distribution of lymphocyte subpopulations in multiple sclerosis plaques versus autoimmune demyelination lesions. *Springer Seminars in Immunopathology*, **8**, 71–95

TRAUGOTT, U., REINHERZ, E. L. and RAINE, C. S. (1983) Multiple sclerosis: distribution of T cells, T cell subsets and Ia-positive macrophages in lesions of different ages. *Journal of Neuroimmunology*, **4**, 201–221

TROIANO, R., HAFSTEIN, M., RUDERMAN, M., DOWLING, P. and COOK, S. (1984) Effect of high-dose intravenous steroid administration on contrast-enhancing computed tomographic scan lesions in multiple sclerosis. *Annals of Neurology*, **15**, 257–263

VANGURI, P., KOSKI, C. L., SILVERMAN, B. and SHIN, M. L. (1982) Complement activation by isolated myelin: activation of the classical pathway in the absence of myelin-specific antibodies. *Proceedings of the National Academy of Science, USA*, **79**, 3290–3294

VISSCHER, B. A., SULLIVAN, C. B. and DETELS, R. (1981) Measles antibody titers in multiple sclerosis patients and HLA-matched and unmatched siblings. *Neurology*, **31**, 1142–1145

WILLIAMS, A., ELDRIDGE, R., McFARLAND, H., HOUFF, S., KREBS, H. and McFARLIN, D. (1980) Multiple sclerosis in twins. *Neurology*, **30**, 1139–1147

7
The pathophysiology of multiple sclerosis
W. I. McDonald

INTRODUCTION

The introduction of nuclear magnetic resonance imaging (NMRI) to the investigation of multiple sclerosis (MS) has highlighted something which has long been known: that there is a discrepancy between the number and extent of lesions and their clinical expression. Pathologically, demyelinating lesions are occasionally found at post-mortem in patients in whom MS was not suspected during life; it is common to find evoked potential evidence of involvement of sensory pathways without corresponding symptoms; and there are extensive periventricular abnormalities at NMRI in almost all cases of MS and in at least half the patients with apparently isolated optic neuritis and acute brainstem lesions (Ormerod *et al.*, 1985) (*see* Chapter 2). Nevertheless there is a good correlation between the development of acute symptoms in MS (e.g. optic neuritis) and the appearance of electrophysiological abnormalities, and between major clinical deficits and the findings at post-mortem.

These discrepancies raise important questions about the mechanism of symptom production and remission, and the relationship between abnormalities and structure and function in central nerve fibres.

PATHOLOGY

The essential lesion in multiple sclerosis is the plaque — a more or less circumscribed lesion varying in size from a few cubic millimetres to many cubic centimetres in advanced cases. The small plaques are easily seen to be orientated around venules. This relationship is harder to see in very large plaques, but the systematic study by Fog (1965) established that virtually all the lesions in the cerebral hemispheres are perivenular in distribution (*see* Chapter 6).

The characteristic changes in the plaque itself are destruction of myelin with relative preservation of axon continuity, and gliosis (*Figure 7.1*). In considering the pathological background to symptomatology, it is important to appreciate that the nature and severity of the clinical deficit will be influenced not only by the position of the plaque and the proportion of the nerve fibres subserving a particular function

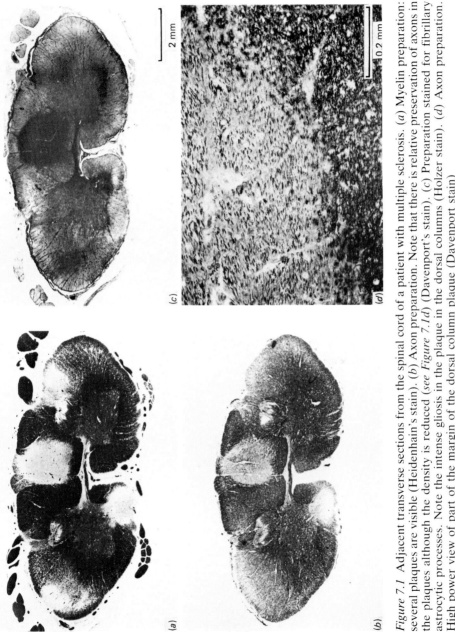

Figure 7.1 Adjacent transverse sections from the spinal cord of a patient with multiple sclerosis. (*a*) Myelin preparation: several plaques are visible (Heidenhain's stain). (*b*) Axon preparation. Note that there is relative preservation of axons in the plaques although the density is reduced (*see Figure 7.1d*) (Davenport's stain). (*c*) Preparation stained for fibrillary astrocytic processes. Note the intense gliosis in the plaque in the dorsal columns (Holzer stain). (*d*) Axon preparation. High power view of part of the margin of the dorsal column plaque (Davenport stain)

which are involved by it, but also by the details of the structural alterations within it. The study of experimental demyelinating lesions has established that within any one lesion there may be marked variations in the form and extent of demyelination on adjacent fibres, or along the length of an individual fibre (Harrison, McDonald and Ochoa, 1972; Harrison *et al.*, 1972; Ohlrich and McDonald, 1974; Mastaglia *et al.*, 1976; Gledhill and McDonald, 1977). Full thickness demyelination may be confined to the paranodal region, or may extend over one or many consecutive internodes. Partial thickness demyelination producing tapering of the internode towards the node is common. All these features have been recognized in MS (Prineas and Connell, 1979).

Characteristically, continuity is preserved in the majority of axons. However, there is always some axonal loss which may be detected even after the first clinical attack of optic neuritis when it is reflected in the ophthalmoscopically visible loss of bundles of nerve fibres (Frisén and Hoyt, 1974; *see* Chapter 1). In advanced cases at post-mortem, axonal loss may be extensive (*Figure 7.1b,d*).

Remyelination is observed at post-mortem, but is limited in extent and is predominantly confined to the edges of the plaques (Prineas and Connell, 1979). Whether it may be more extensive early in the course of the disease, or in younger patients, is unknown, although the possibility that this may be the case is raised — but certainly not established — by the observation that the incidence of restoration to normal or delayed evoked potentials in patients with optic neuritis is much higher in childhood (greater than 50%) than in adult life (approximately 10%) (McDonald, 1983).

Another striking feature of the plaque is intense astrocytic gliosis (*Figure 7.1c*). In chronic lesions fibrillary astrocytic processes largely fill the spaces between the axons created by myelin loss and the variable amount of Wallerian-type degeneration. There is also evidence of a diffuse increase in astrocyte numbers in the normal-appearing white matter beyond the edges of the plaques (Allen, 1984).

A number of other features may be seen. In small lesions, and at the edges of some large lesions, there is often evidence of myelin breakdown products both intracellularly and extracellularly. Lymphocytes, predominantly T cells, are seen within the lesion and in the adjacent normal-appearing white matter (Traugott, Reinherz and Raine, 1983). Perivenular cuffing with lymphocytes and plasma cells is commonly seen in and beyond lesions showing evidence of active myelin breakdown. Oedema is usually obvious in such 'active' lesions.

DISORDERED PHYSIOLOGY

It is to be expected that many of the morphological changes in the plaque of multiple sclerosis will influence the physiological properties of the nerve fibres traversing it. The changes in conduction produced by demyelination are well established from investigations carried out initially on experimental lesions in the peripheral nervous system. All the defects found there have been observed in the central nervous system when they have been looked for, although the possibilities of conduction in persistently demyelinated fibres and of ephaptic cross-excitation have not yet been examined directly. In keeping with the variety of structural changes, a range of abnormalities may be found in different individual fibres traversing a single lesion. The precise relationship between particular structural and functional changes is, for the most part, not established by direct experiment, although computer simulation of conduction in demyelinated nerve has given some insights into the mechanisms probably involved (Koles and Rasminsky, 1972). In the discussion which follows, the term 'demyelination' is used without implying any particular form of it, unless specifically stated.

Complete conduction block

It has long been known that complete conduction block is common in demyelinating lesions of the peripheral and central nervous system (Denny-Brown and Brenner, 1944; McDonald and Sears, 1970). The necessary morphological prerequisites for the development of complete conduction block are incompletely understood. There is no doublt that it is more common in large lesions than in small lesions. In peripheral nerve, there is evidence that it can occur with paranodal demyelination alone (Gilliatt, 1982; Lafontaine *et al.*, 1982); the mechanisms are discussed by Lafontaine *et al.* (1982). Evidence for conduction block in the human central nervous system comes from the study of evoked potentials. In optic neuritis for example, the visual evoked potential is absent when there is profound reduction in acuity, but returns with recovery of vision (*Figure 7.2*) (Halliday, McDonald and Mushin, 1973).

The role of conduction block in producing a functional deficit is easily understood when all the fibres subserving a particular function are involved. The

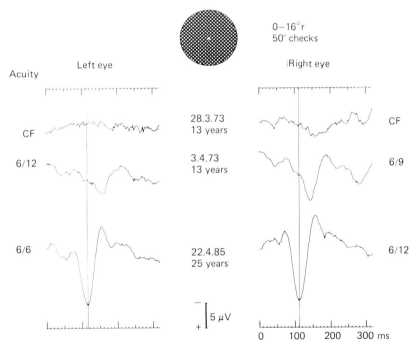

Figure 7.2 Visual evoked potentials to pattern reversal recorded from a girl aged 13 at presentation, 3 days, 9 days and 12 years after onset of an attack of acute bilateral optic neuritis. (Courtesy of Dr A. M. Halliday and Dr A. Kriss)

detailed interpretation of the relationship between incomplete lesions and symptomatology is more difficult even in the peripheral nervous system, because of the difficulty of determining physiologically the proportion of fibres blocked from the amplitude of the compound action potential which is determined by contributions from fibres of different sizes. It is even more difficult to make such an interpretation from a cerebral evoked potential which is generated after multiple synaptic relays. A second problem is the relative insensitivity of most clinical tests. It is nevertheless reasonable to suggest that the development of a clinical abnormality is influenced by the number of fibres subserving the particular function and the proportion which are blocked by the lesion. It is obvious that factors such as these contribute to some of the apparent discrepancies seen between evoked potentials and the clinical state of the patient.

Intermittent conduction block

In experimental demyelinating lesions, individual nerve fibres may show impairment of the ability to conduct trains of impulses at physiological frequencies. Alternation of response to suprathreshold stimuli at frequencies as low as 1 Hz can be seen in peripheral demyelinating lesions, both experimentally induced and naturally occurring (R.W. Gilliatt, P. Rudge and W.I. McDonald, unpublished observations; McDonald, 1982b). Evidence for intermittent conduction block in multiple sclerosis has been obtained by recording the somatosensory evoked potential in response to median nerve stimulation. Sclabassi, Namerow and Enns (1974) showed that the cortical response was able to follow at 100 Hz in normal individuals but that in patients with sensory loss in the hand, failure of transmission occurred down to 40 Hz, the severity of the abnormality being greater in those with more severe sensory loss. From the general applicability of studies on peripheral demyelinated fibres to central fibres, it seems likely that failure occurs at lower frequencies too.

A second type of intermittent conduction block has been observed experimentally both in peripheral and central fibres. With continuous stimulation above a critical frequency the refractory period increases until conduction is completely though reversibly blocked (McDonald and Sears, 1970; Rasminsky and Sears, 1972).

The inability of demyelinated fibres to transmit faithfully trains of impulses at physiological frequencies is likely to impair those functions which depend on the delivery of precisely timed bursts of impulses, for example the appreciation of vibration. It is also likely to contribute to weakness. Strong, smooth muscle contraction depends on the maintenance of a tetanus in motor units and the inability of fibres to sustain trains of impulses is likely to result in a failure of fusion, producing both weakness and intermittency of contraction manifested as the irregular tremor seen in weak muscles. The longer periods of conduction failure seen in some fibres probably contribute to the progressive increase in weakness seen during maintained exercise in patients with demyelinating lesions of the motor pathways and to the intermittent, though short lived, episodes of impairment of visual acuity experienced by some patients after optic neuritis. A recent patient recovering from an episode of optic neuritis reported that when she first looked at the Snellen chart it appeared blurred; after two to three seconds it was clear for one to two seconds then blurred again for a further three to four seconds, then clear again for a shorter period. This cycle was repeated with shorter periods of clarity until the vision became persistently fogged for several minutes. During the clear periods the vision was 6/12 (20/40).

Thermolability

The blocking temperature for conduction in demyelinated nerve fibres is reduced (Davis and Jacobson, 1971), and Rasminsky (1973) has shown that changes of as little as 0.5°C within the physiological range may convert intermittent to complete conduction block in individual fibres.

The exacerbation of symptoms in MS by a hot bath or exercise has been known since Uhthoff's description at the end of the last century. Persson and Sachs (1981)

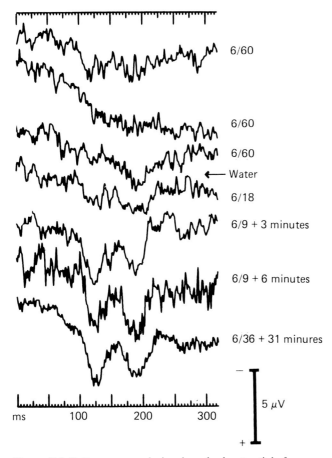

6/60

6/60

6/60

← Water

6/18

6/9 + 3 minutes

6/9 + 6 minutes

6/36 + 31 minures

5 μV

ms   100   200   300

Figure 7.3 Pattern reversal visual evoked potentials from a patient with multiple sclerosis. The visual acuities are given at the end of each trace. There is no consistent response in the top three traces. At the arrow, the patient drank a litre of ice-cold water over the course of 7 min. Subsequent records show the appearance of a delayed VEP which persisted for approximately 1 h. Note the difference in the time course of the changes in the evoked potentials and the visual acuity. (Courtesy of Dr A. Kriss and Dr B. Lecky)

have shown that impairment of acuity induced by exercise is accompanied by a reduction in amplitude of visual evoked potential without a change in latency, indicating that conduction block had developed. Recovery of acuity was accompanied by restoration of the evoked potential amplitude. Improvement in clinical function is often reported by patients following a cold bath. We observed a patient recently who reported an improvement in vision whenever he drank cold water. This patient was investigated by Dr A. Kriss and Dr B. Lecky, and the sequence of changes in acuity and evoked potentials is shown in *Figure 7.3*. Initially, there was no detectable response to pattern reversal stimulation but after drinking one litre of ice cold water, the acuity improved and an evoked potential was detectable. Both subsequently declined, although as can be seen from *Figure 7.3*, the time relations were not precise. This discrepancy, together with the rarity with which patients complain of exacerbation of symptoms in association with demyelinating peripheral neuropathy, suggests that the mechanisms involved in thermolability may be more complex than might seem at first sight.

Slowed conduction

One of the most striking physiological consequences of demyelinating lesions is slowing of conduction (McDonald, 1962, 1963; McDonald and Sears, 1970; Rasminsky and Sears, 1972). In keeping with the varying degrees of demyelination seen on different fibres within the same lesion, a range of reductions in velocity is found in single fibre studies. Evidence that slowing occurs in MS is derived from the study of evoked potentials. Delays in the P100 of the visual evoked potential are found in 90% of patients with optic neuritis, the mean being approximately 30–35 ms (Halliday, McDonald and Mushin, 1972, 1973; Shahrokhi, Chiappa and Young, 1978). Delays in the auditory and somatosensory evoked potentials are much shorter, of the order of 5–10 ms, which is more in keeping with the delays seen in peripheral demyelination (Robinson and Rudge, 1977; S.J. Jones, personal communication).

The mechanisms of the very long delays in the visual evoked potential are not established. The first question to be answered is whether they are real, in view of the much shorter delays encountered in the auditory and somatosensory evoked potentials. Certainly they are functionally relevant in some patients since the mean interocular difference in perception time for simple visual stimuli is of the same order (approximately 30 ms) as the mean delays in the visual evoked potential (Heron, Regan and Milner, 1974). It should be noted however that the visual evoked potential delay is sometimes more apparent than real, the major positive wave being formed by the normal P135 arising from the paramacular area which dominates the response when the macular fibres are blocked (Halliday *et al.*, 1979). Selective stimulation of different parts of the retina nevertheless suggests that true delays occur (Halliday *et al.*, 1979).

From what is known of conduction in experimentally demyelinated nerve, it is highly likely that slowed conduction contributes to the delay in the visual evoked potential, but whether it can account for the whole delay is another matter. The degree of slowing across individual internodes and the total length of demyelination on individual fibres are obviously relevant. Crude measurements at post-mortem reveal lengths of demyelination of 3 mm to 3 cm in the optic nerve (McDonald, 1976). The total lengths are likely to be much greater: even at presentation, patients with isolated optic neuritis may show clinically unsuspected abnormalities in the optic radiation at NMRI (*see Figure 2.10a*) (Ormerod *et al.*, 1985). A 25-fold increase in internodal conduction time has been observed in demyelinating peripheral nerve fibres (Rasminsky and Sears, 1972), but while it seems likely that slowing of a similar order can occur in the central nervous system, it is rather unlikely that slowing of this degree could be sustained over the 30 or 40 consecutively damaged internodes which are probably present in a plaque 1 cm long (McDonald, 1976). The biophysical mechanisms which produce slowing .in demyelinated fibres are discussed by Koles and Rasminsky (1972) and in the volume edited by Waxman and Ritchie (1981).

Another contributing factor might be slowed conduction in completely demyelinated segments if, as seems likely, it occurs in the central nervous system (*see below*). The range of conduction velocities in human optic nerve is unknown. The peak frequency in the fibre diameter spectrum is probably about 1.2 µm (*see* Ogden and Miller's (1966) discussion of Chacko's (1948) observations). The Hursh factor for primate optic nerve is 3.2 (Ogden and Miller, 1966) and if this is applied to the corrected human data the mean conduction velocity would be about 3.8 ms. To account for a delay of 30 ms over a plaque 1 cm long, the conduction velocity would have to be about one-thirteenth of the normal velocity, a reduction rather less than that observed in demyelinated fibres in the peripheral nervous system (Bostock and Sears, 1978; Smith, Bostock and Hall, 1982). The fibres in the optic nerve are much smaller than the peripheral fibres so far studied and it remains to be seen whether this degree of slowing actually occurs.

There may be other factors contributing to the delay in the visual evoked potentials. There could be a delay in the generation of the cortical response as a result of conduction block in a proportion of the incoming fibres or as a result of dispersion of the afferent volley from unequal slowing in different fibres. Plant and Hess (1986) have argued that cortical delays do occur but their magnitude is uncertain. A contribution from retinal delays has also been suggested (Heron, Regan and Miller, 1974), but no evidence for this has been forthcoming either in studies of the pattern electroretinogram (ERG) (Plant, Hess and Thomas, 1986) or in the psychophysical experiments of Patterson, Foster and Heron (1982). It is unlikely that selective block of the faster fibres makes a significant contribution to the delays.

In summary, there are a number of mechanisms which *could* account for the delays seen in the visual evoked potential, but the contribution of each is uncertain.

Turning now to the relevance of slowing of conduction to the genesis of symptoms, Brindley (1970) in another context has pointed out that probably 'the exact value of the interval between an impulse and its nearest neighbour is of little importance, but the time occupied by a group of half a dozen or so impulses is highly significant'. Thus slowing of conduction may be rather unimportant in the genesis of many symptoms. There are however certain circumstances in which a disturbance of timing may be relevant. One is the perception of vibration where unequal slowing (as well as intermittent conduction failure) in different fibres would be expected to lead to distortion or loss of the normal pattern of grouped discharges. Another is the effect of disparity in arrival time in the two hemispheres of information transmitted from the two eyes. This phenomenon can be demonstrated in normal individuals by placing a neutral density filter over one eye while observing a pendulum swinging in one plane; the pendulum appears to describe an ellipse (the Pulfrich effect — Pulfrich, 1922). The same phenomenon can be demonstrated readily following an attack of unilateral optic neuritis (Frisén *et al.*, 1973; Rushton, 1975) and the illusion can be abolished by placing a neutral density filter over the *good* eye. It is likely that this class of abnormality underlies the difficulty that some patients experience following an attack of optic neuritis, in judging the direction of moving objects, e.g. in playing tennis and in crossing the road in moving traffic. These difficulties too may be diminished by placing a neutral density filter over the good eye (A.C. Bird, personal communication).

Increased excitability

Abnormal excitability is readily demonstrated in demyelinated and dysmyelinated nerve fibres in the peripheral nervous system of animals and man (Howe, Loeser and Calvin, 1977; Rasminsky, 1978; Nordin *et al.*, 1984). In a single unit study of demyelinated central nerve fibres, Smith and McDonald (1982) found a range of abnormalities within a single lesion in the posterior column. Some fibres were continuously active over many hours with a strikingly regular discharge pattern. Some showed grouped discharges, two or three impulses at approximately 100 Hz recurring two or three times per second. Many fibres were mechanically very sensitive at the site of the lesion, small deformations (less than 1 mm) producing an increase in discharge frequency in spontaneously active fibres or bursts of activity which adapted over a few seconds, in silent fibres (*Figure 7.4a*).

These physiological abnormalities provide a sufficient explanation for a number of symptoms commonly encountered in MS. In sensory fibres, prolonged continuous spontaneous discharges are likely to account for sustained paraesthesiae. The time course of the discharges induced by mechanical deformation at the site of the lesion is similar to that of the surge of paraesthesiae induced by neck flexion (Lhermitte's symptom) and, indeed, Nordin *et al.* (1984) have recently demonstrated that it is possible to record bursts of impulses in peripheral nerve during this manoeuvre in a patient with MS (*Figure 7.4b*). A similar mechanism is likely to account for the phosphenes induced by eye movement which are experienced by up to one-third of patients with optic neuritis (Davis *et al.*, 1976; McDonald, 1983). The grouped discharges from experimental central lesions bear a striking resemblance to those recorded by Matthews (1966) and Hjorth and Willison (1973) in facial myokymia in MS.

Ephaptic cross activation

Rasminsky (1978) first convincingly demonstrated that ephaptic cross activation could occur in the circumstances of naturally occurring disease. He showed that impulses arising spontaneously in dysmyelinated fibres of the 'dystrophic' mouse could activate adjacent fibres and then propagate both centrifugally and centripetally. The appropriate experiment has not yet been performed in the central nervous system, but for the reasons already given it seems likely that the phenomenon occurs there too. The slow spread of ephaptic excitation has been

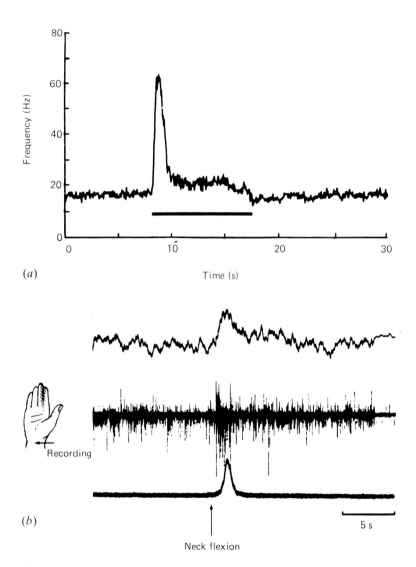

Figure 7.4 (*a*) A plot of discharge frequency of a single unit traversing an experimental demyelinating lesion in the cat induced by the direct microinjection of lysophosphatidylcholine into the dorsal column. Note the increase in discharge frequency when the lesion was depressed 0.75 mm for 10 s (bar) by a glass rod (Smith and McDonald, 1982). (*b*) Recording from the right median nerve of a skin fascicle with receptive field indicated. At the moment indicated by the arrow, the patient flexed her neck which elicited Lhermitte's phenomenon. The moment for the abnormal sensation was indicated by a grip force signal shown in the lower trace. Above is seen the multi-unit burst in the neurogram and the integrated neurogram. (Time constant 0.5 s). (From Nordin *et al.*, 1984, courtesy the Editor and Publishers, *Pain*)

proposed as the mechanism underlying such paroxysmal phenomena in MS as painful tonic seizures and episodic dysarthria (Matthews, 1975; *see* Chapter 10). Such a mechanism is plausible, but nothing is known of the factors which might determine the self-limited cycles of increased liability to cross activation which must underlie the intermittency of the symptoms.

Conduction in persistently demyelinated axons

There is now clear experimental evidence that axonal conduction can develop in the absence of myelin in the peripheral nervous system both in the congenitally dysmyelinated fibres of the 'dystrophic' mouse (Rasminsky *et al.*, 1978), and in adult nerve fibres demyelinated by diphtheria toxin or lysophosphatidylcholine (Bostock and Sears, 1978; Smith, Bostock and Hall, 1982). In adult demyelinated fibres, conduction develops about 6 days after induction of the lesion, and appears to be commoner in smaller than in larger diameter fibres. The conduction velocity is reduced to approximately 1 m/s (2.5–5% of the normal velocity). The form of conduction is different in the two models of toxin-induced demyelination. In the diphtheria toxin lesion it appears to be continuous and in this respect resembles conduction in normal unmyelinated fibres (Bostock and Sears 1978). In the lysophosphatidylcholine lesion conduction is saltatory between regularly spaced sites ('physiological' nodes) on the demyelinated segment of axon (Smith, Bostock and Hall, 1982).

There is an important change in the nature of conduction in the demyelinated segment (Bostock, Sears and Sherratt, 1981). Evidence derived from electrophysiological experiments, saxitoxin binding experiments and cytochemical staining have established that in the normal mammalian peripheral nerve fibre there are important inhomogeneities in the distribution of sodium and potassium channels (*see* review by Ritchie and Chiu, 1981). At the nodes there is a high density of sodium channels but few potassium channels. The converse is true for the internodal axon. During propagation of the impulse in normal fibres there are no changes in potassium conductance because of the inaccessibility of the internodal potassium channels to the extracellular fluid. The same is true for central nerve fibres (Kocsis and Waxman, 1981). Following demyelination in peripheral nerve fibres, sodium channels appear in the internodal axon (whether by insertion of new channels or by redistribution of existing channels is unknown). Propagation of the impulse then involves sequential changes of sodium and potassium conductance similar to those of normal unmyelinated and amphibian myelinated fibres.

There has not been so far a crucial experiment to determine whether continuous conduction can develop following central demyelination. There is however strong clinical evidence that some form of conduction must develop in persistently demyelinated fibres. Wiśniewski, Oppenheimer and McDonald (1976) had the opportunity to examine the optic nerves of a 40-year-old woman who died from a massive pulmonary embolus 4 days after the visual acuity had been measured by two separate examiners. She was able to count fingers with each eye and to read with telescopes (McDonald, 1976). At post-mortem both optic nerves were exhaustively examined by light and electron microscopy. At one level in one nerve a montage of a complete transverse section of the nerve was constructed from electron micrographs. Many intact axons were present in each nerve. Myelin sheaths were however completely absent in one nerve and in the other were confined to a small group of fibres over a length of about 3 mm at one edge. The total observed length of demyelination was 27 mm in one nerve and 30 mm in the other.

The nature of conduction in demyelinated central nerve fibres and the factors influencing its development remain unknown. If fibre size is relevant, as it is in the peripheral nervous system, it is perhaps not surprising that remission is so frequent (early in the course of the illness) after involvement of the optic nerves or pyramidal tracts in MS, since in both these pathways 90% of the fibres are probably less than 4 μm in diameter (Lassek, 1942; Chacko, 1948; Oppel, 1963; Ogden and Miller, 1966).

Conduction in remyelinated nerve

The properties of remyelinated peripheral nerve fibres are well known. Smith, Blakemore and McDonald (1981) showed that conduction was restored to demyelinated central fibres following remyelination by oligodendrocytes, the time course of restoration of conduction corresponding with the time course of remyelination. The refractory period of transmission was rapidly restored to normal, implying that the remyelinated fibres would be capable of carrying trains of impulses at physiological frequencies.

Conclusive evidence that restoration of conduction by remyelination occurs in MS is lacking, although the occasional recovery of normal latency of the visual evoked potential in adults, and the more frequent recovery in children following optic neuritis is consistent with the assumption that it does (*see Figure 7.2*) (McDonald, 1983).

Consequences of Wallerian-type degeneration

It is important to remember that Wallerian-type degeneration is always present in the lesions of MS, and though of relatively little importance to some, particularly in those interpreted as being 'early' lesions because of their small size and the presence of recent myelin breakdown products, it is a striking feature of many lesions in advanced cases (*see Figure 7.1*). It is therefore appropriate to consider the functional consequences of axonal loss.

Jacobson, Eames and McDonald (1979) investigated the time course of recovery of visual acuity and contrast sensitivity in cats following stereotactically induced incomplete degenerative lesions of the intracranial optic nerve. An example is illustrated in *Figure 7.5*. The animal had been trained to recognize stripes of different sizes. The percentage of correct responses (x-axis) to randomly presented vertical gratings of different spatial frequencies (y -xis) is plotted against time (z-axis). After many months of training, at the time indicated by the arrow in the z-axis, a lesion of one intracranial optic nerve and the adjacent part of the chiasm was made. In this particular experiment, fibre counts after its completion showed that 77% of the fibres of the nerve had been destroyed. There was an initial rapid recovery of response to medium spatial frequencies in the first week, during which parallel histological studies had shown that the striking oedema of the early lesion was resolving. The response to the large stripes (low spatial frequency) returned during the first month, and thereafter there was a more gradual recovery of

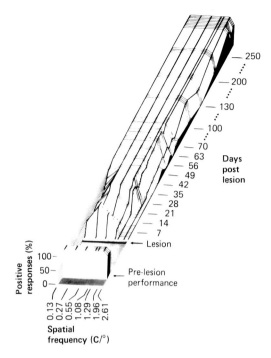

Figure 7.5 Frequency-of-seeing curves for a cat in which a predominantly degenerative lesion had been induced in the right optic nerve and adjacent parts of the optic chiasm and optic tract by the stereotactic injection of diphtheria toxin; x-axis: spatial frequency (c/degree); y-axis: per cent correct responses; z-axis: time after induction of lesion. (From Jacobson, Eames and McDonald, 1979, courtesy the Editor and Publishers, *Experimental Brain Research*)

response to fine gratings — despite the destruction of three-quarters of the fibres. Contrast sensitivity also recovered. The mechanism of the slower phases of recovery is unknown, but since there are no alternative anterior pathways for vision it must involve adaptive synaptic changes centrally, and/or in the retina. Other possible mechanisms are discussed by Jacobson, Eames and McDonald (1979). The clinical implications of the response to Wallerian-type degeneration are considered further in the discussion of remission.

Humoral influences on conduction

It has often been suggested that in experimental and clinical demyelinating disease there may be circulating factors which influence conduction in nerve fibres (normal or partially demyelinated), across synapses, or both (*see* reviews by Schauf and Davis, 1981; Seil, 1977, 1981). There is now clear experimental evidence for the production of conduction block *in vivo* in peripheral nerve fibres within 1 h of intraneural injection of anti-galactocerebroside serum, and there is electrophysiological evidence that the block is caused by paranodal demyelination (Lafontaine *et al.*, 1982). In central nerve fibres, anti-galactocerebroside serum injected directly into the optic nerve initiates demyelination within 1–2 h, but its effects on conduction have not been studied (Sergott *et al.*, 1984).

The evidence in relation to the existence of a humoral blocking factor in the serum of patients with MS is however conflicting. In the only investigation employing an *in vivo* system (rat cortex) the effect was not specific; some sera both from patients with MS and normal human volunteers attenuated the direct cortical response (Seil, Leiman and Kelly, 1976). Seil's (1977) summary puts the case precisely: 'The role of serum neuroelectrical block factors, specific or non-specific, in the pathogenesis of human or experimental demyelinating disease remains undefined.'

Finally, it should be noted that almost nothing is known of the effects on conduction of increased water content and changes in ionic composition produced by oedema and myelin breakdown. Possible pressure effects of oedema are discussed below.

The role of the astrocyte

Gliosis is one of the cardinal features of the plaque of MS, and the question thus arises whether the astrocyte might have a role in the symptomatology of multiple sclerosis. The functions of this cell are still incompletely understood and it is therefore impossible at present to define its role in pathophysiology. Nevertheless, it is worth considering the possible relevance to the development of symptoms of those properties which are known.

It has been shown recently that in tissue culture the astrocyte can act as an antigen presenting cell (Fontana, Fierz and Wekerle, 1984) and it is possible, though not established, that it may play a role in the pathogenesis of demyelination in MS. Fontana *et al.* (1982) also showed that astrocytes in culture produce large quantities of interleukin-1. When astrocyte-derived interleukin-1 is injected intraventricularly into rats, slow wave activity in the sleep EEG is significantly enhanced (Tobler *et al.*, 1985). The question thus arises whether the extraordinary sense of fatigue (out of proportion to physical effort and in the absence of depression) so common in patients with MS might be related to the diffuse astrocytic proliferation which occurs within and beyond the lesions.

The similarity of the organization of astrocytic processes at the central node to that of the Schwann cell at the peripheral node (Hildebrand and Waxman, 1984) suggests that the astrocyte may have a role in normal conduction, although what this might be is uncertain. In the plaque of MS the fibrillary astrocytic processes enter into an intimate relationship with the demyelinated axons, and a variety of axo-glial membrane specializations has been described (Soffer and Raine, 1980). It is possible that a sufficient change in resistance and capacitance might be produced by this ensheathment to influence the restoration of conduction in persistently demyelinated fibres. There is also evidence that the astrocyte may play a buffering role in relation to potassium (Orkand, 1982) and might thereby influence conduction in demyelinated fibres in which, at least in the peripheral nervous system, changes in potassium conductance are important.

These suggestions are highly speculative. Their validity can only be assessed when the properties of the astrocyte and its interrelationship with the axon are better understood.

MECHANISM OF REMISSION

In the foregoing account I have considered the physiological consequences of the structural abnormalities which are present in the plaque of multiple sclerosis. It is now appropriate to consider the mechanisms which underlie remission. It is convenient to do so in relation to optic neuritis, a condition in which quantitation of changes in function with time can be recorded fairly readily thus facilitating comparison with recovery curves obtained from animals with experimental lesions.

In childhood particularly, recovery can begin and progress rapidly. The patient illustrated by *Figure 7.2* was first seen 3 days after the onset of bilateral optic neuritis when the visual acuities were reduced to counting fingers in both eyes. Visual evoked potentials were undetectable at this stage, but 6 days later, when the acuities had risen to VR 6/9 (20/30) and VL 6/12 (20/40) well-formed though delayed responses were present. The absence of evoked potentials at the early stage and their presence later provides evidence for recovery of conduction block between the two recording sessions. The factors involved in the production of acute conduction block have not been fully elucidated. On the basis of what is known in the peripheral nervous system they probably include ischaemia (Lewis, Pickering and Rothschild, 1931) and paranodal detachment of myelin lamellae (Lafontaine *et al.*, 1982), as well as frank demyelination (Denny-Brown and Brenner, 1944; McDonald, 1963; Gilliatt, 1982). The membrane attack complex of complement may also be implicated (Morgan, Campbell and Compston, 1984).

Compression of central nerve fibres produces conduction block which is rapidly reversible by decompression and is probably dependent on ischaemia (McDonald, 1982a). This effect may well be important in optic neuritis in which the acute demyelinating lesion is probably associated with oedema and swelling of the optic nerve which can be detected occasionally with the CT scan (*see* Chapter 2). It seems likely that oedema in regions of tight constriction such as the scleral and optic canals might produce a sufficient local rise in intraneural pressure not only to produce the swelling of the optic disc which is so common in optic neuritis, but also conduction block in partially damaged or even normal nerve fibres. Rapid dispersal of oedema with relief of compression could then result in rapid restoration of conduction.

The usual time course of remission is however rather longer. In the patient illustrated in *Figure 7.6*, there was an initial fairly rapid period of improvement in the few weeks after the visual acuity reached its lowest level, followed by more gradual recovery over many months. This biphasic course has its counterparts in the restitution of conduction by central remyelination (Smith, Blakemore and McDonald, 1981) and in the adaptive mechanisms operating in animals with incomplete destruction of one optic nerve (Jacobson, Eames and McDonald, 1979). Both these mechanisms are likely to contribute to recovery in MS. The development of conduction in persistently demyelinated fibres may well turn out to be of equal of greater importance, but at present its role cannot be assessed because the frequency of its occurrence, the factors influencing its development and its time course are unknown.

These conjectures about mechanism can be regarded only as tentative. There are many gaps in our knowledge: it is for example unknown whether changes in the extracellular fluid during demyelination influence conduction and whether detached myelin lamellae might be rapidly reattached in the acute phase. There is

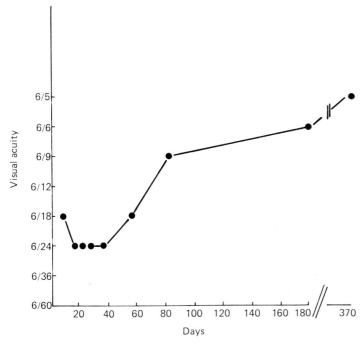

Figure 7.6 Recovery curve of visual acuity (y-axis) in a patient with acute unilateral optic neuritis. The time after the onset of symptoms is plotted in days on the x-axis. (From McDonald, 1983, courtesy the Editor and Publishers of *Transactions of the Ophthalmologic-al Societies of the United Kingdom*)

little doubt however that all of the processes described above contribute to recovery, but the relative importance of each at different ages and in different stages of evolution of the lesion remains to be established.

The 'silent' lesion

To what extent can we account for the 'silent' lesion detected by evoked potentials or imaging or found unexpectedly at post-mortem?

Several factors must be taken into account. At the simplest level there is the question whether the particular patient was sufficiently troubled to complain. The symptoms may have occurred so long ago that he may have forgotten about them; an episode of minor sensory disturbance is particularly vulnerable in this respect. There is also the problem of whether the appropriate questions have been asked of the patient and whether the appropriate clinical assessment has been made. It is remarkable for example that phosphenes induced by eye movement, now commonly noted, were rarely recorded until 10 years ago: patients infrequently complain of them but often respond positively and characteristically to direct questioning. Loss of the sense of smell is generally held to be rare in MS, yet extensive demyelination may be found in the olfactory tract at post-mortem (personal observations), and Pinching (1977) found that 15 out of 22 patients with

MS had significant abnormalities on critical testing. The existence of the Pulfrich effect and its consequent symptoms in optic neuritis was unrecognized until Frisén *et al.* (1973) predicted that it would be present in conditions in which there was a difference in brightness of images or in nerve conduction between the two eyes. The frequency of defects of memory early in the course of multiple sclerosis was not appreciated until specifically sought (*see* Chapter 8). The substantial delays in perceptual time in optic neuritis were not detected until looked for using refined psychophysical techniques (Heron, Regan and Milner, 1974).

There are other lesions which may be identified, for example by NMRI, for which corresponding functional deficits have not yet been found. In many cases this probably reflects the fact that the appropriate assessments have not been made. Neural factors too must contribute to apparent silence. There is considerable 'redundancy' in some pathways and until a critical proportion of the fibres subserving a particular function are impaired, a functional deficit will not appear. The speed of development of the lesion too is probably relevant. It is common in ophthalmological clinics to see patients who have discovered accidentally severe unilateral vision loss due, for example, to tumour. The same degree of impairment developing acutely would give rise to severe symptoms. It seems likely that slowly progressive affection of nerve fibres in MS would allow the development of compensatory mechansms such as those described above, thereby delaying or preventing the achievement of the critical level of involvement necessary for the appearance of a functional deficit.

'Severity' and 'activity'

The notions of clinical severity and activity of multiple sclerosis are complex. The former term is usually employed loosely to refer to the degree of functional disability and the frequency of relapses, and the latter to indicate the occurrence of a relapse or of progressive deterioration. Pathological activity is said to be present where there is evidence of recent myelin breakdown and it may be seen in two rather different contexts — at the edge of a chronic plaque, and throughout a smaller perivenular lesion when it is usually regarded as being evidence of 'recent' acute damage. The acute lesion, for reasons already mentioned, is perhaps more likely to be associated with the development of symptoms. Pathological activity at the edge of a chronic plaque may well not be associated with any symptoms at all: only a small number of fibres is affected and because of the disposition of fibres in tracts (clustering of those subserving the same function in a limited anatomical region) the critical number necessary for the emergence of a deficit may not be reached. For example: activity at one part of the margin of a large plaque in the cervical dorsal column (*see Figure 7.1*) may involve fibres from the arm, at another, fibres from the leg, and at yet another propriospinal fibre.

From the foregoing discussion it is clear that the clinical condition of the patient at any time is only crudely related to the total volume of abnormal tissue in the brain and whether active myelin breakdown is occurring. For example, a patient with extensive periventricular lesions may never have complained of neurological symptoms (*Figure 7.7*). Conversely, when a deficit is due to conduction block at one level in a pathway, e.g. in the corticospinal tract in the spinal cord, clinical expression of additional proximal lesions involving the same fibres is impossible.

The mechanism of accumulation of fixed deficit in multiple sclerosis is poorly understood. Several factors are likely to contribute. First, there will be increasing amounts of Wallerian degeneration each time a new plaque develops. Second, the length of certain individual pathways, e.g. the corticospinal tract, renders them particularly vulnerable since as Rasminsky (1973) has pointed out: 'Just as a chain is only as strong as its weakest link, a demyelinated fibre is only as functional as its most severely affected internode.' There is thus a statistically greater chance of loss

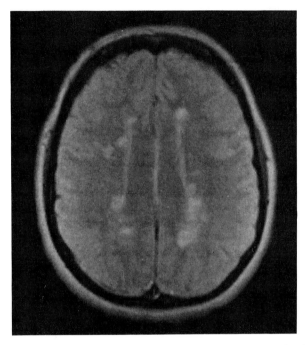

Figure 7.7 NMR image from an apparently healthy individual. Spin echo sequence. Note the extensive periventricular abnormalities

of function in very long fibres than in short fibres. Third, the effectiveness of compensatory mechanisms may change with time. The possibility of a greater capacity for remyelination in childhood has been mentioned already. It is also conceivable, although there is no evidence bearing on the point, that repeated damage at the same site could impair the capacity of remyelination through increasing loss of oligodendrocytes, exhaustion of the supply of their precursors (if they exist in the human adult central nervous system as they do in the rat – G. Wolswijk and M. D. Noble, unpublished observations) or impairment of the migration of oligodendrocytes or their processes by tissue disorganization. The factors influencing the structural integrity of axons subjected to demyelination are poorly understood, and it is conceivable that both the total length of demyelination and the occurrence of repeated episodes of demyelination at a single level might increase the chance of axonal disintegration.

Steadily progressive versus relapsing and remitting disease

It is a striking fact that some patients show steady progression from the onset of their illness, others experience relapses and remissions throughout the course, and yet others enter a progressive phase after some years of remitting disease. The pathophysiological basis of these variants is unknown. One obvious suggestion is that in the relapsing and remitting cases there are cycles of activity and quiescence of the pathogenetic process. The periodic changes in the T suppressor/helper ratio in peripheral blood (*see* Chapter 5) are consistent with this hypothesis and the failure of such changes to be accompanied on every occasion by clinical change (e.g. Compston, 1983) is not against it – indeed it is what would be expected. In the progressive cases it might be supposed that the immunopathogenetic process is continually active. Though likely, however, it remains to be established that there is a necessary connection between myelin breakdown and the immunological abnormalities so far demonstrated in multiple sclerosis.

It is also possible that when there is a substantial fixed deficit in a particular function, small additional increases which might occur as the remaining intact fibres are affected, even episodically, may not be detectable individually by the patient or the neurologist. These considerations and the present inaccessibility to clinical testing of many parts of the cerebral white matter emphasize the importance for the monitoring of therapy, of developing independent measures of the amount of abnormal tissue in the central nervous system, and of whether or not active myelin destruction is taking place. Advances in imaging techniques are likely to help, although the present methods are still relatively crude.

References

ALLEN, I. M. (1984) Demyelinating diseases. In *Greenfield's Neuropathology*, 4th edn, edited by J. H. Adams, J. A. N. Corselis and L. W. Duchen, pp. 338–384. London: Edward Arnold

BOSTOCK, H. and SEARS, T. A. (1978) The internodal axon membrane: electrical excitability and continuous conduction in segmental demyelination. *Journal of Physiology*, **280**, 273–301

BOSTOCK, H., SEARS, T. A. and SHERRATT, R. M. (1981) The effects of 4-aminopyridine and tetraethylammonium ions on normal and demyelinated mammalian nerve fibres. *Journal of Physiology*, **313**, 301–315

BRINDLEY, G. S. (1970) *Physiology of the Retina and Visual Pathway*. p. 90. London: Edward Arnold

CHACKO, L. W. (1948) An analysis of fibre size in the human optic nerve. *British Journal of Ophthalmology*, **32**, 457–461

COMPSTON, D. A. S. (1983) Lymphocyte subpopulations in patients with multiple sclerosis. *Journal of Neurology, Neurosurgery and Psychiatry*, **46**, 105–114

DAVIS, F. A. and JACOBSON, S. (1971) Altered thermal sensitivity in injured and demyelinated nerve: a possible model of temperature effects in multiple sclerosis. *Journal of Neurology, Neurosurgery and Psychiatry*, **34**, 551–561

DAVIS, F. A., BERGEN, D., SCHAUF, C., McDONALD, W. I. and DEUTSCH, W. (1976) Movement phosphenes in optic neuritis: a new clinical sign. *Neurology*, **26**, 1100–1104

DENNY-BROWN, D. and BRENNER, C. (1944) Lesion in peripheral nerve resulting from compression by spring clip. *Archives of Neurology and Psychiatry*, **52**, 1–19

FOG, T. (1965) The topography of plaques in multiple sclerosis. *Acta Neurologica Scandinavica*, **41**, (Suppl. 15), 7–16

FONTANA, A., KRISTENSEN, F., DUBS, R., GEMSA, D. and WEBER, E. (1982) Production of prostaglandin-E and interleukin-1 like factors by cultured astrocytes and C6 glioma cells. *Journal of Immunology*, **129**, 2413–2419

FONTANA, A., FIERZ, W. and WEKERLE, H. (1984) Astrocytes present myelin basic protein to encephalitogenic T-cell lines. *Nature*, **307**, 273–276

FRISÉN, L. and HOYT, W. F. (1974) Insidious atrophy of retinal nerve fibres in multiple sclerosis. *Archives of Ophthalmology*, **92**, 91–97

FRISÉN, L., HOYT, W. F., BIRD, A. C. and WEALE, R. A. (1973) Diagnostic uses of the Pulfrich phenomenon. *Lancet*, **2**, 385–386

GILLIATT, R. W. (1982) Electrophysiology of peripheral neuropathies—an overview. *Muscle and Nerve*, **5**, S108–S116

GLEDHILL, R. F. and McDONALD, W. I. (1977) Morphological characteristics of central demyelination and remyelination: a single-fiber study. *Annals of Neurology*, **1**, 552–560

HALLIDAY, A. M., McDONALD, W. I. and MUSHIN, J. (1972) Delayed visual evoked response in optic neuritis. *Lancet*, **1**, 982–985

HALLIDAY, A. M., McDONALD, W. I. and MUSHIN, J. (1973) Delayed pattern-evoked responses in optic neuritis in relation to visual acuity. *Transactions of the Ophthalmological Societies of the United Kingdom*, **93**, 315–324

HALLIDAY, A. M., BARRETT, G., BLUMHARDT, L. D. and KRISS, A. (1979) The macular and paramacular subcomponents of the pattern evoked response. In *Human Evoked Potentials*, edited by D. E. Lehmann and E. Callaway, pp. 135–151 New York: Plenum Publishing

HARRISON, B. M., McDONALD, W. I. and OCHOA, J. (1972) Remyelination in the central diphtheria toxin lesion. *Journal of the Neurological Sciences*, **17**, 293–302

HARRISON, B. M., McDONALD, W. I., OCHOA, J. and OHLRICH, G. D. (1972) Paranodal demyelination in the central nervous system. *Journal of the Neurological Sciences*, **16**, 489–494

HERON, J. R., REGAN, D. and MILNER, B. A. (1974) Delay in visual perception in unilateral optic atrophy after retrobulbar neuritis. *Brain*, **97**, 69–78

HILDEBRAND, C. and WAXMAN, S. G. (1984) Postnatal differentiation of rat optic nerve fibers: electron microscopic observations on the development of nodes of Ranvier and axoglial relations. *Journal of Comparative Neurology*, **224**, 25–37

HJORTH, R. J. and WILLISON, R. G. (1973) The electromyogram in facial myokymia and hemifacial spasm. *Journal of the Neurological Sciences*, **20**, 117–126

HOWE, J. F., LOESER, J. D. and CALVIN, W. H. (1977) Mechanosensitivity of dorsal root ganglia and chronically injured axons: a physiological basis for the radicular pain of nerve root compression. *Pain*, **3**, 25–41

JACOBSON, S. G., EAMES, R. A. and McDONALD, W. I. (1979) Optic nerve fibre lesions in adult cats: pattern of recovery of spatial vision. *Experimental Brain Research*, **36**, 491–508

KOCSIS, J. D. and WAXMAN, S. G. (1981) Action potential electrogenesis in mammalian central axons. In *Demyelinating Diseases. Basic and Clinical Electrophysiology*, edited by S. G. Waxman and J. M. Ritchie, pp. 299–312. New York: Raven Press

KOLES, Z. J. and RASMINSKY, M. (1972) A computer simulation of conduction in demyelinated nerve fibres. *Journal of Physiology*, **227**, 351–364

LAFONTAINE, S., RASMINSKY, M., SAIDA, T. and SUMNER, A. J. (1982) Conduction block in rat myelinated fibres following acute exposure to anti-galactocerebroside serum. *Journal of Physiology*, **323**, 287–306

LASSEK, A. M. (1942) The human pyramidal tract. IV. A study of the mature myelinated fibres of the pyramid. *Journal of Comparative Neurology*, **76**, 217–225

LEWIS, T., PICKERING, G. W. and ROTHSCHILD, P. (1931) Centripetal paralysis arising out of arrested blood flow to limb, including notes on form of tingling. *Heart*, **16**, 1–32

MASTAGLIA, F. L., McDONALD, W. I., WATSON, J. V. and YOGENDRAN, K. (1976) Effects of X-radiation on the spinal cord: an experimental study of the morphological changes in central nerve fibres. *Brain*, **99**, 101–122

MATTHEWS, W. B. (1966) Facial myokymia. *Journal of Neurology, Neurosurgery and Psychiatry*, **29**, 35–39

MATTHEWS, W. B. (1975) Paroxysmal symptoms in multiple sclerosis. *Journal of Neurology, Neurosurgery and Psychiatry*, **38**, 617–623

McDONALD, W. I. (1962) Conduction in muscle afferent fibres during experimental demyelination in cat nerve. *Acta Neuropathologica*, **1**, 425–432

McDONALD, W. I. (1963) The effects of experimental demyelination of conduction in peripheral nerve: a histological and electrophysiological study. II Electrophysiological observations. *Brain*, **86**, 501–524

McDONALD, W. I. (1976) Conduction in the optic nerve. *Transactions of the Ophthalmological Societies of the United Kingdom*, **96**, 352–354

McDONALD, W. I. (1982a) The symptomatology of tumours of the anterior visual pathways. The 1981 Silversides Lecture. *Canadian Journal of Neurological Sciences*, **9**, 381–390

McDONALD, W. I. (1982b) Clinical consequences of conduction defects produced by demyelination. In *Abnormal Nerves and Muscles as Impulse Generators*, edited by W. J. Culp and J. Ochoa, pp. 253–270. New York: Oxford University Press

McDONALD, W. I. (1973) Doyne lecture. The significance of optic neuritis. *Transactions of the Ophthalmological Societies of the United Kingdom*, **103**, 230–246

McDONALD, W. I. and SEARS, T. A. (1970) The effects of experimental demyelination on conduction in the central nervous system. *Brain*, **93**, 583–598

MORGAN, B. P., CAMPBELL, A. K. and COMPSTON, D. A. S. (1984) Terminal component of complement (C9) in cerebrospinal fluid of patients with multiple sclerosis. *Lancet*, **2**, 251–254

NORDIN, M., NYSTRÖM, WALLIN, U. and HAGBARTH, K.-E. (1984) Ectopic sensory discharges and paraesthesiae in patients with disorders of peripheral nerves, dorsal roots and dorsal columns. *Pain*, **20**, 231–245

OGDEN, T. E. and MILLER, R. F. (1966) Studies of the optic nerve of the Rhesus monkey: nerve fibre spectrum and physiological properties. *Vision Research*, **6**, 485–506

OHLRICH, G. D. and McDONALD, W. I. (1974) Demyelination in the central nervous system of the cat studied by single fibre isolation. *Proceedings of the Australian Association of Neurologists*, **11**, 77–87

OPPEL, O. (1963) Mikroskopische Untersuchungen über Die Anzahl und Kaliber der markhaltige Nervenfasern im Fasiculus opticus des Menschen. *Graefes Archiv für Ophthalmologie*, **160**, 19–27

ORKAND, R. K. (1982) Signalling between neuronal and glial cells. In *Neuronal-Glial Interrelationships*, edited by T. A. Sears, pp. 147–157. Berlin: Springer-Verlag

ORMEROD, I. E. C., McDONALD, W. I., DU BOULAY, G. H. *et al.* (1985) Disseminated lesions at presentation in patients with optic neuritis. *Journal of Neurology, Neurosurgery and Psychiatry* (in press)

PATTERSON, V. H., FOSTER, D. H. and HERON, J. R. (1982) Rod- and cone-mediated visual function in multiple sclerosis. *Journal of the Neurological Sciences*, **57**, 385–393

PERSSON, H. E. and SACHS, C. (1981) Visual evoked potentials elicited by pattern reversal during provoked visual impairment in multiple sclerosis. *Brain*, **104**, 369–382

PINCHING, A. (1977) Clinical assessment of olfaction reassessed. *Brain*, **100**, 377–388

PLANT, G. T. and HESS, R. F. (1986) The electrophysiological assessment of optic neuritis. In *Optic Neuritis*, edited by R. F. Hess and G. T. Plant, pp. 192–229. Cambridge: Cambridge University Press

PLANT, G. T., HESS, R. F. and THOMAS, S. J. (1986) The pattern evoked electroretinograms in optic neuritis: a combined psychophysical and electrophysiological study. *Brain* (in press)

PRINEAS, J. and CONNELL, L. F. (1979) Remyelination in multiple sclerosis. *Annals of Neurology*, **5**, 22–31

PULFRICH VON, C. (1922) Die Stereoskopie im Dienste der isochromen unt heterochromen Photometrie. *Naturwissenschaften*, **10**, 553–564, 569–574, 596–601, 714–722, 735–743, 751–761

RASMINSKY, M. (1973) The effects of temperature on conduction in demyelinated single nerve fibres. *Archives of Neurology*, **28**, 287–292

RASMINSKY, M. (1978) Ectopic generation of impulses and cross talk in spinal nerve roots in 'dystrophic' mice. *Annals of Neurology*, **3**, 351–357

RASMINSKY, M. and SEARS, T. A. (1972) Internodal conduction in undissected demyelinated nerve fibres. *Journal of Physiology*, **227**, 323–350

RASMINSKY, M., KEARNEY, R. E., AGUAYO, A. J. and BRAY, G. M. (1978) Conduction of nervous impulses in spinal roots and peripheral nerves of dystrophic mice. *Brain Research*, **143**, 71–85

RITCHIE, J. M. and CHIU, S. Y. (1981) Distribution of sodium and potassium channels in mammalian myelinated nerve. In *Demyelinating Diseases. Basic and Clinical Electrophysiology*, edited by S. G. Waxman and J. M. Ritchie, pp. 329–342. New York: Raven Press

ROBINSON, K. and RUDGE, P. (1977) Abnormalities of the auditory evoked potentials in patients with multiple sclerosis. *Brain*, **100**, 19–40

RUSHTON, D. (1975) Use of Pulfrich pendulum for detecting abnormal delay in the visual pathway in multiple sclerosis. *Brain*, **98**, 283–296

SCHAUF, C. L. and DAVIS, F. A. (1981) Circulating toxic factors in multiple sclerosis: a perspective. In *Demyelinating Diseases. Basic and Clinical Electrophysiology*, edited by S. G. Waxman and J. M. Ritchie, pp. 267–280. New York: Raven Press

SCLABASSI, R. J., NAMEROW, N. S. and ENNS, N. F. (1974) Somatosensory response to stimulus trains in patients with multiple sclerosis. *Electroencephalography and Clinical Neurophysiology*, **37**, 23–33

SEIL, F. J. (1977) Tissue culture studies of demyelinating disease: a critical review. *Annals of Neurology*, **2**, 345–385

SEIL, F. J. (1981) Tissue culture studies of neuroelectric blocking factors. In *Demyelinating Diseases. Basic and Clinical Electrophysiology*, edited by S. G. Waxman and J. M. Ritchie, pp. 281–288. New York: Raven Press

SEIL, F. J., LEIMAN, A. L. and KELLY, J. M. (1976) Neuroelectric blocking factors in multiple sclerosis and normal human sera. *Archives of Neurology*, **33**, 418–422

SERGOTT, R. C., BROWN, M. J., SILBERBERG, D. H. and LISAK, R. P. (1984) Antigalactocerebroside serum demyelinates optic nerve *in vivo*. *Journal of the Neurological Sciences*, **64**, 297–303

SHAHROKHI, F., CHIAPPA, K. H. and YOUNG, R. R. (1978) Pattern shift visual evoked responses. *Archives of Neurology*, **35,** 65–71

SMITH, K. J., BLAKEMORE, W. F. and McDONALD, W. I. (1981) The restoration of conduction by central remyelination. *Brain*, **104,** 383–404

SMITH, K. J., BOSTOCK, H. and HALL, S. M. (1982) Saltatory conduction precedes remyelination in axons demyelinated with lysophosphatidylcholine. *Journal of the Neurological Sciences*, **54,** 13–31

SMITH, K. J. and McDONALD, W. I. (1982) Spontaneous and evoked electrical discharges from a central demyelinating lesion. *Journal of the Neurological Sciences*, **55,** 39–47

SOFFER, D. and RAINE, C. S. (1980) Morphologic analysis of axo-glial membrane specialisations in the demyelinated central nervous system. *Brain Research*, **186,** 301–313

TOBLER, I., BORBELY, A. A., SCHWYZER, N. and FONTANA, A. (1985) Interleukin-1 derived from astrocytes enhances slow wave activity in sleep EEG of the rat. *European Journal of Pharmacology*, **104,** 191–192

TRAUGOTT, U., REINHERZ, E. C. and RAINE, C. (1983) Multiple sclerosis: distribution of T-cell subsets within active chronic lesions. *Science*, **219,** 308–310

WAXMAN, S. G. and RITCHIE, J. M. (EDS) (1981) *Demyelinating Diseases. Basic and Clinical Electrophysiology*. New York: Raven Press

WISŃIEWSKI, H., OPPENHEIMER, D. and McDONALD, W. I. (1976) Relation between myelination and function in MS and EAE. *Journal of Neuropathology and Experimental Neurology*, **35,** 327

8
Neuropsychological and psychiatric disturbances in multiple sclerosis

Igor Grant

INTRODUCTION

Neuropsychological and psychiatric disturbances commonly occur in multiple sclerosis (MS). Disturbances in affect, personality, reality testing, and cognitive function have all been reported. Occasionally it has been suggested that emotional upheavals occasioned by severe life stresses may contribute to exacerbation of symptoms and even that they may lead to the first clinical expression of the disease. The object of this chapter is to review the nature and prevalence of neuropsychological and psychiatric disturbances in multiple sclerosis and to consider which are integral parts of the evolving disease process and which constitute adaptations to chronic disease. I shall concentrate on recent research findings and shall touch on the older literature only insofar as it is necessary to achieve an historical perspective. Readers who are interested in a more thorough treatment of the earlier literature will find reviews by Pratt (1951), Surridge (1969), and Trimble and Grant (1982) to be of value.

NEUROPSYCHOLOGICAL AND PSYCHIATRIC PHENOMENA POSSIBLY RELATED TO CEREBRAL LESIONS

Affective disorders

The term affective disorder describes a substantial and relatively persistent disturbance of mood. When that mood shift is in the direction of sadness, pessimism, hopelessness, and accompanied by lack of energy, sleep disturbance, weight loss, and general loss of interest, a person is said to be suffering from a depressive episode. Upward shifts in mood characterized by abnormal optimism, elation, grandiosity, irritability, and excessive energy describe a manic episode. Persons who have bouts of mania and depression are termed bipolar (manic-depressive). Those whose mood is persistently somewhat dysphoric, but rarely sufficiently depressed to qualify for a major depressive episode, are termed dysthymic (American Psychiatric Association, 1980). In reviewing the literature on the association of MS and affective disturbance, readers would do well to keep

134

these modern definitions in mind, since much of the disagreement between studies might have less to do with the effect of MS on mood, than with inconsistent and imprecise terminology.

There is a convergence of evidence that depression is a prevalent neuropsychiatric concomitant of MS. Interestingly, depression has only come to be acknowledged as an important factor in MS relatively recently. For example, Charcot (1877), Moxon (1875, quoted by Pratt, 1951), and Gowers (1893) did not give any emphasis to depression in their clinical descriptions. Indeed, with the possible exception of the study by Braceland and Giffin (1950), virtually all references to depression in MS come from literature of the 1970s and 1980s. Again, this perhaps reflects more the progress that has been made in the classification and identification of the affective disorders in the past two decades, than some secular shift in the presenting features of multiple sclerosis.

As noted above, Braceland and Giffin (1950) appear to have been the first to observe an increased prevalence of depression in a controlled investigation. Of their 75 patients with MS, 20% were depressed. This rate is comparable with that reported 20 years later by Kahana, Leibowitz and Alter (1971). These authors found that 18% of patients with cerebral MS were depressed, and that their rate of suicide (8 out of 295 patients) was 14 times higher than that in the general population of Israel, the country in which this study was conducted.

A small but carefully designed study was conducted by Whitlock and Siskind (1980). These authors compared 30 patients with MS with an equal number of patients who had other neurological diseases which produced similar levels of physical disability. The average age of the subjects was 45, and the typical patient with MS had a duration of illness of 5–9 years. There were 12 men and 18 women. The study design called for clinical interviews which gathered historical information on the possible presence of depression prior to onset of neurological symptoms, the number of episodes since the disease was diagnosed, and current level of depression. The latter was also assessed using a standardized instrument, the Beck Depression Inventory.

The authors found that at the time of interview patients with MS tended to have higher Beck Depression Scores than neurological controls. For example, eight of 30 patients with MS and only one of the controls scored 15 or higher on the Beck Inventory (a score of 15 indicates moderate depression). Furthermore, the authors found that approximately one-half of the patients with MS (as compared with approximately one-sixth of the neurological controls) had suffered from episodes of depression since their diagnosis was made. Equally important was Whitlock and Siskind's observation on the qualitative features of the affective disorder. The depressions of the patients with MS were frequently characterized by the presence of 'endogenous' signs – that is vegetative changes and diurnal variations in mood and energy. Such a symptom complex is currently thought to be more suggestive of a 'psychobiological' rather than 'reactive' depression.

If one assumes depression to be more prevalent among patients with multiple sclerosis than in non-patient controls, then the question of specificity becomes pertinent. Put another way, is depression simply a reaction to chronic disease and disability, or is there something inherent in the disease process which places patients with MS at even greater risk for affective disturbance?

The study by Surridge (1969) compared 108 patients with MS and 39 patients with muscular dystrophy. Although the MS group had a higher prevalence of depression (27% vs 13%), this difference was not statistically significant. Pratt

(1951), who performed one of the other large controlled studies (100 patients with MS compared to 100 patients with other neurological diseases, matched for level of disability), did not specifically comment on the presence of affective disorder in either group.

The results of a large retrospective study of case records was recently reported by Schiffer and Babigian (1984). These authors identified inpatients carrying the diagnosis of multiple sclerosis, temporal lobe epilepsy, and amyotrophic lateral sclerosis who had been inpatients at the Strong Memorial Hospital, Rochester, New York, between 1965 and 1978. These records were then matched to the Monroe County (New York) Psychiatric Register for the period 1960–1978. The authors found that 19.3% of the patients with MS had contact with psychiatric facilities in that period. Comparable rates for patients with temporal lobe epilepsy (TLE) and for amyotrophic lateral sclerosis (ALS) were 22.9 and 4.8% respectively. When the nature of the psychopathology was compared, then patients with MS and TLE had similar rates of all types of disorders except for depression. In this instance, 62% of those patients with MS who had a psychiatric contact were treated for depression, as compared with 42% for TLE. Overall, these results suggest that psychiatric disorder in chronic neurological disease is not simply a product of seriousness or chronicity of illness (since patients with ALS had relatively few psychiatric contacts). The two neurological groups that had the most psychiatric contacts suffered from diseases that impaired cerebral function in addition to being physically disabling. Even here, differences appeared, suggesting that patients with MS were particularly vulnerable to depression.

Several case reports provide further evidence that at least in some instances depression in MS may have a 'neurological' as well as a 'reactive' basis. According to Whitlock and Siskind (1980), Pommé, Girard and Planche (1963) were among the first to observe that some patients developed depression before the onset of their neurological signs, and that such depresion was responsive to drug treatment. Whitlock and Siskind also took note of a report by O'Malley (1966) which described a patient who developed suicidal depression 4 years prior to the onset of MS.

More recently, Young, Saunders and Ponsford (1976) described five cases of patients with various mental disturbances which preceded the development of overt neurological signs. In two instances these psychiatric phenomena included depression. Similarly, Goodstein and Ferrell (1977) presented three case reports of patients experiencing profound depressions several years prior to neurological confirmation of MS. In one instance the patient had been diagnosed as having 'polyneuritis' of 4 weeks duration 20 years previously; in the other two cases, there were no neurological antecedents whatever.

The archival investigation by Schiffer and Babigian (1984), which involved matching of independently obtained neurological and psychiatric clinical records, permitted an assessment of timing of onset of neurological and psychiatric symptoms for 71 patients with multiple sclerosis. For 52 of these (73%) neurological symptoms clearly preceded psychiatric phenomenology; in 12 (17%) the psychiatric symptoms came first; and for seven (10%) the timing could not be established with certainty. For the comparison group of patients with temporal lobe epilepsy, the antecedent rate of psychopathology was even higher – 30% of patients had psychiatric treatment before receiving their neurological diagnosis, whereas 51% had onset of neurological symptoms first. The timing was unclear in 18%. A second neurological comparison group, consisting of patients with ALS, had too few psychiatric contacts to ascertain the timing of psychiatric and neurological symptoms.

In sum, the study by Schiffer and Babigian strongly suggests that approximately one-fifth of patients with MS will experience psychiatric disturbances of sufficient severity to require treatment; further, of those that need treatment perhaps one-sixth will experience the onset of psychopathology *before* definite neurological signs appear. These findings indicate that in a small number of patients (probably less than 5%) psychiatric signs, depression in particular, will constitute the first symptom of the disease process.

Whereas depressive episodes appear to occur with relative frequency in the course of multiple sclerosis, frank manic episodes and bipolar disorder seem to be uncommon. It is important here to distinguish between mania, an affective disorder characterized by a prominent and relatively persistent elevated, expansive, or irritable mood coupled with symptoms such as increase in activity, talkativeness, racing thoughts, inappropriately inflated self esteem, reduced need for sleep, and excessive involvement in grandiose activities, from the terms 'euphoria' and 'lability of affect' that have sometimes been associated with MS. Mania, as the term is used in this chapter, describes a distinct psychiatric disorder which is usually part of bipolar affective illness. Mania can also occasionally occur as a secondary phenomenon complicating drug intoxications, or various disease states. Thus, the term mania describes a phenomenon that goes considerably beyond inappropriate cheerfulness or denial of illness, which is what the term 'euphoria' is usually meant to convey.

Frank manias appear to be rare in multiple sclerosis. Mapelli and Ramelli (1981) presented a patient in whom mania occurred in association with MS. These authors suggested that this patient suffered from 'secondary mania' since there was no evidence of a bipolar affective disorder. Kellner *et al.* (1984) presented two cases of rapidly cycling bipolar disorder in patients who were diagnosed as having MS. The authors suggested that MS be considered in the differential diagnosis of patients who had affective disorders and associated with minor and apparently non-specific neurological complaints.

Euphoria, eutonia, and lability of affect

As indicated above, the term euphoria is used here to describe an inappropriate cheerfulness, out of keeping with the patient's physical and social circumstances. Eutonia connotes an inappropriate sense of physical well-being, while lability of affect describes sudden, dramatic, and inexplicable shifts in mood, for example, sudden bursts of laughter or tearfulness the origin of which the patient has difficulty in explaining.

A sense of inappropriate well-being has been commented upon virtually from the time MS became delineated as a clinical entity. Charcot (1877), Moxon (1875), and Gowers (1893) all remarked on it. Cottrell and Wilson (1926) found euphoria, eutonia, and affective lability in the majority of their patients, and suggested that these three symptoms constituted a diagnostic triad for multiple sclerosis.

More recent observations have tended to reduce the salience of these mood alterations in MS. For example, Pratt's (1951) controlled investigation showed that seven of his 100 patients with MS experienced an elevation of mood since onset (vs none of the neurological controls), that six of 100 patients with MS exhibited a tendency to laugh easily (vs one of the controls) and that 29 patients with MS reported a tendency to cry easily (vs 17 controls). Only the first two comparisons reached statistical significance. Pratt noted that the tendency to laugh inapprop-riately was found more in patients rated clinically as having a greater degree of organic mental impairment. Braceland and Giffin (1950) also found euphoria in a minority (10%) of their patients. Surridge (1969) found a somewhat higher rate of euphoria (18.5%). Surridge also found that 31% of patients with MS had impaired awareness of the extent of their physical disability and 11% exhibited complete anosognosia. Exaggeration of emotional expression was found in 10% of cases, and this finding seemed most evident in patients with intellectual deterioration.

Schiffer, Rudick and Herndon (1983) estimated that approximately 30% of their patients experienced short, sudden shifts in affective expression which are not consonant with underlying feelings. They noted that such 'emotional incontinence' can be very disturbing to the patients as well as to their families. These authors commented that frank euphoria was an uncommon syndrome in their population (although they did not provide statistics) and that it was their impression that this symptom coexists with diffuse cerebral involvement.

My own experience, based on interviews with patients in connection with a neuropsychological study (Grant *et al.*, 1984), suggests that euphoria, eutonia, and lability of affect are uncommon in early and middle phases of this disease. For example, only one of 43 patients was frankly euphoric, and only two exhibited some degree of lability. Several patients, on careful interviewing, did admit to a sense of 'disconnection' between their inner experience of affect and their outward expression of it. This was observed most commonly during inquiries about depression. These patients commented that they felt sad or depressed, but their facies and body language did not express this. Whether this disconnection represents the presence of lesions in the brainstem, producing a pseudobulbar picture, or interruption of connections between the limbic lobe and cerebral cortex, is unclear at this time.

Psychosis

Psychotic symptoms (thought disorder, hallucinations, bizzare behaviour) are not prominent in multiple sclerosis. None of Pratt's 100 patients was psychotic, and his review of 544 other patients seen or traced in the years 1948–1950 uncovered only one patient who developed definite psychosis. This incidence of psychosis in MS was slightly less than that expected in the general population of the UK during a comparable period of time (Pratt, 1951). Surridge (1969) reported that only one of 108 patients with MS exhibited a non-affective functional psychosis. In Schiffer and Babigian's (1984) record study, 24% of patients with MS who had contact with a psychiatric facility were diagnosed as having a 'major psychotic episode'. Since approximately 19% of all patients with MS studied had a psychiatric diagnosis assigned to them during the period in question (1960–1978), it can be estimated that approximately 5% of patients with MS followed for an extended period of time will develop psychotic symptoms.

Although it is arguable whether the incidence of psychosis in MS is significantly higher than that in the general population, several case reports suggest that psychotic features can wax and wane with the course of the demyelinating disorder

(Schmalzbach, 1954; Parker, 1956; Geocaris, 1957; Drake, 1984). Furthermore, several case studies suggest that psychosis can be the initial presenting feature in MS (Parker, 1956; Geocaris, 1957; Hollender and Steckler, 1972; Matthews, 1979).

Hysteria

Hysterical symptoms are still thought to be associated with multiple sclerosis. For example, a recent edition of *Brain's Diseases of the Nervous System* states, 'It is not rare…for a patient to develop hysterical symptoms in addition to those of MS and an hysterical overlay present in the early stages when physical signs are minimal often causes difficulty in initial diagnosis' (Walton, 1977). Although many neurologists go along with this statement, hard data demonstrating such an association simply do not exist. Much of the difficulty arises from the imprecise usage of 'hysteria'. The term has come to embrace conversion phenomena, dissociations, a personality style, and a multi-system symptom complex (Briquet's syndrome). Sometimes patients who exaggerate their symptoms, or are overly dramatic about them are called hysterical. In many instances the designation of hysteria says more about how physicians feel about their patients than what they can scientifically infer from objective evidence.

The fact that the early symptoms of MS can have strong subjective elements with few objective findings except on very careful examination, that the symptoms can come and go, and that the disease has a penchant for afflicting young women, appears to have increased the likelihood that hysterical phenomena and neurological symptoms become confused. Almost a century ago, Thomas Buzzard delivered 'a clinical lecture on insular sclerosis and hysteria' at the National Hospital, London. The observations he made then have currency today:

> 'I take it that we have all of us at various times given the name hysteria to an early stage of insular sclerosis. One reason for the common fallacy in diagnosis appears to be that we have somehow failed to remember that insular sclerosis does not spring suddenly into existence in a typical form. Like most other chronic or sub-acute ailments, it has to go through a budding period, during which the aspect presented differs much from that of the fullblown disease. Several years ago I expressed the opinion that 'many symptoms which have come to be considered characteristic of hysteria will, if examined by the light of improved knowledge and experience, be relegated to disseminated sclerosis.' In the case just shown you there are illustrations of this. The sudden loss of power in a limb, occurring after mental shock in an otherwise healthy girl and passing off completely in a month, is a symptom which is practically certain to be set down to hysteria. And so with the dimness of vision in one eye of temporary character, recovering without treatment; and, again, the dragging of a leg, which felt "numbed like a log of wood".' (Buzzard, 1897).

Wilson (1940) agreed with Buzzard that the apparent association of hysterical phenomena with MS represented a misinterpretation of the meaning of early symptoms. He believed that genuinely hysterical phenomena were rare in MS, and that instances of their coexistence were coincidental. Pratt (1951) found only two cases of hysterical symptomatology in his 100 patients, a rate that was no different than that found in his comparison group of neurological patients with other disorders.

A contrasting theme was struck by Langworthy (1950). Based on clinical psychiatric evaluations and, in some cases, years of psychotherapy with patients, Langworthy and associates concluded not only that hysterical symptoms were prevalent in MS but also that conversion hysterics and patients with MS might have similar psychodynamic makeups. It was suggested, for example, that many MS patients were 'rather passive individuals caught in entangling emotional relationships with the mother'. Furthermore, patients with MS were said to 'have shown a tendency to conversion of anxiety over sexual problems' (Langworthy, 1950). This close interweaving of the psychodynamic and neurological was further articulated by Grinker, Ham and Robbins (1950) who believed that the majority of patients with MS had psychoneurotic difficulties anteceding (and predisposing to) neurological onset. More recently, Aring (1965) gave renewed expression to this unitary view by suggesting the existence of a 'multiple sclerosis–conversion hysteria complex'. This notion is clearly a rejection of the separationist views of Buzzard and Wilson; it emphasizes that symptoms of conversion and multiple sclerosis frequently coexist and are, for all practical purposes, often indistinguishable. Further, since most of the treatment the physicians have to offer consists of understanding, support, and exhortation, such psychotherapy is best administered by someone well versed with the patient's unique psychodynamics.

Caplan and Nadelson (1980) have attempted to strike a middle ground between the 'splitters' and 'lumpers'. They note that hysterical symptoms can coexist with a wide variety of physical illnesses. Further, they suggest that, beyond its negative aspects, illness can provide, for some patients, a sense of purpose, self-worth, and means of exerting control over others. For patients who have such needs, it seems possible that their close personal familiarity with the phenomenology of MS might facilitate augmentation of existing complaints, or even generation of psychogenic symptoms that mimic those of MS. Left unanswered by Caplan and Nadelson's analysis is the thorny question of whether there is some *unique* link between conversion phenomena and multiple sclerosis. As an example, some patients with epilepsy are known at times to have 'hysterical fits'. Further, there is an increased prevalence of conversion phenomena in patients who are depressed (Chodoff, 1974), and depression, as we have seen, is common in MS.

In summary, there is no definitive evidence on the question of increased prevalence of conversion phenomena in patients with multiple sclerosis. To the extent that such an association might exist, it probably reflects the operation of two processes. The first has to do with mislabelling of prodromal and early neurological symptoms as hysteria; the second involves unconsciously motivated augmentation or exacerbation of previous neurological symptoms by patients who have a need to use bodily symptoms to communicate their wishes, fears, and conflict to others. This second process, the true conversion, is probably more prevalent in patients with MS than in the general population. It is not known if it is any more frequent in MS than in other chronic diseases, or in other patients with depression.

NEUROPSYCHOLOGICAL AND PSYCHIATRIC PHENOMENA AS POSSIBLE REACTIONS TO CHRONIC NEUROLOGICAL DISEASE

Hysterical symptoms, which I suggest can represent both aggravations of neurological complaints and symbols of inner conflict constitute for discussion purposes a convenient transition between neuropsychiatric phenomena, which are probably caused by the demyelinating process *per se* (i.e. endogenous depression, euphoria and lability of affect, reactive mania, acute psychosis), and those behavioural symptoms which can better be regarded as adaptive responses to a major illness.

Some of the stages of psychological response to multiple sclerosis have been articulated most eloquently by professionals who were themselves victims. According to Burnfield (1984), a psychiatrist who developed MS as a medical student, patients generally go through several stages of adjustment.

The first stage is one of shock, disbelief, and fright when the diagnosis is first revealed or suspected. Some physicians are not candid with their patients either because they are unsure of their diagnosis or feel they need to 'protect' the patient. Such lack of candour can lead to greater uncertainty and fear on the part of the patient. The patient might undertake his own library research and glean from this, inappropriately, that he is doomed to paralysis, incontinence, and dementia.

After the first emotional shock has passed, a period of denial may ensue. Kinley (1980), a nurse who developed MS, reported that her denial was characterized by insistence on continuing work and home activities at the same pace despite weakness and fatigue. Burnfield comments that some patients both deny and are embarrassed by their symptoms, and may go to great lengths to conceal them.

Burnfield suggests that depression is a common next phase of adaptation, especially during periods of exacerbation. At this stage patients may be grieving over their loss of health and productivity. Kinley observes that additional responses can include regression – feeling totally overwhelmed and becoming excessively dependent on others – and marked irritability. Sometimes the irritability is related to treatment with ACTH. ACTH appears capable of provoking such irritability both directly and by interfering with sleep.

A later stage, achieved by a large majority of patients, is that of acceptance, or at least some relative adjustment to the multiple sclerosis. Such acceptance is particularly true of patients who experience relatively long periods of quiescence. According to Kinley (1980), acceptance in many patients is facilitated by involvement in self-help groups and religious activities.

There have been several eforts to paint a more objective picture of adaptive changes in MS. Dalos *et al.* (1983) employed the General Health Questionnaire (GHQ) to detect changes in emotional state. This is a self-administered instrument which has been widely used to detect emotional disturbance in various groups. Sixty-four patients with multiple sclerosis and 23 with spinal cord injuries completed the GHQ on a minimum of two occasions (the exact number of repititions is not specified, but questionnaire responses were averaged). The authors compared responses from patients with MS who completed questionnaires during exacerbation, patients who completed questionnaires during remission, and the spinal cord injury patients. Disease exacerbation was strongly associated with a rise in emotional distress as measured by the GHQ. The patients with MS who were in remissions had scores indicating slightly more disturbance than patients with spinal cord injury, and 39% of the former group were thought to have abnormal scores (usually in the mild range) as compared with approximately 15% of the spinal cord injury patients. The authors did not report a significant association between emotional disturbance and age, sex, duration or severity of disease, or degree of disability (Kurtzke score). The authors concluded that severe emotional disturbances were uncommon in patients with MS in remission, but were very prevalent (estimated at 90%) among those experiencing an exacerbation.

Maybury and Brewin (1984) also used the GHQ in a study of 36 patients with MS. Since there was no comparison group, we cannot discern what the absolute rate of emotional disturbance was; nevertheless the authors did attempt to relate GHQ to a number of predictors. Like Dalos *et al.* they were unable to find a relationship between level of physical disability (Kurtzke), length of time since diagnosis, or demographic factors and GHQ-measured emotional disturbance. These authors did not partition their sample into exacerbation/remission.

Several studies have focused on more specific aspects of coping in relation to the progress of MS. Brooks and Matson (1982) administered a self-concept measure to 103 patients with MS 7 years apart. These were largely middle-aged women (68% female; average age, 52) whose duration of illness since diagnosis was approximately 17 years, and of whom 56% were ambulatory, 34% chairbound and 10% bedfast. The authors found no overall change in self-concept and also very little change in physical disability. However, among those who had a large number of episodes of exacerbation, there tended to be a reduction in self-concept. Zeldow and Pavlou (1984) attempted to predict several dimensions of psychosocial adjustment from a combination of demographic variables, length of time since disease was diagnosed, and physical disability status. They found that a composite score thought to reflect social poise, self assurance, and interpersonal adequacy was adversely influenced by declining physical status. Furthermore, persons who were more physically disabled reported an increased emotional reliance on other people. In contrast, Maybury and Brewin (1984) did not find a significant association between a measure of self-esteem and the Kurtzke disability score. They did find an association between number of contacts patients reported with able-bodied persons and self-esteem. Although the authors introduced some statistical adjustments into their analyses, it is not clear whether disability status was partly influencing self-esteem, since those who had more 'able-bodied contact' were also younger, working, and had lower Kurtzke scores.

It was noted in the previous section that patients with MS appear to have an increased prevalence of depression when they are compared with other disabled groups. Furthermore, at least some patients with MS who are depressed exhibit 'endogenous' signs suggestive of a psychobiological affective disorder. Even if this is true, it is theoretically possible that an additional source of depression in MS (beyond that being produced directly by brain disease) lies in other characteristics of the disease (e.g. level of disability), or other characteristics in the environment (e.g. presence or absence of social supports). McIvor, Riklan and Reznikoff (1984) endeavoured to tease these influences apart by examining a group of 120 non-hospitalized patients with spinal multiple sclerosis. Using the Beck Depression Inventory as a measure of depression, these authors attempted to predict Beck scores from a combination of age, length and course of illness, Kurtzke disability status score, and perceived social support. Using multiple regression to model their data they found that older, more disabled persons with unremitting illness and who had a low level of perceived social support were more depressed. Although one cannot be sure that these patients did not, in fact, have cerebral lesions as well (no CT or nuclear magnetic resonance imaging (NMRI) results are given), this study gives preliminary support to the view that at least some of the depression in MS has to do with a combination of degree of disability and negative aspects of the social environment. In a similar vein, Baretz and Stephenson (1981) noted a tendency for increased depression in bedridden patients with MS. Parenthetically, approximately three-quarters of Baretz and Stephenson's 40 patients had some degree of depression; of these, 33% were thought to be 'overtly' depressed, and 48% to have 'concealed' depression.

In summary, beyond those neuropsychiatric changes which it is suggested might be direct products of the disease process, patients with multiple sclerosis experience more general disturbances in psychological adaptation in relation to progression of their disease. More specifically, exacerbations of illness are accompanied by major emotional disturbances of various kinds, especially depression; and negative changes in self-esteem, self-concept, mood, and personal effectiveness are related to increased physical disability.

COGNITIVE DECLINE IN MULTIPLE SCLEROSIS

Observers from Charcot onwards have agreed that intellectual decline occurs in at least some patients with MS. With the introduction of standardized neuropsychological tests in the middle of the 20th century it became practicable to begin delineating the prevalence and qualitative features of neuropsychological deficit in this disorder. Several years ago the neuropsychological research findings in MS up to 1980 were reviewed (Trimble and Grant, 1982). At about the same time Marsh (1980) reviewed the use of the Wechsler Adult Intelligence Scale (WAIS) in MS. Since readers interested in this earlier work can easily consult one of these two reviews, I shall limit my present remarks to a brief overview of earlier findings while emphasizing newer research emerging since 1980.

Estimates of the prevalence of cognitive disturbance in MS have varied widely. Brown and Davis (1922) and Cottrell and Wilson (1926) reported few cases of intellectual deterioration. Ombredane (1929) and Surridge (1969) both estimated that about two-thirds of their patients were impaired, whereas Pratt (1951) reported a range of 15–28%. Schiffer, Rudick and Herndon (1983) stated that about one-half of their clinic patients showed cognitive impairment on 'careful testing', but they did not specify their method of ascertainment. This rate is comparable to the 55% impairment reported by Bertrando and Maffei (1983); and to the figure of 51% scoring in the impaired range on the Category test, a sensitive measure of abstracting ability, reported by Peyser *et al.* (1980). These disparities doubtless reflect differences in patient population (ranging from deteriorated institutionalized patients to others who remained ambulatory despite a number of years of disease), and also variability in methods of assessing neuropsychological decline. For example, Peyser *et al.* (1980) found that of patients judged clinically by neurologists to have intact mentation, 49% were impaired on the Category test.

In 1955 Ross and Reitan performed the first comprehensive neuropsychological study of a small number of patients with MS. They found that patients with MS had severe difficulties in tasks stressing motor speed, strength, and coordination; had preserved verbal abilities; and exhibited intermediate difficulties in abstracting and concept formation (Ross and Reitan, 1955). Much of the work in the 25 years that followed served in various ways to confirm these observations (Trimble and Grant, 1982). In addition, Jambor (1969), Beatty and Gange (1977) and Staples and Lincoln (1979) showed that patients with fairly long established multiple sclerosis exhibited difficulties in learning and recall of verbal and non-verbal material.

One direction of recent neuropsychological research has been to characterize the memory difficulties of patients with MS with greater precision. For example, a recent study explored aspects of learning and short- and long-term memory for verbal and spatial material in a group of 43 patients who were generally in the early or middle phases of their disease (Grant *et al.*, 1984). There were 27 women and 16 men in the sample, their typical age was late 30s, and the average patient had experienced 4 years of active disease at the time of examination (years of active disease was defined as the number of years in which a patient had a minimum of 7 days of significant symptomatology). In this sample 31 patients had clinically definite MS, 11 had probable MS and one carried the diagnosis of early progressive MS.

Short-term memory was assessed through presentation of consonant trigrams using the Brown-Peterson technique. In brief, patients were required to look at cards inprinted with three consonants. After 2 s of exposure, the cards were removed and the patient was expected to say what was on the card. For some card presentations, patients had to give an immediate recall. For other presentations they were allowed a 2 or 4 s 'consolidation'. For still other presentations a 'distractor' technique was introduced. The distractor consisted of having patients perform subtractions out loud for a period of 3–18 s before being required to recollect the consonant trigram. Thus, it was possible to measure the efficiency of short-term memory with and without a delay period, and also in the face of having to perform tasks designed to disrupt memory consolidation. It was found that patients and controls both performed very well in the 'easy' condition – that is the requirement simply to recall a trigram without any interference. Also, it was immaterial whether or not a 2 or 4 s delay before recall was introduced. Patients did experience progressively greater difficulty when compared to controls in remembering in the face of interference. The longer they were required to perform subtractions, the more divergent their performance became from that of controls. This portion of the experiment suggested that patients who were in a relatively early stage of their multiple sclerosis could encode verbal material reasonably well so long as competing information was excluded. In the face of interference, however, patients became markedly inefficient. Furthermore, although controls were able to cope better with interference if they were provided with a 2 to 4 s 'consolidation' period, patients with MS did not realize such a benefit.

Another test of verbal memory consisted of a short story from the Wechsler Memory Scale. Subjects were read a prose passage, consisting of approximately 22 bits of information, asked to repeat the story directly, and again after a 45-minute delay. If a subject did not reach a criterion score (a minimum of 15 bits of information) then the story was repeated until this criterion level was reached, or until at least five trials were administered. This method allowed assessment of immediate verbal recall, verbal learning, and delayed verbal recall.

We found that patients with MS learned fewer bits of information in the first instance, required more trials to reach the criterion score and, despite greater exposure to the material, still forgot more than did controls.

A similar paradigm was used for non-verbal learning and recall. Figures from the Wechsler Memory Scale were presented initially, an immediate reproduction was required, and a 45 min delayed reproduction was also scored. A trials to criterion approach was again used. The results for spatial learning were similar to those for verbal learning: patients remembered less in the first place, needed more trials to reach criterion, and forgot more at 45 min. In general, their spatial learning was somewhat less impaired than their verbal learning, at least based on these techniques.

The second part of the study was to determine whether certain characteristics of the patients were especially predictive of impairment. In particular were considered the possible joint effects of age, years of active disease, education level, and whether the patient was in exacerbation or remission. Using a multiple regression technique it was found that performance on the Brown-Peterson test was significantly related to age, years of active disease, and acute-quiescent status. In a separate analysis it was not possible to show an effect for current medications (i.e. ACTH or prednisone), but this may be because prescription of such drugs was heavily correlated with being assigned to the 'acute' condition.

In summary, the study showed that even patients who are in relatively early phases of their disease can manifest substantial difficulties in learning and remembering of both verbal and non-verbal material. It appears that older patients who have had more years of active disease will have more severe memory impairment; at the same time, patients tested during a period of exacerbation will perform less well than those who are in remission.

Another interesting study was reported recently by Rao *et al.* (1984). These investigators examined 44 patients with chronic progressive MS, and compared their performance on tests of verbal and spatial recall to that of 23 patients with pain syndromes and 15 hospital worker controls. The patients with MS consisted of 29 women and 15 men who were typically in their early 40s, who experienced their first symptom about 10 years prior to examination, and whose diagnosis was established roughly 7 years previously. The average Kurtzke disability score was 6.6 with a range from 4 to 9. Forty-five per cent of patients were described as taking 'psychoactive medications', but the type of drugs used was not specified. A comparable proportion of the pain-patient controls was also taking psychoactive medications.

The verbal free recall test required that subjects memorize a list of words through a series of five presentations, thereby defining a learning curve. After being exposed to a list of distractor words, subjects were then expected to perform a free recall of the original word list, as well as to identify these words intermixed with other unfamiliar ones. Finally, a 30 min delayed free recall of the word list was demanded. A spatial memory test was also given using a similar paradigm. Patients with MS and control pain patients (but not the healthy controls) were also administered the standard Wechsler Memory Scale and a cognitive screening examination which consisted mostly of tests of sensori-motor functioning.

As in the study by Grant *et al.* (1984), Rao and associates found that patients with MS had difficulty in learning and recalling prose passages. They were also less efficient than normal controls in learning the word list and recalling it after a delay. Interestingly, however, there were fewer statistically significant differences on the free verbal recall test when patients with MS and patients with pain were compared. It may be that the latter patients were performing suboptimally because many of them were receiving psychotropic medications. On spatial recall patients with MS performed significantly worse than either pain controls or the non-patients. In sum, the results of the study by Rao *et al.* suggest that patients with MS experienced particular difficulty in recalling verbal information in the face of interference, but that simple acquisition of verbal information, although also compromised to some degree, was less severely impaired than free recall or recognition recall.

These findings are congruent with those reported by Grant *et al.* (1984). Rao *et al.* did find, however, that patients with MS had more difficulty with spatial learning when compared to another patient group. This finding is consistent with the earlier report by Staples and Lincoln (1979) who showed that patients with MS were impaired in immediate recall of Wechsler figures, but not of stories. On the other hand, the patients investigated by Grant *et al.* (1984) suggested substantial deficiencies in both verbal and non-verbal memory, whereas a recent study by Carroll, Gates and Roldan (1984) showed patients with MS to be inferior on a verbal recognition test but not on perceptual memory or picture recognition.

The study by Carroll *et al.* (1984) probed more deeply into the nature of verbal memory deficiency in MS. These investigators found that patients had difficulty identifying words which were seen before as 'familiar', but did not differ in identifying words which were 'unfamiliar'. Carroll *et al.* (1984) have suggested that the defect here was one of 'relational processing', i.e. that patients had difficulty forming semantic categories to help them recognize familiar and related words; further, even when such categories were formed, these were not as helpful as they were among controls – indeed, they sometimes resulted in inter-item semantic encoding confusion.

Beyond exploring the details of memory deficit in multiple sclerosis, another direction of neuropsychological research has involved an attempt to create useful subgroups of patients by utilizing a combination of medical, psychological and functional descriptors. The work of Peyser, Edwards and Poser (1980) exemplifies this approach. Using the technique of cluster analysis, these investigators attempted to develop groupings of patients based on a combination of the following descriptors: sex, age, length of disease, age at diagnosis, Purdue Pegboard Score (a measure of manipulative dexterity), Kurtzke Disability Scale Score, Category Test Score (a neuropsychological test sensitive to defects in abstracting ability), and scores from the Minnesota Multiphasic Personality Inventory (MMPI – a standardized self report instrument which is sensitive both to current psychological reaction or 'state', and more enduring personality characteristics or 'trait').

Peyser, Edwards and Poser (1980) identified six clusters of patients with differing psychoneurological and demographic characteristics. Cluster 1 consisted of patients who had had the disease for a long time (18 years), were moderately disabled (Kurtzke score, approximately 6), were fairly impaired cognitively, and whose MMPI indicated very substantial psychiatric disturbance which included bizzare ideation. Cluster 2 were mostly young women with a brief duration of illness (5 years), little disability (Kurtzke approximately 1.5), intact neuropsychological functioning, and essentially normal MMPI (with the exception of a tendency to deny illness). Cluster 3 were largely older women (average age, 49) with an intermediate duration of illness (11 years), moderate disability (Kurtzke approximately 4), intact neuropsychological functioning, and an MMPI profile suggestive of worry, depression and somatic concerns. Cluster 4 were mostly women who were in their early 40s, had an intermediate duration of illness (12 years), who were mildly disabled (Kurtzke approximately 2), but who had serious neuropsychological deficits. These patients had essentially normal MMPI profiles, suggesting the possibility that these patients' cognitive impairment might be causing them inappropriately to report few concerns of a psychological nature. Cluster 5 had only three patients averaging 39 years old. This group was interesting in that, despite only mild disability (average Kurtzke 1.7) and normal neuropsychological functioning these patients had elevations in the first three scales of the MMPI, with a scale configuration that has sometimes been called the 'Conversion V' – i.e. patients who report many somatic complaints, have a tendency to express psychological difficulty in physical terms, to repress their conflicts, and not to report sadness or depression that would be consistent with their other complaints. These few patients might be candidates for the 'multiple sclerosis–conversion hysteria' proposed by Aring (1965) and discussed in an earlier section of this chapter. Cluster 6 consisted of younger (average age, 31) mildly to moderately disabled (Kurtzke 2.6) men who had a relatively brief length of illness (4 years), who were cognitively intact, but who reported a major degree of psychological distress on the MMPI. Presumably, these were patients who had relatively rapid progress of illness with an acute psychological reaction as a concomitant.

Rao *et al.* (1984) employed a somewhat different approach to patient classification. Their cluster analysis was based on the results of selected memory tests, adjusted for demographic variables. Rao *et al.* identified three clusters of patients who differed markedly in memory functioning but had roughly comparable Kurtzke disability scores (approximately 6.5). Cluster 1 had normal memory performance, cluster 2 slightly impaired, and cluster 3 were the most impaired. Patients identified by differences in memory were then compared in terms of their demographic characteristics, length of disease, medication status, performance on certain perceptual motor tests, and MMPI profile. There were no striking differences between the clusters in terms of age, education, reported length of illness, age of symptom onset, or age of diagnosis, except that cluster 3 patients (those with the greatest memory impairment) were about 4 years older than patients with no memory impairment. Results from additional tests suggested that cluster 3 patients had a broad array of neuropsychological deficits beyond their memory problems. MMPI analyses showed that both cluster 1 and cluster 2 patients expressed somatic concerns beyond those of cluster 3, but that cluster 2 (mild memory impairment) patients also reported more depression. Cluster 3 patients had slight elevations in the so-called 'psychotic' scales, suggesting more severe psychological disturbance. Many patients in cluster 2 were taking psychoactive medications at the time of testing, and this differentiated them from the other two clusters. In summary, results from the study by Rao *et al.* (1984) seems to suggest that patients with the greatest degrees of memory impairment are also those who show the most deviant psychological profiles as measured by the MMPI, and also have more global neuropsychological deterioration. At the same time, there appears to be a subgroup of patients whose mild memory disturbance might be related at least in part to experiencing moderate depression and being medicated with psychoactive drugs.

These studies by Peyser, Edwards and Poser (1980a) and Rao *et al.* (1984) must be regarded as provocative but preliminary. Sample sizes were small, and the stability of these 'clusters' is in some doubt. Nevertheless, this work does suggest one avenue of research, whereby data from several domains – neurological, psychological, cognitive, social functioning – might be combined into meaningful groupings which might help clinicians in planning treatment.

An important missing link in the neuropsychological study of MS has been the absence of neuroradiological and the neuroanatomical correlates to observed cognitive disturbances. We do not have systematic data on distribution of plaques of demyelination in relation to pattern of neuropsychological decline. Furthermore, until recently neuroradiological techniques lacked sensitivity and resolution power with respect to localizing small plaques. NMRI shows promise as a sensitive technique for mapping lesions. Although there are scattered preliminary reports of improvement in function paralleling change in NMRI such findings must be considered speculative at this time. Nevertheless, it seems certain that NMRI will open new and important possibilities for future studies of brain behaviour relationships in multiple sclerosis.

LIFE STRESS AND SYMPTOMS IN MULTIPLE SCLEROSIS

Since the first documented description of the onset of symptoms of multiple sclerosis in Augustus d'Este (1782–1846) was associated with attending the funeral of a father figure (Warren, Greenhill and Warren, 1982), clinicians and patients alike have speculated that adverse life events could influence both the onset and exacerbation of symptoms. The middle of the 20th century brought forth a group of studies with contradictory conclusions. Several groups of investigators believed that major changes in life circumstances, traumatic experiences, and difficult interpersonal situations were all contributory to the onset and exacerbation (Langworthy, 1948; Brickner and Simons, 1950; Grinker, Ham and Robbins, 1950; Philippopoulos, Wittkower and Cousineau, 1958; Groen, Prick and Bastiaans, 1967; Mei-Tal, Meyerowitz and Engel, 1970). Ranged against these positive studies were the negative findings of Braceland and Giffin (1950) and Alter, Antonovsky and Leibowitz (1968). A careful inquiry by Pratt (1951) revealed some increase in stressful events preceding symptomatology in patients with MS compared with a group of other neurological patients, but the difference between the groups did not reach statistical significance.

Recently, our group completed a detailed set of interviews with 40 patients with MS using the life events methodology developed by Brown and Harris (1978). Approximately 70% of patients with MS reported experiencing a markedly threatening life event or severe difficulty in the year prior to the onset of major symptoms. This rate significantly exceeded the number of sociodemographically matched controls who reported similar events, and is substantially higher than the rate of approximately 20% of markedly threatening events that Brown and Harris have noted in their community surveys. Our rate of patients with MS experiencing threatening events is consistent with recent findings by Warren, Greenhill and Warren (1982) who found that 79% of their patients with MS reported substantial increases in stress.

The issue of life stress in MS has been reviewed in detail elsewhere (Grant, 1985; Grant *et al.*, 1986). It can be concluded that the link between adversities and symptom onset or exacerbation has yet to be demonstrated unequivocally. Clearly, stresses aggravate symptoms in a number of patients; however, the precise nature of the stress, the exact characteristics of the host, and the regularity with which stress–symptom relationship obtains, remain poorly understood.

CONCLUDING REMARKS

This review has considered the current state of our knowledge regarding the neuropsychological and psychiatric phenomena in MS. It has been noted that depression is prevalent in MS, and might have two aetiologies. There is evidence that patients with MS, in common with others who have chronic debilitating illness, are subject to periods of dysphoria. Such episodes of dysphoria occur more often in patients who have greater disability or more frequent exacerbations. At the same time, the research suggests that patients with MS may have a greater tendency to develop affective disorders than do other chronically medically ill persons. For example, the rate of depression in MS exceeds that found in other neurological groups. Such observations lead to the possibility that an affective disorder can be provoked directly by the disease process. Future research involving NMRI should help clarify whether persons with plaques in limbic structures are more likely to have affective disorder than patients with lesions distributed elsewhere.

Whatever the cause of increased depression in MS, recent evidence suggests that such depressions are treatable. Schiffer, Rudick and Herndon (1983) recommend a combination of antidepressant drugs and supportive therapy. In terms of the former, they recommend the use of tricyclic antidepressants, particularly where there might be a side benefit from their anticholinergic effects. Supportive therapy is administered through a combination of practically oriented individual counselling and group treatment.

Recently, Larcombe and Wilson (1984) published a provocative study, the results of which suggest that cognitive-behaviour therapy might be effective in the treatment of the depression associated with MS. Cognitive-behavioural therapy is modelled after the work of A.T. Beck (Beck *et al.*, 1979) who has shown that depressed psychiatric patients respond to an active-structured form of psychother-apy that focuses on a negative view of self, others, and the future. Pessimistic and defeatist ideas are identified, challenged and the patient is helped to replace these with others that might be more useful. These cognitive aspects of treatment are coupled with behavioural assignments designed to have patients structure their lives in such a way that there is a better likelihood for getting 'rewards' out of the environment. The pilot study by Larcombe and Wilson (1984) indicated that 6 weeks of cognitive-behavioural treatment can lead to substantial decrease in depression, when compared with patients not receiving such treatment.

Fatigue, general demoralization, and decline in self-image are other common correlates of the progression of MS. Once again, empathetic but reality-based interventions, either by the physician or by lay support groups, can be most effective.

Neuropsychological decline occurs variably in MS although most patients will experience some cognitive dysfunction as the disease progresses into its later stages. Deficiency in learning and recall appear to be commonplace, and sometimes are in evidence even in patients who have been ill for only a relatively short period of time. Disturbances in abstracting ability occur somewhat later, and are often sufficiently subtle that only sensitive neuropsychological tests will uncover them. Deficiencies in sensori-motor performance are, of course, commonplace and these may be coupled with perceptual difficulties, as well. Although dysarthria is common, aphasia is not.

There is now good evidence that the so-called euphoria of MS is not a characteristic sign but rather a correlate of more advanced brain disease. Although the more severe forms of lability, euphoria, and eutonia tend to be late stage phenomena, there is evidence that at least some patients in the middle phases of their illness experience a 'disconnection' between inner experience of emotion and outward expression of affect.

Neuropsychological and psychiatric phenomena appear to be related in part to exacerbations and remissions. In periods of exacerbation, depression, neuro-psychological deficits and, on occasion, psychosis can be evident. It is also known that some of the treatments of MS are in themselves capable of producing psychiatric disturbance. For example, ACTH can produce irritability, hostility, paranoia, and mania in some patients. Occasionally, patients respond to this drug with depression. Prednisone and other steroid drugs can have similar effects.

The years immediately ahead promise to accelerate our understanding of the aetiology and pathogenesis of neuropsychological and psychiatric change in multiple sclerosis. Advanced imaging techniques should help to establish how the distribution, number, and evolution of plaques are related to these phenomena. At the same time, research which employs improved methodology for studying life events, coping styles, and social supports, and combines these with newer measures of neuroimmunological functioning should provide better answers to the possible link between stress and exacerbation of multiple sclerosis.

Acknowledgements

This work was supported, in part, by a Veterans Administration Medical Research Service award (MRIS 3240) to Igor Grant. I would like to express special thanks to Ms Joanne McCoy for assisting in the preparation of this manuscript.

References

ALTER, M., ANTONOVSKY, A. and LEIBOWITZ, V. (1968) Epidemiology of multiple sclerosis in Israel. In *The Epidemiology of Multiple Sclerosis*, edited by M. Alter and J. Kurtzke, pp. 83–109. Springfield: Thomas

AMERICAN PSYCHIATRIC ASSOCIATION (1980) *DSM III: Diagnostic and Statistical Manual of Mental Disorders*. Washington, DC: APA Press

ARING, C. D. (1965) Observations on multiple sclerosis and conversion hysteria. *Brain*, **88**, 663–674

BARETZ, R. M. and STEPHENSON, G. R. (1981) Emotional responses to multiple sclerosis. *Psychosomatics*, **22**, 117–127

BEATTY, P. A. and GANGE, J. J. (1977) Neuropsychological aspects of multiple sclerosis. *Journal of Nervous and Mental Disease*, **164**, 42–50

BECK, A. T., RUSH, A. J., SHAW, B. F. and EMERY, G. (1979) *Cognitive Therapy of Depression*. New York: Guilford Press

BERTRANDO, B. and MAFFEI, C. (1983) A study of neuropsychological alterations in multiple sclerosis. *Acta Psychiatrica Belgica*, **1**, 13–21

BRACELAND, F. J. and GIFFIN, M. E. (1950) The mental changes associated with multiple sclerosis (an interim report). *Proceedings of the Association for Research in Nervous and Mental Diseases*, **28**, 450–455

BRICKNER, R. and SIMONS, B. (1950) Emotional stress in relation to attacks of multiple sclerosis. *Proceedings of the Association for Research in Nervous and Mental Diseases*, **28**, 143

BROOKS, N. A. and MATSON, R. R. (1982) Social-psychological adjustment to multiple sclerosis. A longitudinal study. *Social Science and Medicine*, **16**, 2129–2135

BROWN, S. and DAVIS, T. K. (1922) The mental symptoms of multiple sclerosis. *Archives of Neurology and Psychiatry*, **7**, 629–634

BROWN, G. W. and HARRIS, T. (1978) *Social Origins of Depression: a Study of Psychiatric Disorders in Women*. London: Tavistock

BURNFIELD, A. (1984) Doctor-patient dilemmas in multiple sclerosis. *Journal of Medical Ethics*, **1**, 21–26

BUZZARD, T. A. (1897) A clinical lecture on insular sclerosis and hysteria. *Lancet*, **1**, 1–4

CAPLAN, L. R. and NADELSON, T. (1980) Multiple sclerosis and hysteria. *Journal of the American Medical Association*, **243**, 2418–2421

CARROLL, M., GATES, R. and ROLDAN, F. (1984) Memory impairment in multiple sclerosis. *Neuropsychologia*, **22**, 297–302

COTTRELL, S. S. and WILSON, S. A. K. (1926) The affective symptomatology of disseminated sclerosis. A study of 100 cases. *Journal of Neurology and Psychopathology*, **25**, 1–30

CHARCOT, J. M. (1877) *Lectures on the Diseases of the Nervous System.* London: New Sydenham Society

CHODOFF, P. (1974) The diagnosis of hysteria: an overview. *American Journal of Psychiatry,* **131,** 1073–1078

DALOS, N. P., RABINS, R. V., BROOKS, B. R. and O'DONNELL, P. (1983) Disease activity and emotional state in multiple sclerosis. *Annals of Neurology,* **13,** 573–577

DRAKE, M. E. (1984) Acute paranoid psychosis in multiple sclerosis. *Psychosomatics,* **25,** 60–65

GEOCARIS, K. (1957) Psychotic episodes heralding the diagnosis of multiple sclerosis. *Bulletin of the Menninger Clinic,* **21,** 107–116

GOODSTEIN, R. K. and FERRELL, R. B. (1977) Multiple sclerosis presenting as depressive illness. *Diseases of the Nervous System,* **38,** 127–131

GOWERS, W. R. (1893) *A Manual of Diseases of the Nervous System,* 2nd edn. London: Churchill

GRANT, I. (1985) The social environment and neurologic disease. In *Advances in Psychosomatic Medicine,* edited by M. Trimble, pp. 26–48. Basel: S. Karger AG

GRANT, I., McDONALD, W. I., PATTERSON, T. L. and TRIMBLE, M. R. (1986) Life events and multiple sclerosis. In *Life Events and Illness: Studies of Psychiatric and Physical Disorders,* edited by G. W. Brown and T. Harris. New York: Guilford Press (in press)

GRANT, I., McDONALD, W. I., TRIMBLE, M. R., SMITH, E. and REED, R. (1984) Deficient learning and memory in early and middle phases of multiple sclerosis. *Journal of Neurology, Neurosurgery and Psychiatry,* **47,** 250–255

GRINKER, R. R., HAM, G. C. and ROBBINS, F. P. (1950) Some psychodynamic factors in multiple sclerosis. *Proceedings of the Association for Research in Nervous and Mental Diseases,* **28,** 456–460

GROEN, J. J., PRICK, J. J. G. and BASTIAANS, J. (1967) *Multiple Sclerosis.* Haarlem: De Erven F. Bohn, NV

HOLLENDER, M. H. and STECKLER, P. P. (1972) Multiple sclerosis and schizophrenia: a case report. *Psychiatry in Medicine,* **3,** 251–257

JAMBOR, K. L. (1969) Cognitive functioning in multiple sclerosis. *British Journal of Psychiatry,* **115,** 765–775

KAHANA, E., LEIBOWITZ, V. and ALTER, M. (1971) Cerebral multiple sclerosis. *Neurology,* **21,** 1170–1176

KELLNER, C. H., DAVENPORT, Y., POST, R. M. and ROSS, R. J. (1984) Rapidly cycling bipolar disorder and multiple sclerosis. *American Journal of Psychiatry,* **141,** 112–113

KINLEY, A. E. (1980) Multiple sclerosis: from shock to acceptance. *American Journal of Nursing,* **80,** 274–275

LANGWORTHY, O. R. (1948) Relation of personality problems to onset and progress of multiple sclerosis. *Archives of Neurology and Psychiatry,* **59,** 13–28

LANGWORTHY, O. R. (1950) A survey of the maladjustment problems in multiple sclerosis and the possibilities of psychotherapy. *Proceedings of the Association for Research in Nervous and Mental Diseases,* **28,** 598–611

LARCOMBE, N. A. and WILSON, P. H. (1984) An evaluation of cognitive-behaviour therapy for depression in patients with multiple sclerosis. *British Journal of Psychiatry,* **145,** 366–371

MAPELLI, G. and RAMELLI, E. (1981) Manic syndrome associated with multiple sclerosis: secondary mania? *Acta Psychiatrica Belgica,* **81,** 337–349

MARSH, G. (1980) Disability and intellectual function in multiple sclerosis. *Journal of Nervous and Mental Disease,* **168,** 758–762

MATTHEWS, W. B. (1979) Multiple sclerosis presenting with acute remitting psychiatric symptoms. *Journal of Neurology, Neurosurgery and Psychiatry,* **42,** 859–863

MAYBURY, C. P. and BREWIN, C. R. (1984) Social relationships, knowledge and adjustment to multiple sclerosis. *Journal of Neurology, Neurosurgery and Psychiatry,* **47,** 372–376

McIVOR, G. P., RIKLAN, M. and REZNIKOFF, M. (1984) Depression in multiple sclerosis as a function of length and severity of illness, age, remissions, and perceived social support. *Journal of Clinical Psychology,* **40,** 1028–1033

MEI-TAL, V., MEYEROWITZ, S. and ENGEL, G. L. (1970) The role of psychological process in a somatic disorder: multiple sclerosis. *Psychosomatic Medicine,* **32,** 67–86

O'MALLEY, P. O. (1966) Severe mental symptoms in disseminated sclerosis. *Journal of the Irish Medical Association,* **55,** 115–127

OMBREDANE, A. (1929) *Sur les Troubles Mentaux de la Sclerose en Plaques.* Thèse de Paris. Quoted by Surridge, D. (1969)

PARKER, N. (1956) Disseminated sclerosis representing as schizophrenia. *Medical Journal of Australia,* **1,** 405–407

PEYSER, J. M., EDWARDS, K. R. and POSER, C. M. (1980) Psychological profiles in patients with multiple sclerosis. *Archives of Neurology,* **37,** 437–440

PEYSER, J. M., EDWARDS, K. R., POSER, C. M. and FILSKOV, S. B. (1980) Cognitive function in patients with multiple sclerosis. *Archives of Neurology,* **37,** 577–579

PHILIPPOPOULOS, G. S., WITTKOWER, E. D. and COUSINEAU, A. (1958) The etiologic significance of emotional factors in onset and exacerbations of multiple sclerosis. *Psychosomatic Medicine*, **20**, 458

POMMÉ, B., GIRARD, J. and PLANCHE, R. (1963) Forme dépressive de début d'une sclérosis en plaques. *Annales Medico Psycholiques* (Paris), **121**, 133

PRATT, R. T. C. (1951) An investigation of the psychiatric aspects of disseminated sclerosis. *Journal of Neurology, Neurosurgery and Psychiatry*, **14**, 326–336

RAO, S. M., HAMMEKE, T. A., McQUILLEN, M. P., KHATARI, B. O. and LLOYD, D. (1984) Memory disturbance in chronic progressive multiple sclerosis. *Archives of Neurology*, **41**, 625–631

ROSS, A. T. and REITAN, R. M. (1955) Intellectual and affective functions in multiple sclerosis. *Archives of Neurology and Psychiatry*, **73**, 663–677

SCHIFFER, R. B. and BABIGIAN, H. M. (1984) Behavioral disorders in multiple sclerosis, temporal lobe epilepsy, and amyotrophic lateral sclerosis. *Archives of Neurology*, **41**, 1067–1069

SCHIFFER, R. B., RUDICK, R. A. and HERNDON, R. M. (1983) Psychologic aspects of multiple sclerosis. *New York State Journal of Medicine*, **83**, 312–316

SCHMALZBACH, O. (1954) Disseminated sclerosis in schizophrenia. *Medical Journal of Australia*, **1**, 451–452

STAPLES, D. and LINCOLN, N. B. (1979) Intellectual impairment in multiple sclerosis. *Rheumatological Rehabilitation*, **18**, 153–160

SURRIDGE, D. (1969) Investigation into some psychiatric aspects of multiple sclerosis. *British Journal of Psychiatry*, **115**, 749–764

TRIMBLE, M. R. and GRANT, I. (1982) Psychiatric aspects of multiple sclerosis. In *Psychiatric Aspects of Neurologic Disease, Vol II*, edited by D. F. Benson and D. Blumer, pp. 279–299. New York: Grune and Stratton

WALTON, J. N. (1977) *Brain's Diseases of the Nervous System*, p. 556. London: Oxford University Press

WARREN, S., GREENHILL, S. and WARREN, K. G. (1982) Emotional stress and the development of multiple sclerosis. Case-control evidence of a relationship. *Journal of Chronic Disease*, **35**, 821–831

WHITLOCK, F. A. and SISKIND, M. M. (1980) Depression as a major symptom of multiple sclerosis. *Journal of Neurology, Neurosurgery and Psychiatry*, **43**, 861–865

WILSON, S. A. K. (1940) *Neurology*. London: Arnold

YOUNG, A. C., SAUNDERS, J. and PONSFORD, J. R. (1976) Mental change as an early feature of multiple sclerosis. *Journal of Neurology, Neurosurgery and Psychiatry*, **39**, 1008–1012

ZELDOW, P. B. and PAVLOU, M. (1984) Physical disability, life stress, and psychosocial adjustment in multiple sclerosis. *Journal of Nervous and Mental Disease*, **172**, 80–84

9

Treatment aimed at modifying the course of multiple sclerosis

George W. Ellison

INTRODUCTION

Over the past 10 years numerous treatments have been used which have sought to change the course of multiple sclerosis (MS) (Ellison and Myers, 1978, 1980; Hallpike, 1980; International Federation of Multiple Sclerosis Societies, 1982; Alter, 1983; Confavreux, 1983; Hughes, 1983; Leibowitz, 1983; Tourtellotte *et al.*, 1983; Waksman, 1983; Ellison *et al.*, 1984; Miescher and Beris, 1984; Raine, 1984). Most of these attempt to affect the putative immunopathogenesis of the disorder (*see* Chapters 5 and 6).

Most of the discussion which follows is based upon studies for which no adequate control group exists or for which only a single well-controlled study can be quoted. In the next 5–10 years we shall sort out the various treatments and discover which, if any, are useful. But, in the meantime, the patient and the physician will agonize uncertainly over the decision whether to treat or not. Even after the decision is made to treat, which agent(s) (alone or in combination), route, dose, and what duration of treatment must be considered. Many of the drugs and agents tried carry significant risks of toxicity and may have complications such as cancer occurring 10–15 years later.

GOALS OF TREATMENT

Charcot (1877) recognized two clinical phenomena in multiple sclerosis – exacerbations and progression. Exacerbations (relapses or bouts) are sudden changes in neurological signs which last more than 24 hours and are not explained by infections, or other extraneous conditions (*see* Chapter 1) (Schumacher *et al.*, 1965). Progression implies a more gradual change in signs usually occurring over several months. In general, most cases begin with an exacerbating–remitting course but, in the majority, progression eventually occurs (McAlpine and Compston, 1952; McAlpine, 1961, 1965; Bauer, Firnhaber and Winkler, 1965; Poser, Wikstrom and Bauer, 1979; Confavreux, Aimard and Devic, 1980). Thus, the general approach for therapeutic interventions which would modify the course would be to decrease the frequency of exacerbations (i.e. to prevent them; *see* US

Department of Health, Education and Welfare, 1974), to decrease their intensity, to shorten their duration, or to enhance recovery from them (Schumacher *et al.*, 1965; McAlpine, 1965; Brown, 1979; Hallpike, 1980). On the other hand, physicians have attempted to halt or even reverse the steady progression and deterioration of the neurological signs and symptoms (Weiner and Ellison, 1983; Weiner, 1985). In the medical literature both frequent exacerbations and the inexorable progression have been called 'activity' and the reader is cautioned to read clinical trial reports carefully to discern exactly what type of course has been studied.

Because we do not know the cause of MS, it may be wise to think about it as a syndrome rather than as a single disease entity. If MS is a syndrome, then some patients may respond to a particular therapy, but others with a different pathogenesis may not. An analagous situation may be the treatment of anaemia, in which there are several differing mechanisms of disease with the same overall label. Furthermore, even though we separate courses into exacerbating–remitting, progressive, and exacerbating–remitting then progressive (Confavreux, Aimard and Devic, 1980), recent studies with magnetic resonance imaging indicate that the MS process may be constant in many patients. The clinical phenomena upon which we are forced to rely as measures in clinical trials may be poor indicators of the biochemical and biophysical causes of the signs and symptoms of MS (*see* Chapter 7).

THE DESIGN OF CLINICAL TRIALS

In the USA, clinical trials have been divided into several phases (US Department of Health, Education and Welfare, 1977). In phase I, normal subjects are studied to determine the toxicity and potential pharmacological effect of an agent. However, early trials in patients may also be considered part of a phase I study. Pharmacodynamic and pharmacokinetic studies are usually incorporated into phase I studies. For patients with multiple sclerosis the most important studies are phase II. These studies consist of controlled clinical trials for the demonstration of efficacy. Usually 100–200 patients are studied. If the drug appears to be effective and relatively safe, a phase III expanded controlled study is used to detect subgroups of patients which may or may not be responsive, and for the definition of drug-related toxicity. Phase IV (post-marketing clinical trials) have not been carried out in MS.

An alternative classification of clinical trials was developed by the National Advisory Commission on Multiple Sclerosis (USA) (US Department of Health, Education and Welfare, 1974). Studies are divided into preliminary, pilot, and full. Uncontrolled, non-randomized studies are classified as preliminary. Trials in which patients serve as their own controls, or in which a group of patients seen in the past (historical controls) are studied, are also 'preliminary'. Investigations of a total of 100–200 patients with random assignment to treatment or placebo groups and with a concurrent control population are pilot studies. The terms 'pilot' and 'preliminary' studies are often used interchangeably in the neurology literature. Clinical trials with randomized, concurrent placebo or positive treatment control groups involving 500–600 patients are called 'full'.

In the past decade, there has been increasing use of random assignment of patients to placebo or potentially active treatment. Many past studies involved only the putative therapeutic drug or a biological agent, and not placebos. If a control group was included at all, either the courses of the patients themselves were contrasted before and after treatment, or there was an historical control group. In general, these approaches have been unsatisfactory because of the lack of a control group; MS has extreme variability: there is a tendency for exacerbations to decrease in frequency and a tendency for the rate of progression to slow as time passes or there is an increasing difficulty in recognizing progression (*see* Chapter 7). In addition, an unconscious bias in interpretation of the results by both the investigators and their subjects comes into play when all are aware that only the active treatment is used. Furthermore, the 'placebo effect' of any intervention whatsoever (including an enthusiastic physician) appears to change the course for an unknown length of time. The omission of the placebo has been justified on the ethical imperative to give the most effective treatment to the individual patient. Unfortunately, we cannot detect less than 100% effectiveness without an adequate treatment control population of randomly assigned, concurrent patients. Moreover, the placebo-treated group may receive substantial benefit for reasons we do not understand, and these individuals have not been exposed to the substantial risks that some of the drugs pose. In my opinion, we have no other choice but to continue with well-designed trials including sufficient numbers of patients followed for an appropriate length of time. Randomization to treatment or placebo group is absolutely necessary given the types of agents we have available. These trials will be difficult for all concerned.

Hommes, Lamers and Reekers (1980) make a strong case for selecting patients who have entered the progression phase for clinical trials, using prognostic indicators such as HLA tissue type (DR2), homozygous, short duration of disease, early age at onset, and a low neurological dysfunction score. They found that a decrease in cerebrospinal fluid IgG was an indicator that the treatment had affected the desired component of the immune response. But no one has been able consistently to change oligoclonal band patterns. Treatment with corticotropin will also change the IgG level but does not seem to be an effective treatment in the long run. It may be that elevated CSF IgG is an epiphenomenon and its significance remains unknown.

Additional problems with therapeutic trials aimed at modifying the course are: (1) measurement tools are inexact when applied to the neurological assessment, and (2) laboratory tests such as spinal fluid IgG or other immune parameters may not reflect the important pathogenetic process. All in all, the treatment of multiple sclerosis has been and remains highly empirical (International Federation of Multiple Sclerosis Societies, 1982).

In spite of these problems, there is evidence that the course can be modified with agents which affect the immune system.

TREATMENT AIMED AT MODIFYING AN EXACERBATING–REMITTING COURSE

Historically, adrenocorticosteroids (initially as corticotropin and subsequently as synthetic hormones) were the first anti-inflammatory or immunosuppressive treatments used to treat exacerbations (reviewed by Ellison and Myers, 1978, 1980). A double-blind placebo-controlled trial of ACTH showed a slightly more rapid improvement in the month following the institution of treatment (Rose *et al.*,

1970). However, it is not known if the long-term recovery of function is any different whether one gives steroids or not (Rose *et al.*, 1970; Henderson *et al.*, 1978).

More recently, higher doses of synthetic steroids (methylprednisolone) have been claimed to reverse clinical signs, or lesions demonstrated by computer-assisted tomography (Dowling, Bosch and Cook, 1980; Buckley, Kennard and Swash, 1982; Newman, Saunders and Tilley, 1982; Goas, Marion and Missoum, 1983; Stevens, 1983; Troiano *et al.*, 1984; Barnes *et al.*, 1985a). Synthesis of immunoglobulins in the cerebrospinal fluid may be diminished by steroid treatment (Trotter and Garvey, 1980) but the oligoclonal band patterns are minimally affected (Tourtellotte *et al.*, 1982). A well-designed therapeutic trial of these agents would be welcome.

Although used initially to correct suspected unsaturated fatty acid deficits in patients with MS, linoleic or linolenic acid has now been used to induce immunosuppression (Martin, 1984). Recently, data on the use of linoleic acid in three trials were combined and reanalysed by Dworkin *et al.* (1984). The reanalysis was conducted on 87 patients treated with linoleic acid; 85 patients treated with oleic acid, a control preparation; and treatment was at least 1 year in duration. Relapses were scored for frequency, severity, and duration. The authors concluded that patients treated with linoleic acid had lower relapse scores than did patients in the control group. They further noted that people entering with lower disability scores benefited most from the treatment. Since this treatment seems relatively innocuous, some American practitioners are recommending sunflower seed oil (two tablespoonfuls) each day. This therapy is expensive but it appears to be a satisfactory temporizing measure.

In 1982 Jacobs *et al.* (1982) claimed a dramatic reduction in frequency of exacerbations in patients with multiple sclerosis who were given intrathecal β-interferon. It was postulated that MS is a viral disease and that interferon would 'interfere' with viral replication. Now it is recognized that the interferons have substantial effects upon the immune system. Although there are numerous studies underway to determine the efficacy and toxicity of this treatment, there has been resistance by physicians to the use of the intrathecal route. This method has not reached the level of development that it can be recommended for widespread use.

Knobler *et al.* (1984) reported that exacerbation rates were reduced in patients receiving α-interferon therapy given by intramuscular injections. This preparation from human lymphoid cells or a comparable placebo was given for 6 months in a double-blind crossover experimental design. The investigators believed that the crossover design would control for spontaneous remissions. Twenty-four patients were treated. Exacerbation rates appeared to be reduced in both interferon and placebo treatment groups. However, the reduction occurred in the placebo-treated group following interferon use, perhaps indicating a carry-over effect or a reduction in relapse rate with the passage of time. Other evidence of possible efficacy was detected in the severity of the exacerbations. Those treated with interferon had fewer moderate and no severe exacerbations, in contrast to those receiving placebo treatment. The statistical analysis revealed a borderline mathematical probability that the interferon was better than the placebo. It was disquieting that patients who had a relapsing–remitting (exacerbating–remitting) and then subsequently progressive course appeared to deteriorate during the interferon treatment. Fog (1980) in early work with interferon also felt that one of his patients deteriorated with interferon treatment. Currently there is a large double-blind study of systemic interferon underway (K.P. Johnson, 1984, personal communication). We await the results before recommending general use of interferon or the interferon inducer polyinosinic polycytidilic acid polylysine (poly ICLC) (Bever *et al.*, 1984).

The immunosuppressive alkylating agent cyclophosphamide was given as a 'pulse' of several weeks duration by Gonsette, Demonty and Delmotte (1977). The authors claimed a dramatic reduction in the frequency of subsequent exacerbations. Thus, if effective, this treatment would approach the goal of prevention of future relapses. Unfortunately, long-term use of oral cyclophosphamide has the risk of bladder cancer or leukaemia (Mougeot-Martin *et al.*, 1978; Casciato and Scott, 1979; Plotz *et al.*, 1979; IARC, 1981; Krause, 1982; Baltus *et al.*, 1983). The short-term use of cyclophosphamide for the immediate treatment of exacerbations was not effective (Drachman *et al.*, 1975). There is a multicentre trial underway of the combination of corticotropin, cyclophosphamide, and plasmapheresis (H.L. Weiner, 1984, personal communication). It is recommended that practitioners await the trial results before using cyclophosphamide for treatment of relapses.

Although the cause of exacerbations is unknown, there is evidence of a correlation between changes in the immune response measured in blood and the development of neurological signs and symptoms (Hughes, 1983; Khatri, Koethe and McQuillen, 1984) (*see* Chapter 5). In general, prior to and during the exacerbation the level of thymus-derived suppressor cells falls (Antel, Arnason and Medof, 1978; Gonzales, Dau and Spitler, 1979; Huddlestone and Oldstone, 1979, 1982; Bach *et al.*, 1980; Reinherz *et al.*, 1980; Waksman, 1983; Antel, Reder and Oger, 1984). Thymus-derived helper cells, which control the manufacture of immunoglobulins by the bone-marrow-derived B cells, are in relative excess. If one calculates a ratio between the T-helper and T-suppressor cells, MS patients have a higher value than normal subjects. Cyclophosphamide treatment returns that ratio to the normal range. Khatri, Koethe and McQuillen (1984) and Hauser *et al.* (1983a) both comment that return of the T-suppressor cells correlates with the benefit of the treatment. Thus, while these changes in laboratory parameters could merely reflect a more basic phenomenon common to *both* the immunological changes and the neurological change, it is appealing to think that returning the ratio to the normal range, increasing the functional T-suppressor cell population, or decreasing the T-helper/inducer cells actually 'caused' the improvement. There must be investigations with agents (e.g. monoclonal antibodies to specific cell subpopulations) which alter specific subtypes before we conclude a cause and effect relationship.

Azathioprine, an antimetabolite with immunosuppressive properties, has been claimed to decrease the frequency of exacerbations (Aimard *et al.*, 1983, reviewed in Confavreux, 1983; Ellison and Myers, 1980; Hughes, 1983; Lhermitte, 1984; Sabouraud, 1984). Several years of treatment must occur before there is an effect; and the natural history of exacerbations is that they decrease spontaneously (Mickey *et al.*, 1983). A double-blind placebo-controlled, randomized therapeutic trial to address the utility of azathioprine in MS is underway in England (J. G. Mertin, 1984, personal communication). Since there may be an increased risk for cancer in those taking azathioprine, I prefer to recommend that the results of this trial be awaited before treating with this drug.

In summary, there are several potential therapies for reducing the intensity, duration, or frequency of exacerbations in MS. Unfortunately, most must be carefully tested in well designed and executed therapeutic trials before they can be recommended.

THERAPY AIMED AT SLOWING THE RATE OF PROGRESSION

There is evidence that cyclophosphamide with adrenocorticosteroids (Hommes, Lamers and Reekers, 1980; Hauser *et al.*, 1983a) and plasmapheresis (Khatri *et al.*, 1985) alter the rate of progression in some but not all patients. This combination is especially appealing because it fits with the current theory that the decreased thymus-derived T-suppressor cells account for the immunoregulatory defect observed in the blood of MS patients. It is posited that B cells are manufacturing demyelinating antibodies because they are not held in check by the suppressor cells. Plasmapheresis removes the antibodies and the immunosuppressive treatment destroys the antibody-producing cells (Jones, 1978). However, Weiner (1985) in an editorial accompanying the paper of Khatri *et al.* (1985) posited that immunosuppressant drugs by themselves might be just as effective over the long term. We know that the demyelinating factors are not specific for MS (Seil, 1977; Hirayama, Lisak and Silberberg, 1984) and we know that there are demyelinating factors other than antibodies in blood (Grundke-Iqbal and Bornstein, 1980; Silberberg, Manning and Schreiber, 1984). Plasmapheresis to remove circulating factors or antibodies is expensive and cumbersome. Nevertheless, Khatri *et al.* (1985) are to be congratulated on the adequacy of their clinical trial. Their accomplishment stands as a target for others to match or exceed. If similar results are found by other investigators with a larger number of patients, there will be a strong impetus to use plasmapheresis. Since it is not clear at this time whether or not the combination of drugs and plasmapheresis are needed or if the drugs alone are sufficient, I still would consider these therapies experimental.

Although they did not use plasmapheresis in their open, uncontrolled therapeutic trials of patients with rapid progression, Hommes, Lamers and Reekers (1980) claimed dramatic interruption of progression and reversal of signs in the majority of patients treated with prednisone (100 mg day) and sufficient cyclophosphamide intravenously to produce a leukopenia over 2–3 weeks. Hommes' careful analysis of the results is convincing, even though he uses historical controls from the literature.

In a randomized, controlled, early pilot study with 20 patients in each treatment arm, Hauser *et al.* (1983b) confirmed stabilization or improvement of the progressive course in 18 out of 20 patients followed for 1 year after treatment with intravenous ACTH tapered over 21 days, and cyclophosphamide (400–500 mg) given intravenously daily in four divided doses until the white blood cell count fell to 4×10^9 (4000/mm^3). Although the patients were randomly assigned to treatment with the above regimen, to ACTH alone, or to ACTH with low dose cyclophosphamide and with plasmapheresis, double-blinding was not felt to be feasible. Since eight of the 20 patients treated with ACTH alone did respond by the 6-month evaluation and failed to maintain their improvement at the 12 month assessment, seven of the 18 treated by plasma exchange responded at 12 months, and 18 of the 20 patients treated with high-dose cyclophosphamide were still better at the 1 year assessment, it appears that the combination of ACTH and high dose cyclophosphamide is effective in halting the progression for some rapidly progressing patients.

The investigators in these studies of cyclophosphamide (Gonsette, Demonty and Delmotte, 1977; Hommes, Lamers and Reekers, 1980; Weiner, 1985) point out that the treatment does not work in all patients, and that there is return of progression 1–2 years after the cessation of treatment. Therefore, repeated 'pulses' or chronic maintenance therapy may be considered. Will this increase the risk of cancer to the point where the treatment is more dangerous than the MS? As with all putative therapies, the patient will have to participate fully in the decision to treat or not if such a dilemma occurs. Some patients will elect treatment in order to 'have a few good years' and accept the risk of death from cancer in the distant future. Other patients will want no part of the treatment.

In summary, the use of cyclophosphamide with or without steroids and/or plasmapheresis epitomizes the dilemma of treatment for MS. We really do not know the dose, duration, or pharmacological interactions of the permutations and combinations of the treatments. To clarify them in phase II–III trials is beyond our resources. The practitioner, faced with a patient rapidly deteriorating, must do something. I feel the regimen devised by Khatri *et al.* (1985) has the most supporting evidence to warrant its use. There must be absolute honesty between the physician and the patient with the acknowledgement that the intervention is experimental and is used under pressure as a 'last ditch effort'.

It is interesting and important that the patients who appeared to respond best to the above interventions with cyclophosphamide were those whose T-suppressor cells rose during treatment (Hauser *et al.*, 1983b; Khatri, Koethe and McQuillen, 1984). These observations support the claim for a correlation between clinical state and the immunological state as reflected in the blood lymphocytes. Furthermore, Hommes, Lamers and Reekers (1980) have discussed the association between the HLA system and response to therapy. Since our genes determine our immune response and the way in which we metabolize drugs, the link between genetics, immunology, and therapeutics may be very important in MS.

Thus, there is indirect evidence that therapeutic interventions which change immunological parameters in the blood must eventually change the immune response within the white matter of the brain and spinal cord. Such changes are associated with stabilization or improvement of clinical signs and symptoms. Do they indicate a causal relationship? Are they manifestations of a direct effect of the drug upon neurological function?

Azathioprine is less toxic than cyclophosphamide (and less carcinogenic), but it does not seem as efficacious for slowing or halting the progression phase of MS. There are several studies of 5 or more years' treatment where claims are made that the course of MS is stabilized (Aimard *et al.*, 1983; Lhermitte *et al.*, 1984; Sabouraud *et al.*, 1984). Unfortunately these are poorly controlled and could even be misleading. The most reliable study is that of Patzold, Hecker and Pocklington (1982). In a randomized, but open non-blinded protocol, these investigators treated patients with a fixed dose of azathioprine, 2 mg/kg for 2 years. The control population received a diet high in polyunsaturated acids. The investigators found little change in relapse rate but a slowing of the progression rate of patients with the exacerbating–remitting then progressive type of MS. Those progressive from the beginning did not receive benefit.

Currently Ellison *et al.* are in the latter half of a 3 year study of methylprednisolone and azathioprine for progressive MS. This trial is double-blind, randomized, and placebo-controlled. The results are expected in April 1986. In England, a multicentre double-blind controlled trial of azathioprine is in progress (J. G. 1984, Mertin, personal communication). With the results of these two studies, we expect to know what role there is for azathioprine in the treatment of MS. As before, I prefer not to recommend azathioprine at this time.

OTHER TREATMENTS

Hyperbaric oxygen has been advocated by Neubauer (1983) for several years. Although his experience is anecdotal on selected patients, Fischer, Marks and Reich (1983) in a randomized, placebo-controlled pilot study found supporting evidence for stabilization and improvement. A registry has been established in the USA to try to collect the results of several trials, some of which are pilot trials, and some of which are uncontrolled. There is a connection to the immune system. Monocytes (macrophages), which could play a role in the pathogenesis of MS, are affected by the treatment.

Hyperbaric oxygen therapy has been used widely on an uncontrolled basis in the UK. A number of placebo-controlled double-blind control studies have however been initiated and the results of one have been published (Barnes *et al.*, 1985b). No short-term benefit was found. The patients are still being followed, but as the authors point out, there is no satisfactory evidence that the therapy can influence the disease in the long term without there being some initial improvement during the treatment. Although the risks involved in the treatment are small (Mertin and McDonald, 1984; Barnes *et al.*, 1985b), the treatment cannot be recommended at present for general use.

Transfer factor produced by stimulated leucocytes appears to slow the rate of progression (Basten *et al.*, 1980; Lamoureux *et al.*, 1981). However, the investigators recommended purification of the components of transfer factor before proceeding to new trials. Thymectomy does not seem effective unless azathioprine is added and, in this instance, it is unknown whether the azathioprine alone would have been as satisfactory as the two together (Ferguson *et al.*, 1983). Giordano *et al.* (1982) reported significant improvement in patients treated with removal of both plasma and lymphocytes. Hauser *et al.* (1982) and McFarlin (1983) could not confirm the result. It may be that immunosuppression with azathioprine or cyclophosphamide will be necessary in addition to the physical removal of the plasma and lymphocytes (Hocker *et al.*, 1984). Levamisole, an immunomodulating drug, is not efficacious in MS (Ellison and Myers, 1978; Gonsette *et al.*, 1982). The immunosuppressant cytarabine appears toxic and ineffective in preliminary trials (Tourtellotte *et al.*, 1983; L.W. Myers, 1985, personal communication).

Total lymphoid irradiation, during which lymph nodes are subjected to approximately 3000 cGy, has an understandable theoretical basis. The immunological effects are long lasting, the treatment itself seems relatively well tolerated and non-toxic. However, Gottlieb *et al.* (1983) did not have much success in a preliminary study. Cook *et al.* (1985, personal communication) are conducting a randomized trial to determine the efficacy of the treatment.

If MS is an autoimmune disease, the optimal treatment would be re-establishment of specific immunological tolerance for the inciting antigen. Myelin basic protein was suggested as the antigen and Romine and Salk (1983) attempted unsuccessfully to induce tolerance. Gonsette, Demonty and Delmotte (1977) found little to encourage them in a preliminary study. Bornstein *et al.* (1982) reported encouraging results with a non-encephalitogenic basic protein — copolymer 1. At the American Academy of Neurology Meeting, April 1985, Bornstein *et al.* reported a dramatic decrease in the exacerbation rate in patients with early exacerbating–remitting MS treated with copolymer I compared to a placebo treated control group. There was also slight improvement in the Kurtzke EDSS scores. A 'full' study is in the planning stages.

FUTURE TRIALS

Cyclosporine, a potent immunosuppressant, is especially effective against T-helper cells, and has been used in human transplantation. Unfortunately, there have been reports of a significant number of malignancies and renal complications (Myers *et al.*, 1984). It should be noted that the dosages used in this study are higher than those currently employed in MS trials. The drug is under study in MS in England, West Germany, and in the USA, but the results are not yet available.

Recently Steinman's group altered the course of experimental autoallergic encephalomyelitis, a possible animal model for MS, with mouse monoclonal antibody against T-helper cells (Waldor *et al.*, 1985). Preparations are underway for trials in humans.

CONCLUSIONS

There are several treatments which might prevent relapses – interferons, and linoleic or linolenic acid (as oil of evening primrose). It is appropriate to advance to pilot studies with 100–200 patients with exacerbating–remitting courses. There are several multicentre trials in progress and we should await their results before new trials are begun. Such trials will require the resources of multiple centres and could benefit from participation by practitioners.

High dose methylprednisolone treatment of the acute relapse itself shows more promise but larger studies are necessary before widespread use of the drug is warranted. Patients in the progression phase of their illness have had the progression slowed by the combination therapy of corticotropin or prednisone and cyclophosphamide. The treatment is temporarily (1–2 years) beneficial. More work must be done to define subsequent protocols. Plasmapheresis appears to give additional benefit in an 11-month trial, but longer-term advantages over the immunosuppressant drugs alone remain to be seen.

There is an association between changes in blood immune parameters (functionally determined thymus-derived suppressor cells, thymus-derived helper cells, and their ratio) and the clinical states of patients with multiple sclerosis. This further implicates the immune system in the pathogenesis of the disease. There is evidence for a genetic component also.

In general, immunosuppressive therapy appears to change the course of MS for some people. We need less toxic drugs or agents.

We will require a greater comprehension of the aetiology and pathogenesis of multiple sclerosis before a preventive therapy is found.

Acknowledgements

There have been many lively discussions in The Working Group for Experimental Trials of Multiple Sclerosis organized by Byron H. Waksman, MD of the National Multiple Sclerosis Society (USA) (Chairman, Kenneth P. Johnson, MD). Much information is presented during the public meetings of the group at the American Academy of Neurology meetings. This work was supported by grants NS 08711 and NS 16776 from the US Public Health Service (National Institute of Neurological, Communicative Disorders and Stroke). Ms M. Ellison and Mr Richard Burger helped prepare the manuscript.

References

AIMARD, G., CONFAVREUX, C., VENTRE, J. J., GUILLOT, M. AND DEVIC, M. (1983) Etude de 213 cas de sclerose en plaques traités par l'azathioprine de 1967 à 1982. (Study of 213 cases of multiple sclerosis treated with azathioprine from 1967–1982.) *Revue Neurologique (Paris)*, **139**, 509–513

ALTER, M. (1983) Current medical treatment of multiple sclerosis. *Clinical Therapeutics*, **5**, 455–460

ANTEL, J. P., ARNASON, B. G. W. and MEDOF, M. E. (1978) Suppressor cell function in multiple sclerosis: correlation with clinical disease activity. *Annals of Neurology*, **5**, 338–342

ANTEL, J., REDER, A. and OGER, J. J. F. (1984) Correlations of T-suppressor (Ts) function and immune reactivity in multiple sclerosis (MS). *Neurology (Cleveland)*, **34**, 114

BACH, M. A., PHAN-DINH-TUY, F., TOURNIER, E. *et al.* (1980) Deficit of suppressor T cells in active multiple sclerosis. *Lancet*, **2**, 1221–1223

BALTUS, J. A., BOERSMA, J. W., HARTMAN, A. P. and VANDENBROUCKE, J. P. (1983) The occurrence of malignancies in patients with rheumatoid arthritis treated with cyclophosphamides: a controlled retrospective follow-up. *Annals of the Rheumatic Diseases*, **42**, 368–373

BARNES, M. P., BATEMAN, D. E., CLELAND, P. G. *et al.* (1985a) Intravenous methylprednisolone for multiple sclerosis in relapse. *Journal of Neurology, Neurosurgery and Psychiatry*, **48**, 157–159

BARNES, M. P., BATES, D., CARTLIDGE, N. E. F., FRENCH, J. M. and SHAW, D. A. (1985b) Hyperbaric oxygen and multiple sclerosis: short-term results of a placebo-controlled double-blind trial. *Lancet*, **1**, 297–300

BASTEN, A., McLEOD, J. G., POLLARD, J. D. *et al.* (1980) Transfer factor in treatment of multiple sclerosis. *Lancet*, **2**, 931–934

BAUER, J. H., FIRNHABER, W. and WINKLER, W. (1965) Prognostic criteria in multiple sclerosis. *Annals of the New York Academy of Sciences*, **122**, 542–551

BEVER, C. T., JACOBSON, S., MINGOLI, E. S., McFARLAND, H. F., McFARLIN, D. E. and LEVY, H. B. (1984) Immunologic changes in multiple sclerosis patients treated with poly ICLC. *Neurology*, **34** (Suppl. 1), 112

BORNSTEIN, M. B., MILLER, A., SLAGLE, S. *et al.* (1985) Multiple sclerosis: clinical trials of a synthetic copolymer 1. *Neurology (Cleveland)*, **35** (Suppl. I), 103 (abstract)

BORNSTEIN, M. B., MILLER, A. I., TEITELBAUM, D., ARNON, R. and SELA, M. (1982) Multiple sclerosis: trial of a synthetic polypeptide. *Annals of Neurology*, **11**, 317–319

BROWN, J., BEEBE, G. W., KURTZKE, J. F. *et al.* (1979) The design of clinical studies to assess therapeutic efficacy in multiple sclerosis. *Neurology (New York)*, **29**, 1–23

BUCKLEY, C., KENNARD, C. and SWASH, M. (1982) Treatment of acute exacerbations of multiple sclerosis with intravenous methylprednisolone. *Journal of Neurology, Neurosurgery and Psychiatry*, **45**, 179–180

CASCIATO, D. A. and SCOTT, J. L. (1979) Acute leukemia following prolonged cytotoxic agent therapy. *Medicine (Baltimore)*, **58**, 32–47

CHARCOT, J. M. (1877) *Lectures on Diseases of the Nervous System Delivered at la Saltpetrière* (translation, G. Sigerson). London: The New Sydenham Society

CONFAVREUX, C. (1983) Essais therapeutiques au long cours et sclerose en plaques: un gageure? (Long-term therapeutic trials and multiple sclerosis: the untakable bet?.) *Revue Neurologique (Paris)*, **139**, 431–437

CONFAVREUX, C., AIMARD, G. and DEVIC, M. (1980) Course and prognosis of multiple sclerosis assessed by the computerized data processing of 349 patients. *Brain*, **103**, 281–300

DOWLING, P. C., BOSCH, V. V. and COOK, S. D. (1980) Possible beneficial effect of high-dose intravenous steroid therapy in acute demyelinating disease and transverse myelitis. *Neurology (New York)*, **30**, 33–36

DRACHMAN, D. A., PATERSON, P. Y., SCHMIDT, R. T. and SPEHLMAN, R. T. (1975) Cyclophosphamide in exacerbations of multiple sclerosis. *Journal of Neurology, Neurosurgery and Psychiatry*, **38**, 592–597

DWORKIN, R. H., BATES, D., MILLAR, J. H. and PATY, D. W. (1984) Linoleic acid and multiple sclerosis transverse myelitis. *Neurology (New York)*, **30**, 33–36

DRACHMAN, D. A., PATERSON, P. Y., SCHMIDT, R. T. and SPEHLMAN, R. T. (1975) Cyclophosphamide in exacerbations of multiple sclerosis. eurology (*Minneapolis*), **28**, 132–139

ELLISON, G. W. and MYERS, L. W. (1980) Immunosuppressive drugs in multiple sclerosis: pro and con. *Neurology (New York)*, **30**, 28–32

ELLISON, G. W., VISSCHER, B. R., GRAVES, M. C. and FAHEY, J. L. (1984) Multiple sclerosis. *Annals of Internal Medicine*, **101**, 514–526

FERGUSON, T. B., CLIFFORD, D. B., MONTGOMERY, E. B., BRUNS, K. A., McGREGOR, P. J. and TROTTER, J. L. (1983) Thymectomy in multiple sclerosis. Two preliminary trials. *Journal of Thoracic and Cardiovascular Surgery*, **85**, 88–93

FISCHER, B. H., MARKS, M. and REICH, T. (1983) Hyperbaric-oxygen treatment of multiple sclerosis. A randomized, placebo-controlled, double-blind study. *New England Journal of Medicine*, **308**, 181–186

FOG, T. (1980) Interferon treatment of multiple sclerosis patients. A pilot study. In *Search for the Cause of Multiple Sclerosis and Other Chronic Diseases of the Central Nervous System*, edited by A. Boese, pp. 490–493. Weinheim: Verlag Chemie

GIORDANO, G. F., MASLAND, W., KETCHEL, S. J. *et al.* (1982) Lymphocytapheresis in multiple sclerosis: a preliminary report. *Progress in Clinical and Biological Research*, **106**, 255–262

GOAS, J. Y., MARION, J. L. and MISSOUM, A. (1983) High dose intravenous methyl prednisolone in acute exacerbations of multiple sclerosis (letter). *Journal of Neurology, Neurosurgery and Psychiatry*, **46**, 99

GONSETTE, R. E., DEMONTY, L. and DELMOTTE, P. (1977) Intensive immunosuppression with cyclophosphamide in multiple sclerosis. Follow up of 110 patients for 2–6 years. *Journal of Neurology*, **214**, 173–181

GONSETTE, R. E., DEMONTY, L., DELMOTTE, P. *et al.* (1982) Modulation of immunity in multiple sclerosis: a double-blind levamisole-placebo controlled study in 85 patients. *Journal of Neurology*, **228**, 65–72

GONZALES, R. L., DAU, P. C. and SPITLER, L. E. (1979) Altered regulation of mitogen responsiveness by suppressor cells in multiple sclerosis. *Clinical and Experimental Immunology*, **36**, 78–84

GOTTLIEB, M. S., ELLISON, G. W., FAHEY, J. L., TESLER, A. and MYERS, L. W. (1983) Treatment of chronic progressive multiple sclerosis with total lymphoid irradiation. *Annals of Neurology*, **14**, 113

GRUNDKE-IQBAL, I. and BORNSTEIN, M. B. (1980) Multiple sclerosis: serum gamma globulin and demyelination in organ culture. *Neurology* (New York), **30**, 749–754

HALLPIKE, J. F. (1980) New treatments for multiple sclerosis. *British Journal of Hospital Medicine*, **23**, 63–64, 66, 68

HAUSER, S. L., FOSBURG, M., KEVY, S. and WEINER, H. L. (1982) Plasmapheresis, lymphocytapheresis, and immunosuppressive drug therapy in multiple sclerosis. *Progress in Clinical and Biological Research*, **106**, 239–254

HAUSER, S. L., DAWSON, D. M., LEHRICH, J. R., BEAL, M. F., KEVY, S. V. and WEINER, H. L. (1983a) Immunosuppression and plasmapheresis in chronic progressive multiple sclerosis. Design of a clinical trial. *Archives of Neurology*, **40**, 687–690

HAUSER, S. L., DAWSON, D. M., LEHRICH, J. R. *et al.* (1983b) Intensive immunosuppression in progressive multiple sclerosis. A randomized, three-arm study of high-dose intravenous cyclophosphamide, plasma exchange, and ACTH. *New England Journal of Medicine*, **308**, 173–180

HENDERSON, W. G., TOURTELLOTTE, W. W., POTVIN, A. R. and ROSE, A. S. (1978) Methodology for analyzing clinical neurological data: ACTH in multiple sclerosis. *Clinical Pharmacology and Therapeutics*, **24**, 146–153

HIRAYAMA, M., LISAK, R. P. and SILBERBERG, D. H. (1984) *In vitro* studies of serum-mediated oligodendrocyte cytotoxicity in multiple sclerosis (MS). *Neurology* (Cleveland), **34**, 114–115

HOCKER, P., STELLAMOR, V., SUMMER, K. and MANN, M. (1984) Plasma exchange (PE) and lymphocytophoresis (LCA) in multiple sclerosis (MS). *International Journal of Artificial Organs*, **7**, 39–42

HOMMES, O. R., LAMERS, K. J. and REEKERS, P. (1980). Effect of intensive immunosuppression on the course of chronic progressive multiple sclerosis. *Journal of Neurology*, **223**, 177–190

HUDDLESTONE, J. R. and OLDSTONE, M. B. A. (1979) T suppressor lymphocytes fluctuate in parallel with changes in the clinical course of patients with multiple sclerosis. *Journal of Immunology*, **123**, 1616–1618

HUDDLESTONE, J. R. and OLDSTONE, M. B. A. (1982) Suppressor T cells are activated *in vivo* in patients with multiple sclerosis coinciding with remission from acute attacks. *Journal of Immunology*, **129**, 915–917

HUGHES, R. A. C. (1983) Immunological treatment of multiple sclerosis. *Journal of Neurology*, **230**, 73–80

IARC WORKING GROUP (1981) Some antineoplastic and immunosuppressive agents. *IARC Monograph on the Evaluation of The Carcinogenic Risk of Chemicals to Humans*, **26**, 1–387

INTERNATIONAL FEDERATION OF MULTIPLE SCLEROSIS SOCIETIES (1982) *Therapeutic Claims in Multiple Sclerosis*. New York: International Federation of Multiple Sclerosis Societies

JACOBS, L., O'MALLEY, J., FREEMAN, A., MURAWSKI, J. and EKES, R. (1982) Intrathecal interferon in multiple sclerosis. *Archives of Neurology*, **39**, 609–615

JONES, J. V. (1978) Methods of modifying the immune response. *Neurology* (Minneapolis), **28**, 115–118

KHATRI, B. O., KOETHE, S. M. and McQUILLEN, M. P. (1984) Plasmapheresis with immunosuppressive drug therapy in progressive multiple sclerosis. A pilot study. *Archives of Neurology*, **41**, 734–738

KHATRI, B. O., McGUILLEN, M. P., HARRINGTON, G. J., SCHMOLL, D. S. and HOFFMANN, R. G. (1985) Chronic progressive multiple sclerosis: double-blind controlled study of plasmapheresis in patients taking immunosuppressive drugs. *Neurology*, **35**, 312–319

KNOBLER, R. L., PANITCH, H. S., BRAHENY, S. L. *et al.* (1984) Systemic alpha-interferon therapy of multiple sclerosis. *Neurology* (New York), **34**, 1273–1279

KRAUSE, J. R. (1982) Chronic idiopathic thrombocytopenia purpura (ITP): development of acute nonlymphocytic leukaemia subsequent to treatment with cyclophosphamide. *Medical and Pediatric Oncology*, **10**, 61–65

LAMOUREUX, G., COSGROVE, J., DUQUETTE, P., LAPIERRE, Y., JOLICOEUR, R. and VANDERLAND, F. (1981) A clinical and immunological study of the effects of transfer factor on multiple sclerosis patients. *Clinical and Experimental Immunology*, **43**, 557–564

LEIBOWITZ, S. (1983) The immunology of multiple sclerosis. In *Multiple Sclerosis Pathology, Diagnosis and Management*, edited by J. F. Hallpike, C. W. M. Adams and W. W. Tourtellotte, pp. 379–412. Baltimore: Williams and Wilkins

LHERMITTE, F., MARTEAU, R., ROULLET, E., DE SAXCE, H. and LORIDAN, M. (1984) Traitment prolonge de la sclerose en plaques par l'azathioprine a doses moyennes. Bilan de quinze années d'experience. *Revue Neurologique (Paris)*, **140**, 553–558

McALPINE, D. (1961) The benign course of multiple sclerosis. A study of 241 cases seen within three years of onset and followed up until the tenth year or more of the disease. *Brain*, **84**, 186–203

McALPINE, D. (1965) Course and prognosis. In *Multiple Sclerosis: A Reappraisal*, edited by D. McAlpine, N. D. Compston and C. E. Lumsden, pp. 179–196. Edinburgh and London: E. and S. Livingstone Ltd

McALPINE, D. and COMPSTON, N. (1952) Some aspects of the natural history of disseminated sclerosis. *Quarterly Journal of Medicine*, **21**, 135–167

McFARLIN, D. E. (1983) Treatment of multiple sclerosis (editorial). *New England Journal of Medicine*, **308**, 215–217

MERTIN, J. (1984) Omega-6 and omega-3 polyunsaturates and the immune system. *British Journal of Clinical Practice* (Symposium Suppl.), **31**, 111–114

MERTIN, J. and McDONALD, W. I. (1984) Hyperbaric oxygen for patients with multiple sclerosis. *British Medical Journal*, **288**, 957–960

MICKEY, M. R.L). *New England Journal of Medicine*, **308**, 215–217

MERTIN, J. (1984) Omega-6 and omega-3 polyunsaturates and the immune system. *British Journal of Clinical Practice* (Symposium Suppl.mmunosuppressive therapy in the treatment of autoimmune diseases. *Springer Seminars in Immunopathology*, **7**, 69–90

MOUGEOT-MARTIN, M., KRULIK, M., HAROUSSEAU, J. L., AUDEBERT, A. A., CHAOUAT, Y. and DEBRAY, J. (1978) Cases of acute leukaemia following immunosuppressive therapy for disseminated sclerosis and for Behçet's syndrome (author's translation). *Annales de Médecine Interne (Paris)*, **129**, 175–180

MYERS, B. D., ROSS, J., NEWTON, L., LUETSCHER, J. and PERLROTH, M. (1984) Cyclosporine-associated chronic nephropathy. *New England Journal of Medicine*, **311**, 699–705

NEUBAUER, R. A. (1983) A summary of worldwide experience in the treatment of multiple sclerosis with hyperbaric oxygen. Program and abstracts. *First European Conference on Hyperbaric Medicine*, Amsterdam, September 7–9, 1983

NEWMAN, P. K., SAUNDERS, M. and TILLEY, P. J. (1982) Methylprednisolone therapy in multiple sclerosis (letter). *Journal of Neurology, Neurosurgery and Psychiatry*, **45**, 941–942

PATZOLD, U., HECKER, H. and POCKLINGTON, P. (1982) Azathioprine in treatment of multiple sclerosis. Final results of a 4½-year controlled study of its effectiveness covering 115 patients. *Journal of the Neurological Sciences*, **54**, 377–394

PLOTZ, P. H., KLIPPEL, J. H., DECKER, J. L. *et al.* (1979) Bladder complications in patients receiving cyclophosphamide for systemic lupus erythematosus or rheumatoid arthritis. *Annals of Internal Medicine*, **91**, 221–223

POSER, S., WIKSTROM, J. and BAUER, H. J. (1979) Clinical data and identification of special forms of multiple sclerosis in 1271 cases studied with a standardized documentation system. *Journal of the Neurological Sciences*, **40**, 159–168

RAINE, C. S. (1984) Biology of disease. Analysis of autoimmune demyelination: its impact upon multiple sclerosis. *Laboratory Investigation*, **50**, 608–635

REINHERZ, E. L., WEINER, H. L., HAUSER, S. L. *et al.* (1980) Loss of suppressor T-cells in active multiple sclerosis. *New England Journal of Medicine*, **303**, 125–129

ROMINE, J. S. and SALK, J. (1983) A study of myelin basic protein as a therapeutic probe in patients with multiple sclerosis. In *Multiple Sclerosis*, edited by J. F. Hallpike, C. W. M. Adams and W. W. Tourtellotte, pp. 621–630. Baltimore: Williams and Wilkins

ROSE, A. S., KUZMA, J. W., KURTZKE, J. F., NAMEROW, N. S., SIBLEY, W. A. and TOURTELLOTTE, W. W. (1970) Cooperative study in the evaluation of therapy in multiple sclerosis: ACTH vs. placebo. Final report. *Neurology (Minneapolis)*, **20**, 1–59

SABOURAUD, O., OGER, J., DARCEL, F., MADIGAND, M. and MERIENNE, M. (1984) Immunosuppression au long cours dans la sclerose en plaques: evaluation des traitements commencés avant 1972. (Long-term immunosuppression in multiple sclerosis: evaluation of treatments begun before 1972.) *Revue Neurologique (Paris)*, **140**, 125–130

SCHUMACHER, G. A., BEEBE, G., KIBLER, R. E. *et al.* (1965) Problems of experimental trials of therapy in multiple sclerosis: report by the panel on evaluation of experimental trials of therapy in multiple sclerosis. *Annals of the New York Academy of Sciences*, **122**, 552–568

SEIL, F. J. (1977) Tissue culture studies of demyelinating disease: a critical review. *Annals of Neurology*, **2**, 345–355

SILBERBERG, D. H., MANNING, M. C. and SCHREIBER, A. D. (1984) Tissue culture demyelination by normal human serum. *Annals of Neurology*, **15**, 575–580

STEVENS, J. R. (1983) High dose methylprednisolone in acute exacerbations of multiple sclerosis. *Journal of Neurology, Neurosurgery and Psychiatry*, **46**, 99

TOURTELLOTTE, W. W., POTVIN, A. R. M.A, B. I. *et al.* (1982) Isotachophoresis quantitation of subfractions of multiple sclerosis intrablood–brain barrier IgG synthesis modulated by ACTH and/or steroids. *Neurology* (New York), **32**, 261–266

TOURTELLOTTE, W. W., BAUMHEFNER, R. W., POTVIN, J. H., POTVIN, A. R. and POSER, S. (1983) Comprehensive management of multiple sclerosis. In *Multiple Sclerosis,* edited by J. F. Hallpike, C. W. M. Adams and W. W. Tourtellotte, pp. 513–578. Baltimore: Williams and Wilkins

TROIANO, R., HAFSTEIN, M., RUDERMAN, M., DOWLING, P. and COOK, S. (1984) Effect of high-dose intravenous steroid administration on contrast-enhancing computed tomographic scan lesions in multiple sclerosis. *Annals of Neurology*, **15**, 257–263

TROTTER, J. L. and GARVEY, W. F. (1980) Prolonged effects of large-dose methylprednisolone infusion in multiple sclerosis. *Neurology (New York)*, **30**, 702–708

US DEPARTMENT OF HEALTH, EDUCATION AND WELFARE (1974) *National Advisory Commission on Multiple Sclerosis, Report and Recommendations.* Publication no. (NIH) 74-534, pp. 36–38. Washington, DC: US Government Printing Office

US DEPARTMENT OF HEALTH, EDUCATION AND WELFARE, FOOD AND DRUG ADMINISTRATION (1977) *General considerations for the Clinical Evaluation of Drugs.* Publication no. HEW (FDA) 77-3040, pp. 6–11. Washington DC: US Government Printing Office

WAKSMAN, B. H. (1983) Rationales of current therapies for multiple sclerosis. *Annals of Neurology*, **40**, 671–672

WAKSMAN, B. H. and REYNOLDS, W. E. (1984) Multiple sclerosis as a disease of immune regulation. *Proceedings of the Society for Experimental Biology and Medicine*, **175**, 282–294

WALDOR, M. K., SRIRAM, S. *et al.* (1985) Reversal of experimental allergic encephalomyelitis with monoclonal antibody to a T cell subset marker (L3T4). *Science*, **227**, 415–421

WEINER, H. L. (1985) An assessment of plasma exchange in progressive multiple sclerosis. *Neurology (Cleveland)*, **35**, 320–322

WEINER, H. L. and ELLISON, G. W. (1983) A working protocol to be used as a guideline for trials in multiple sclerosis. *Archives of Neurology*, **40**, 704–710

10
Symptomatic management of multiple sclerosis

Charles R. Smith, Mindy L. Aisen and Labe Scheinberg

INTRODUCTION

As is the case for any disease, treatment can be categorized as prophylactic, curative, restorative or symptomatic. For multiple sclerosis (MS) there is no known prophylactic, nor is there any agent that will restore damaged myelin. There is no specific treatment that will reliably interrupt the course of the illness. In recent years, however, advances in our understanding of the pathophysiology of central nervous system (CNS) dysfunction have enabled physicians to improve dramatically the symptomatic management of MS.

TYPES OF SYMPTOMS

The symptoms and signs of MS may be categorized as primary, secondary or tertiary. Primary symptoms indicate the effects of a strategically located lesion. Hence, weakness, spasticity, visual loss, numbness, incontinence, and fatigue may be termed primary symptoms. Secondary symptoms are the complications that arise as a direct result of the primary ones. These include urinary tract infection resulting from urinary retention, fibrous contractures because of sustained muscle spasms, and pressure sores because of immobility and diminished sensation. Tertiary symptoms are the psychological, social, and vocational ramifications of the disease on the patient, family, and community.

 The care of patients with MS requires attention to all categories of symptoms. For this reason, management is optimal in a comprehensive care centre, or its equivalent, with a variety of experienced health professionals including neurologists, physiatrists, urologists, orthopaedists, psychiatrists, specialized nurses, psychologists, physical and occupational therapists and social workers (Scheinberg, Holland and Kirschenbaum, 1981). An MS comprehensive care centre will be able to coordinate effectively the delivery of a uniform standard of care in keeping with up-to-date management guidelines.

PRIMARY SYMPTOMS

Gait dysfunction

Gait disturbance is among the most frequently cited symptoms of MS. In fact, this is the chief complaint of the majority of patients. In the analysis, one or several factors in combination may be responsible for the problem. Weakness, spasticity, ataxia and defective proprioception must each be considered to identify correctly the pathogenesis of the complaint. Only then can the appropriate therapy be provided.

Spasticity

Spasticity is a common primary symptom of MS and is frequently a major contributor to abnormal ambulation. Although precise mechanisms concerning the pathophysiology of spasticity remain unknown (Davidoff, 1978; Young and Delwaide, 1981), effective medical treatment is now available. Baclofen (Lioresal), an analogue of the inhibitory neurotransmitter gamma aminobutyric acid (GABA), is the most useful of the currently available anti-spastic agents. It is thought to act at the spinal level by diminishing the transmission of both monosynaptic extensor and polysynaptic flexor reflexes (Davidoff and Sears, 1974; Fox *et al.*, 1978). Evidence suggests that baclofen may increase presynaptic inhibition by interacting with GABA receptors located on the central terminals of primary afferent fibres (Davidoff, 1985). In addition, baclofen may have a depressive effect on the activity of spinal interneurons (Delwaide, 1985).

Whatever its mechanism of action, both hypertonia and flexor spasms respond readily to this drug and usually at doses that are well tolerated by the majority of patients. The most frequent side-effects are nausea and transient drowsiness. These can usually be prevented by administering the drug with meals, starting with small doses such as 5 mg three times daily and increasing gradually (5 mg/dose every 3–5 days) until the best response is achieved. Other much less frequent side-effects include headache, fatigue, insomnia, hypotension, constipation, urinary frequency and, at high doses, confusion. Rarely, some patients appear to experience a paradoxical response with heightened spasticity for unknown reasons. Elevations of serum transaminases and alkaline phosphatase have been reported to occur in some. Finally, it should be noted that many patients stand on their spasticity, and that excessive use of baclofen may impair gait by unmasking weakness already present. Dosages and responses must be carefully assessed so that maximal benefit with least harmful effects are realized. For this reason, the patient should be given explicit instructions as to the purpose and expected results so that he/she can assist in adjusting his/her own medication.

Many individuals are well managed on 45–80 mg of baclofen daily, but some require substantially higher doses. Occasionally, doses well in excess of the manufacturers advertized limit will be necessary in order to achieve an adequate anti-spastic effect (Kirkland, 1984). It is the response to the drug as perceived by the patient and physician that should determine the dosage.

Diazepam (Valium) is another effective medical treatment for spasticity. This agent enhances GABA-mediated presynaptic inhibition in the spinal cord (Davidoff, 1985; Delwaide, 1985) and may depress activity in the descending lateral reticular formation, thereby inhibiting gamma motor neurons (Ngai, Tseng and

Wang, 1966). This drug may produce all of the side-effects of baclofen. However, therapeutic dosages of baclofen are easier to achieve as it is better tolerated. Diazepam is probably best used in patients who cannot tolerate baclofen for whatever reason, or as an adjunct to baclofen therapy when further increments of baclofen are of no benefit. Although their effect is similar, diazepam and baclofen have different central sites of action and their efficacy may therefore be additive (Delwaide, 1985). As with baclofen, the dose of diazepam should be gradually increased as tolerated. Doses in excess of 30 mg/day are rarely well tolerated because of adverse effects.

Dantrolene sodium (Dantrium) has not been of as much benefit in the management of spasticity secondary to spinal cord disease. Adverse reactions frequently outweigh improvement, if any, and preclude its use in many patients. In addition, this drug has a well known, albeit rare, propensity for inducing potentially serious hepatocellular injury, making it a relatively high risk agent compared to other more effective anti-spastic drugs.

When spasticity is refractory to medical therapy, chemical neurectomy may be necessary. Phenol (5%) may be injected with electromyographic guidance directly into motor nerves or at the site of motor point insertion, producing local neurolysis. Phenol neurectomy is a technically simple procedure which may produce dramatic results. Adductor spasms of the thighs readily respond to obturator nerve blocks, and flexor spasms of the hamstrings can successfully be eliminated by hamstring motor point neurolysis. The effects may last for several months or more and may be repeated if necessary (Moore, 1971).

Some authorities advocate the use of intrathecal Depo-Medrol (methylprednisolone acetate) for refractory spasticity. Some patients experience definite benefit, but, rarely, painful adhesive arachnoiditis may result, especially if the injections are repeated frequently (Nelson, Vates and Thomas, 1973). Late stages of severe spasticity may necessitate intrathecal alcohol administration. This is a last resort that should be entertained only in those patients with severe long-standing urinary retention, severe sensory loss in the lower extremities and paraplegia.

Weakness and ataxia

Both weakness and ataxia are refractory to medical management. Physical therapists, however, are able to provide effective gait training and can instruct patients in the use of aids such as canes, crutches, quadruped walkers and parallel bars when necessary. Their interventions can improve endurance and impart added confidence in those requiring ambulation aids. Orthoses, such as posterior leg splints, are useful for patients with weak ankle dorsiflexors. Less often, other types of ankle and knee braces may be of benefit when gait dysfunction is secondary to weakness. When gait becomes too hazardous even with aids, a wheelchair may be recommended. For some, mechanized wheelchairs (Amigo and others) may permit a degree of independence otherwise impossible. For patients with severe paraparesis and sensory disturbance particular attention should be given to the design of wheelchair cushions. These should be contoured to the individual by careful analysis of pressure points. If, for example, foam cushions are used, appropriate cut outs should be made to ensure that adequate tissue perfusion over bony prominences will be maintained. Finally, the patient should be educated on the prevention of pressure sores by careful attention to chair exercises which periodically relieve pressure (Edberg, Cerny and Stauffer, 1973).

Upper extremities

In the upper extremities, spasticity is less frequently a problem. More difficulty arises from weakness and loss of digital dexterity. These make many activities of daily living virtually impossible, especially when combined with cerebellar tremor. Occupational therapists are often of great help in making available to patients devices to increase independence by accommodating such disturbances and teaching them in their use. Tools for doing up buttons, cutlery with large specially weighted handles, rocker knives, and specially adapted clothing will impart greater independence and improve self-esteem. Many medical professionals fail to appreciate the effects of such apparently less conspicuous problems, such as the ability to button up clothing, on the patient's morale. Often, simple modifications can improve the patient's day-to-day life substantially.

There have been several recent reports on the use of drugs in the management of tremor presumed to be of cerebellar origin. These reports suggest that, depending on the type of tremor, therapeutic responses may be anticipated. Patients with postural cerebellar tremor have been reported to respond to isoniazid 800–1200 mg/day (with pyridoxine supplement) (Sabra *et al.*, 1982; Sabra and Hallett, 1984). Some patients with kinetic tremor have responded to clonazepam (Clonopin) in doses of 1.5–6 mg/day (Scheinberg and Smith, 1985). Although success may occasionally be achieved with these agents, results are usually disappointing (Koller, 1984). A trial may be warranted, however, when tremor is disabling. Propranolol (Inderal) is ineffective in cerebellar tremor (Koller, 1984). Patients with severe tremor may respond to stereotaxic thalamotomy (Cooper, 1960). Bilateral thalamotomy should not be performed because pseudobulbar palsy frequently results.

Urinary symptoms

Almost as frequent as gait disturbance in MS is the involvement of sphincter control (Blaivas *et al.*, 1984). This is not surprising as virtually all levels of the CNS contribute to regulation of bladder function (Hald and Bradley, 1982). Symptoms may reflect neurological impairment, complicating infection or both. Of primary importance in the management of urinary dysfunction is preservation of the integrity of the upper urinary tract. Therefore, initial steps in the evaluation of urological dysfunction should include a urine for culture and microscopic urinalysis. Since the likelihood of bladder infection is associated with excessive post void residual (PVR) urine, all patients with bladder complaints should have a residual urine determination. History alone is inadequate in predicting those patients who are incompletely emptying the bladder (Blaivas, 1980; Philp, Read and Higson, 1981). Reliance solely on history will give rise to an inaccurate analysis in 70% of cases. This may have profound therapeutic implications. The PVR can be determined by catheterization using aseptic technique after the patient has voided or by using a radioisotope-labelled substance completely cleared by the kidney (e.g. [131]I hippurate) (Strauss and Blaufox, 1971). More extensive evaluations such as cystoscopy and urodynamics are less frequently indicated. They should be reserved for patients who fail to respond to the measures described below or for patients in whom complications such as bladder calculi are suspected.

From a practical point of view bladder dysfunction may be categorized as failure to store urine, failure to empty the bladder or a combination of these with detrusor-external sphincter dyssynergia (DESD) (Blaivas, 1980).

The bladder that fails to store urine adequately is characterized by inability to inhibit voluntarily detrusor contractions. The patients generally complain of urgency, frequency, nocturia and urgency incontinence. There may also be symptoms suggestive of obstruction either because volumes expelled may be small due to limited detrusor capacity or because contemporaneous contraction of the external sphincter at the time of detrusor contraction may produce functional obstruction – DESD (Blaivas *et al.*, 1981). In contrast to patients with isolated uninhibited detrusor contractions, patients with DESD have abnormally high residual urines because of functional outlet obstruction and because detrusor contractions are frequently weak and poorly sustained. Isolated inability to empty the bladder without DESD is not as frequent a finding in MS. It may result from demyelination in the sacral spinal cord or in the pons when the pontine facilitatory centre is affected. Occasionally it follows transverse myelitis during the period of spinal shock.

Patients with uninhibited detrusor contractions without significant PVRs are best managed pharmacologically. Anticholinergics, smooth muscle relaxants or drugs which combine both properties may be useful. The most commonly prescribed treatment is propantheline bromide (Pro-Banthine). This drug antagonizes the muscarinic effects of acetylcholine and has little effect at nicotinic receptors. Major side-effects are dryness of the mouth, constipation and visual blurring. It is advisable to instruct patients to consume adequate amounts of fluid and to ensure adequate dietary fibre in order to prevent constipation. Tablets are available in several sizes facilitating accurate titration. The drug should be started at 15 mg three or four times daily and may be rapidly increased, depending on the therapeutic response. Some patients are able to tolerate very large doses such as 300 mg or more daily with excellent control of bladder symptoms and no significant adverse effects.

Although primarily smooth muscle relaxants, both oxybutynin chloride (Ditropan) and dicyclomine hydrochloride (Bentyl) have significant anticholinergic properties. These drugs are probably as effective as propantheline bromide and produce similar side-effects. Typical doses for oxybutynin are 5–10 mg four times daily, and for dicyclomine hydrochloride 20 mg three times daily.

The tricyclic antidepressants, imipramine hydrochloride (Tofranil) and amitriptyline hydrochloride (Elavil) are known to have prominent systemic anticholinergic effects and they are useful in facilitating bladder storage. However, an anti-muscarinic effect on the detrusor has not been documented and these agents may work primarily as adrenergic agents increasing the tone of the primarily adrenergically innervated internal sphincter (Wein, 1980). Doses of 50–150 mg at bedtime, occasionally more, are usually satisfactory in producing day-long control of symptoms, sometimes in conjunction with other agents. Although logical choices, adrenergic agents such as ephedrine sulphate and phenylpropanolamine hydrochloride which would be expected to improve internal sphincter tone, usually produce disappointing results (Blaivas, 1980).

It is important to remember that failure with one medication does not necessarily imply that others will also fail even when of the same pharmacological class. The reasons for this are unclear, but differences in individual metabolism are likely to be important. Sometimes two drugs will work better in alleviating symptoms than either alone. Occasionally, nocturia that has been recalcitrant to other forms of therapy will respond to intranasal desmopressin (DDAVP) 0.1–0.4 ml at bedtime.

When residual urines are abnormally high the treatment of choice is intermittent catheterization (IC) by the clean technique (Lapides *et al.*, 1971). Significant residual urine volumes are defined as greater than 100 ml or greater than 20% of the voided volume. The frequency of intermittent catheterization varies depending on the severity of the problem but a three or four times per day schedule is reasonable, initially at least. More frequent catheterization may lead to urethral irritation and worsening of irritative complaints. With continued intermittent catheterization residual urine volume may fall, allowing for a reduction in the frequency of catheterization. Although considerable resistance still prevails in the general medical community, the value of this technique has been proved by careful studies (Lapides, Diokno and Lowe, 1974; Diokno and Childs, 1985). There is no doubt that bacterial infection is reduced. In patients with DESD, in whom there are irritative symptoms as well as excessive PVRs, application of intermittent catheterization will permit treatment of involuntary detrusor contractions with anticholinergics, reducing complaints.

Obviously, a patient will require adequate manual dexerity, ability to spread the thighs and adequate vision to perform intermittent self catheterization. Otherwise assistance may be necessary. Because of the propensity for infection with excessive PVR, urinary acidifiers such as vitamin C 1g four times daily and urinary antiseptics such as methenamine mandelate (Mandelamine) 1 g four times daily or hexamine hippurate (Hiprex) 1 g twice daily are indicated (Devenport *et al.*, 1984). Patients are also advised to drink cranberry juice as this is the only fruit juice that consistently acidifies the urine. Optimal urine pH should be less than 6.0 to inhibit infection effectively.

Although some physicians advocate the use of cholinergic agents such as bethanechol (Urecholine) to improve detrusor contractions (Lapides, 1974; Diokno and Lapides, 1977) and/or anti-adrenergics such as phenoxybenzamine (Dibenyline) to relax the internal urinary sphincter (Mobley, 1976), no convincing studies exist showing that these agents are useful for any long-term management of neurogenic urinary retention. Anti-spastic agents, however, may be useful in DESD by reducing external sphincter spasm during detrusor contraction. Available evidence suggests that currently available anti-spastic agents, especially baclofen (Lioresal) may be of value in this regard (Wein, 1980). However, effective doses may be higher than those generally tolerated for maximum benefit. There are few studies on the use of these medications in patients with MS and DESD (Roussan *et al.*, 1975).

Surgical procedures such as urinary diversions or artificial sphincters, such as that advocated by Scott, generally produce unsatisfactory results. Frequently, bladder dysfunction changes with the course of the disease and should a patient with a prosthesis develop retention of urine, intermittent catheterization may not be possible. In long-standing urinary retention in a female unable to perform intermittent catheterization a suprapubic vesicotomy may be preferable to an indwelling urethral catheter as hygiene is better maintained, thus reducing the frequency of urinary tract infection. Males with severe DESD and large residual urine volumes who are unable to carry out intermittent catheterization may benefit from sphincterotomy and condom catheter drainage.

Bowel symptoms

In tandem with bladder involvement are complaints referable to bowel and sexual dysfunction. Constipation is the most frequent bowel complaint and usually responds to adequate dietary fibre and hydration. Many patients with irritative bladder symptoms avoid adequate fluid intake, worsening constipation. When necessary, laxatives such as bisacodyl (Dulcolax) oral or rectal preparations, or enemas should be used to ensure regular evacuations every 2–3 days. As with urinary tract infection, constipation, when severe enough, can lead to heightened flexor spasms in the lower extremities simulating an exacerbation of MS.

Sexual dysfunction

Sexual dysfunction is common in MS and may be a source of great frustration especially in males (Barrett, 1977). Both psychological and neurological mechanisms may be responsible. Careful history taking will usually identify contributing factors. A multidisciplinary approach provides the best results. When neurological dysfunction is responsible for impotence in the male, penile implants may be indicated. The expectations should be made very clear to the patient as performance is certainly improved but sensory satisfaction will be unaffected. Anorgasmy, the most frequent complaint in females, may respond to masturbation with electrically operated vibrators (R.T. Schapiro, personal communication, 1984). Patients with MS should be routinely questioned about sexual dysfunction as they may be inhibited from discussing such issues. When appropriate, evaluations by sexual counsellors, psychologists and urologists will help a substantial number of patients (Lilius, Valtonen and Wikstrom, 1976; Lundberg, 1978, Kalb *et al.*, 1984).

Fatigue

After gait and sphincter involvement, most patients with MS cite abnormal fatigue as a major disabling symptom interfering with the activities of daily living (Freal, Kraft and Coryell, 1984). Although this complaint may be confused with depression or the consequences of inefficient gait, it is more commonly a primary manifestation of MS. Most patients clearly describe a diurnal pattern with maximal fatigue occurring in the mid to late afternoon. With warmer weather or after exercise, the sensation is worsened. It is somewhat relieved with rest, but not usually by sleep. Activities possible in the morning may be totally impossible during other times of the day. No generally accepted pharmacological treatment is available, but pemoline (Cylert) (Scheinberg and Smith, 1985) or amantadine (Symmetrel) (Murray, 1984) may be useful. Pemoline 18.75–112.5 mg every morning and amantadine 100 mg twice daily are recommended by their proponents. Whenever possible, daily activities should be scheduled around those times that are most associated with fatigue.

Sensory symptoms

Abnormal sensory function is frequent in MS and may or may not be symptomatic. When painful dysaethesiae occur, treatment may be necessary. Pain of the lancinating type such as tic douloureux responds best to carbamazepine (Tegretol) or phenytoin (Dilantin) and is used in doses similar to those for controlling seizures. Constant burning pain may respond to tricyclic antidepressants such as imipramine or amitriptyline hydrochloride or to monoamine oxidase inhibitors such as phenelzine (Nardil) (Clifford and Trotter, 1984). Occasionally, the combination of a tricyclic antidepressant with a major tranquillizer (e.g. Triavil) may produce the best results. It is important to recognize that coincident depression may be amplifying the complaint of pain and further measures directed against depression may be indicated. Other causes for pain should also be considered. Spasticity may be associated with painful flexor spasms which may be particularly troublesome at night, interfering with sleep. These will respond to anti-spastic agents as already outlined. Coincident arthritis or the radicular pain of herniated intervertebral disc are other common causes of pain.

Visual symptoms

Visual dysfunction is common but is only infrequently severe enough to be a source of significant disability. The sequelae of optic neuritis may include reduced visual acuity and, rarely, blindness. Low vision clinics may help individuals adapt to this. When diplopia interferes with vision a monocular patch may be necessary. Fortunately, many of these visual complaints are self-limited. Patients who are advised to wear a patch should be cautioned about the loss of depth perception which may affect the ability to drive an automobile safely. Oscillopsia, when due to opsoclonus, may respond to clonazepam (Clonopin) as described under the treatment of cerebellar tremor (B. Geisser, personal communication, 1984). Drowsiness is a limiting adverse effect which many patients cannot tolerate. Other causes of oscillopsia such as nystagmus or internuclear ophthalmoplegia do not respond to any medication.

Paroxysmal attacks

A rather unusual but usually remediable phenomenon in MS are the so-called paroxysmal attacks (Matthews, 1975). These include painful tonic seizures, paroxysmal dysarthria and ataxia, paroxysmal diplopia, paroxysmal itching or even paroxysmal hiccups. They are of brief duration, usually seconds or minutes, and may occur many times daily. Carbamazepine and phenytoin are usually effective treatments.

Speech disorders

Disorders of speech usually reflect corticospinal or cerebellar involvement. Although speech therapy is indicated, results are often unsatisfactory. Breath control may help those patients whose speech is hypophonic. Communication devices such as word boards are often helpful when speech is unintelligible. When swallowing difficulties are associated a thorough analysis is necessary. This should include a speech and swallowing assessment by a trained pathologist and radiographic analyses of swallowing patterns (Logeman, 1981). With sufficient information, the proper consistency of food and the appropriate feeding position can be taught to the patient and family; this may be important in preventing serious complications such as aspiration pneumonia. Gastrostomy or other methods of alimentation may be necessary when more conservative measures fail (Ponsky, Gauderer and Stellato, 1983).

Cognitive defects (*see* Chapter 8)

Functionally significant cognitive defects are most often encountered in patients with long-standing, severe, generalized disease. Rarely, these may be presenting features. Although cognitive defects are not amenable to therapy, it is important to distinguish these from the manifestations of depression which may mimic dementia. Depression is by far the most frequent mental disturbance in MS, not euphoria as is commonly believed. When present, euphoria seems to correlate with cognitive dysfunction. Depression, anger and frustration are frequently remedial to therapy, including counselling and, when indicated, antidepressant medications. It is important to remember that some antidepressants have significant anticholinergic effects which may be manifested in bladder and bowel function. These side-effects should be anticipated in patients with urinary retention and in those already complaining of constipation.

SECONDARY FINDINGS

Secondary findings are the medical and surgical complications which develop as a result of the chronic neurological deficits of multiple sclerosis. Bladder infections, urinary tract stones, respiratory infections, decubitus ulcers, tendon contractures, and malnutrition are included in this category.

Urinary tract infections

The infection which most commonly complicates the course of patients with MS is the urinary tract infection (UTI). Dysfunction of the lower urinary tract predisposes to UTI, particularly when there is urinary retention or an indewelling catheter. The urethra is the most common entry route for bacteria (Netto *et al.*, 1978). The urethra and meatus are normally colonized by bacteria; the most common organisms are *Escherichi coli*, enterococci, *Proteus* species, *Klebsiella* species, staphylococci, *Pseudomonas*, and diphtheroids (Hald and Bradley, 1982). The repeated 'wash-out' produced by urination prevents infection in the normal bladder. Bladder neck obstruction, which may occur in patients with MS due to external sphincter hyperactivity, interferes with this bladder defence mechanism by increasing the turbulence of urethral flow. This promotes retrograde movement of bacteria. Urinary retention compounds the likelihood of UTI because stagnant urine serves as an excellent culture medium. Furthermore, vesical distension may promote bladder wall ischaemia, interfering with the local antibacterial properties of the epithelial surface of the bladder (Mehrotra, 1953).

   Lower tract infections may ascend into the ureters and kidneys. The probable mechanism for this is vesicoureteric reflux which may occur when acute cystitis produces oedema and compromise of the valve system, and/or when DESD contributes to excessive intravesicular pressure. As in the development of lower urinary tract infections, flow obstruction in the upper urinary tracts predisposes to turbulence, insufficient wash-out, and retrograde motion of bacteria (Hinmun, 1973). Stones are a common cause of such an obstruction in the patient with MS.

UTI is often a persistent problem. Recurrent UTI refers to relapse with the same bacterial strain after a course of antibiotics has been completed. This may occur in the setting of insufficient antibiotic dosage, with resistant bacterial strains, or when infections originate in the renal medulla. False recurrence refers to reinfection with another bacterial strain shortly after an infection is successfully treated and is very common in the setting of urodynamic dysfunction (Hald and Bradley, 1982). Chronic UTIs are also associated with neurogenic bladder dysfunction, particularly when elevated post void residual urine volumes are present (Shand, Nimmon and O'Grady, 1970). In chronic cystitis, the infection involves deeper layers of the bladder wall. Chronic cystitis increases the risk of developing squamous cell carcinoma of the bladder (Hald and Bradley, 1982).

Acute lower urinary tract infections may be asymptomatic, may produce non-specific symptoms, or may aggravate seemingly unrelated neurological symptoms, such as lower extremity weakness or spasticity. For this reason, frequent surveillance cultures are helpful. Furthermore, any change in neurological symptoms should lead to consideration of UTI. Typically, however, acute urethritis or cystitis will produce pathognomonic local symptoms, including frequency and urgency of urination and burning dysuria. Systemic symptoms, such as fever, myalgias and nausea, usually suggest more extensive spread of infection, for example, to prostate or kidneys (Freedman and Epstein, 1977). The laboratory findings in an acute bacterial lower tract infection include pyuria and bacteriuria. Haematuria may occur in cystitis. Quantitative estimation of bacteria in the urine is a means of distinguishing true infection from contamination. If fewer than 10^4 bacterial colonies can be cultured from voided urine, they are unlikely to be of significance. Greater than 10^5 colonies implies infection (Freedman and Epstein, 1977). When infection occurs, antibiotic treatment is indicated and treatment should be individualized to the organism and its sensitivity. The recommended duration of treatment is controversial (Kunin, 1981). There is mounting evidence that short periods of therapy, perhaps even single-dose therapy, are effective in uncomplicated cystitis (Buckwold *et al.*, 1982). The patient with MS, however, may respond more favourably to the more conventional ten-day course of therapy, in view of the likely concomitant urodynamic abnormalities.

Symptoms of urethritis and pyuria without significant bacteriuria may indicate an acute urethral syndrome. This may be caused by a low grade bacterial infection (10^5 organisms), in which case, conventional antimicrobial therapy will be effective. Alternatively, organisms such as *Chlamydia* or *Mycoplasma*, which do not grow in routine culture media, are frequently the infectious agents (Turck, 1981). Persistent sterile pyuria is an indication for tuberculosis culture. Symptoms of urethritis in the absence of infection may arise from irritation of the lower urinary tract, produced, for example, by repeated catheterization. Treatment with oral phenazopyridine hydrochloride (Pyridium) can provide local analgesia in this setting.

As mentioned, systemic symptoms may signify renal infection. These include fever, rigors, dysuria, nausea, diarrhoea or constipation, myalgias and flank pain. When the infection is severe, urinalysis reveals pyuria, white blood cell casts and bacteriuria. The symptoms may persist for days after instituting antibiotic therapy. Alternatively, symptoms may resolve spontaneously while renal infection and bacteriuria persist. Infections of renal origin, even when asymptomatic, frequently require 4–6 weeks of antimicrobial therapy for cure (shorter courses are associated with frequent relapse with the same strain of bacteria) (Turck, 1981).

Although recurrent infection may reflect an inadequately-treated renal infection, chronic infection may signify structural pathology. Intravenous pyelography may reveal calculi or an abscess; cystoscopy may reveal lesions such as tumour, calculi, or diverticuli. A recurrent UTI in the absence of underlying structural pathology can be effectively managed with chronic low dose antimicrobial prophylaxis (Stamm *et al.*, 1980).

Calculous disease

Recurrent urinary calculi frequently plague the patient with MS. Stones are a significant problem, contributing to chronic infection and renal insufficiency.

Calculogenesis is a complex process, promoted by factors such as urine alkalinity and high solute load. Contributing factors in the MS population include hypercalciuria, due to immobility and bone demineralization, urinary stasis, and infection with urea-splitting bacteria (Malek, 1977; Hald and Bradley, 1982). Urinary tract stones are predominantly composed of calcium oxalate, calcium phosphate, and calcium carbonate with magnesium-ammonium phosphate (struvite). Struvite formation is particularly sensitive to variations in urinary pH. The patient with MS and neurogenic bladder dysfunction may have functional obstruction, which may lead to the retention of preformed microcalculi. Subsequent infection with urea-splitting bacteria (*Proteus*, staphylococci, *Pseudomonas*, *E. coli*) produces an alkaline environment and promotes struvite formation. The situation is aggravated by hypercalciuria which provides a high solute load (Malek, 1977).

Although stones may be asymptomatic, the clinical features associated with urolithiasis are haematuria, recurrent infection, abdominal or flank pain, and renal colic. Azotaemia can complicate upper tract stone disease (Malek, 1977).

Prophylaxis against the formation of stones therefore includes acidifiers, mobilization, and high fluid intake (Boyarsky *et al.*, 1979). Urine must be monitored for evidence of infection, and infections should be promptly treated.

Cystoscopy and intravenous pyelography are diagnostic procedures which allow visualization of the entire urinary tract and allow localization of calculi. Bladder stones can be removed transurethrally. Surgical removal of renal calculi may be necessary, particularly in the setting of infection.

Respiratory infections

The MS population is at increased risk for developing infections of the respiratory tree. Immunosuppressive drug therapies and poor nutrition are factors which alter resistance against bacterial infections. Immobility, diaphragmatic and chest wall weakness, and dysfunction of the pharyngeal musculature may complicate advanced MS. All may interfere with mobilization of secretions contributing to the development of aspiration. Systemic infections, notably urosepsis, may seed the lungs, producing localized pulmonary infections.

Virtually every known pathogenic bacterial organism has been implicated in pneumonia. *Pneumococcus* is the major cause in adults, accounting for 60–80% of bacteriologically proven cases (Tillotson, 1980). Less common organisms include staphylococci, β-haemolytic streptococci, *Klebsiella pneumoniae*, *Haemophilus influenzae*, *Pseudomonas aeruginosa*, *Escherichia coli* and *Legionella pneumophila*. Aspiration pneumonias are usually caused by more than one species of anaerobes, although aerobic bacteria, enteric Gram-negative bacilli, and pseudomonads are also frequently present (Bartlett, Gornbach and Finegold, 1974).

Diagnosis depends upon the recognition of characteristic clinical features of the type of pneumonia, chest X-ray findings, and Gram stain and culture results of appropriately collected sputum samples. Treatment consists of prompt antibiotic therapy, tailored to the presumed infective agent, and aggressive respiratory therapy.

Preventive therapy, vaccination, is warranted in selected patients with MS. A 23-valent pneumococcal vaccine is now commercially available. It appears to be safe and is recommended for patients at risk of a high mortality rate due to pneumococcal bacteraemia. These include people with sickle cell disease, alcoholics, diabetics, those with chronic obstructive pulmonary disease, nephrotic syndrome, and those more than 50 years old. Although the risk of serious pneumococcal infection is increased in patients receiving immunosuppressive drugs, they may not respond to the vaccine (Medical Letter, 1983). The patient with MS at high risk for pneumococcal infection should be immunized, particularly prior to initiating immunosuppressive therapy.

Bacterial pneumonias frequently develop in the setting of resolving acute viral upper respiratory infections, particularly influenza. Vaccination against influenza is recommended for patients at high risk for development of pneumonia (Medical Letter, 1984).

Pressure sores

The pressure ulcer is a common clinical problem in patients with advanced neurological disease. This is readily understood when the risk factors for decubitus ulcer formation are considered. Pressure, shearing forces, friction, and moisture are important local factors, produced by decreased mobility and sensation, spasticity, and incontinence. Nutritional deficiency resulting in hypoproteinaemia and anaemia is a significant systemic factor (Narsete, Orgel and Smith, 1983).

Pressure is the single most important causative element contributing to ulcer formation. Experimental data have confirmed that a constant pressure of 70 mmHg applied to skin for a time period greater than two hours results in irreversible tissue damage; if the pressure is alternated at five-minute intervals, however, damage does not occur (Kosiak, 1959; Dinsdale, 1974). For clinical comparison, pressures measured under the buttocks of a person sitting in a wheelchair are estimated to be greater than 500 mmHg adjacent to the ischial tuberosities (Kosiak *et al.*, 1958).

The pathophysiology of the process relates to the fact that, in skin, the average capillary arteriolar pressure is 32 mmHg. Application of external pressures in excess of this leads to ischaemia, filtration of fluid from capillaries, oedema, and autolysis. Furthermore, external pressure leads to lymphatic obstruction, accumulation of metabolic waste products, and tissue death (Reuler and Cooney,

1981). Shearing forces promote angulation of blood vessels in the dermis and further tissue ischaemia. Friction and moisture contribute to the loss of superficial skin and hasten formation of the ulcer.

For obvious reasons the preponderance of decubitus ulcers develops in the lower part of the body, over bony prominences. The most common sites include sacrum, ischial tuberosities, greater trochanter, medial condyle of the tibia, malleoli, and the heel (Reuler and Cooney, 1981). Pressure sores are conventionally staged by clinical severity (Shea, 1975). Stage I is limited to the epidermis. There is soft tissue discoloration, swelling, and warmth. The lesion resembles an abrasion and is reversible. In a stage II lesion, which is also reversible, the inflammatory response extends through the dermis. A stage III ulcer refers to a full thickness skin defect with extension into the subcutaneous fat. Stage IV involves muscle and bone. Staging of a lesion is performed by physical examination. It is important to remember that a small superficial ulceration may appear over a broadly based deep defect; the extent of the ulcer base must be judged by probing.

Pressure sore prevention is of paramount importance. Frequent repositioning, vigilant attention to vulnerable areas of skin, aggressive anti-spasticity treatment, and maintenance of a dry environment are all crucial. Repositioning should occur at a minimum interval of two hours. Egg-crate cushions, water mattresses, or Clinitron therapy units may help to minimize pressure on sensitive areas. The Clinitron unit is a bed which provides a flotation environment by forcing warm filtered air through a tank filled with soda lime glass beads (Dolezal, Cohen and Schultz, 1985). The Clinitron unit also serves to minimize shearing forces, friction, and moisture, but it is currently limited in its accessibility to most patients because of its weight and cost. Sheepskin bed coverings serve to minimize shear forces and friction and, because of their capacity to absorb moisture, provide a low humidity skin contact surface.

Management of the pressure sore depends on its location and severity. Stage I and II lesions generally respond to local care, while stage III and IV lesions require surgical intervention. In all cases, wound healing is impeded when systemic abnormalities such as hypoproteinaemia and anaemia are present. A high protein diet and correction of significant anaemia through administration of blood or nutritional supplements are therefore indicated.

Medical treatment initially consists of removal of devitalized and infected tissue by debriding the wound. Subsequently, topical antiseptics that penetrate granulation tissue, such as half strength povidone-iodine (Betadine) solution may be applied.

Application of a semi-permeable sterile membrane, such as Opsite or Duoderm, protects the granulation tissue from external friction. The use of these membranes in conjunction with frequent cleansing with sterile saline and antiseptic agents may be quite effective. Most important is the avoidance of any weight bearing on the lesion. Surgical approaches consist of resection of necrotic tissue and bony prominences, followed by closure with myocutaneous flaps. Pedal ulcers may be managed by tight casting after removal of devitalized tissue. This serves to minimize pressure and friction, and promotes granulation by maintaining a moist environment.

Pressure sores may produce serious medical complications (Reuler and Cooney, 1981). Sepsis may occur, and is often polymicrobial in origin, involving Gram-positive, Gram-negative, and anaerobic organisms. Prompt systemic antibiotic therapy is indicated under such circumstances.

As indicated earlier, a relatively small and superficial ulcer may overlie a deep sinus track. Therefore, extension of an infected ulcer into deeper structures including bowel, bladder, bone and joint may lead to chronic life-threatening infections. Radiographic techniques such as computerized tomography or sinography can help to delineate the extent of infection and diagnose osteomyelitis.

Fibrous contractures

Muscle imbalance due to weakness or advanced spasticity may lead to musculoskeletal deformities, adding to the patient's disability. A muscle that is not frequently extended to its full length will develop fibrosis and permanent shortening (Salter, 1978). Muscle contracture can lead to joint pathology, including ankylosis and dislocations. Furthermore, abnormal limb positioning and mobility can promote formation of bedsores and interferes with perineal hygiene.

Such complications can be prevented through aggressive medical management of spasticity, combined with a passive range of movement exercise, performed on a daily basis (Alexander and Abramson, 1984).

When spasticity is severe, medical and physical therapy may be insufficient to overcome muscle contraction; chemical neurectomy or motor point blocks may help distinguish spasticity from contracture. When nerve blocks fail it may be necessary to employ spinal or general anaesthesia to separate severe spasticity from fibrous contractures.

When fibrous contractures produce persistent musculoskeletal deformity, surgical intervention may be warranted. Corrective operations include tenotomy, tendon lengthening, and arthrodesis (Salter, 1978).

Nutrition

Adequate nutrition is often an issue in the chronically ill patient. The patient with MS requires a well balanced, high protein diet, particularly when complications such as decubitus ulcer or infection are present. When neurological dysfunction produces severe dysphagia, an oesophagostomy or gastrostomy may be necessary in order to augment nutrition and to prevent aspiration.

THE TERTIARY COMPLICATIONS

The tertiary complications of multiple sclerosis are the financial, social, and emotional problems which develop during the chronic phase of the illness. They include vocational difficulties, marital and family discord, and social isolation. Problems with obtaining or maintaining employment result from discrimination, physical or mental inability to fulfil job requirements, and architectural barriers. The demands and expense of caring for a dependent disabled individual, coupled with the patient's loss of self-esteem, may result in the breakdown of domestic relationships. Similarly, transportation difficulties, architectural barriers, depression and discrimination all interfere with the development and maintenance of social relationships.

Employment

In most cases MS develops during the most productive years in terms of training and earning potential. Among the causes of disability in adults of working age, MS ranks seventh among causes of severe handicaps (Scheinberg *et al.*, 1981). Studies indicate that 70–80% of patients with MS for more than 20 years are unemployed (Bauer, 1965). Reasons cited for leaving work include spasticity, uncoordination, gait difficulties, visual disturbance, transportation difficulty and fatigue (Bauer, 1978; Scheinberg *et al.*, 1981). The majority of those employed are found to be in white-collar, managerial, or professional positions, probably because the physical demands of such jobs are less than blue-collar or skilled labour occupations.

The physician's role in vocational rehabilitation is manifold. Early in the course of the illness it may be necessary to advise patients to seek education and job skills which will secure them a position in less physically demanding fields. The physician should refer patients to appropriate agencies for vocational rehabilitation, and should maintain contact with agency personnel concerning work abilities and medical intervention which may augment work capacity. The patient's functional potential should be periodically reassessed.

It is often necessary to apply a multidisciplinary approach to this problem, involving social workers, therapists, and rehabilitation counsellors. Legal advice may be required by the patient to obtain disability benefits, remove architectural barriers, and prevent discrimination in employment (Scheinberg *et al.*, 1980). The physician should maintain a referral network to such ancillary personnel. An environment encouraging independence and continued employment should be maintained.

The effect on family life and interpersonal relations

A chronic illness affects a patient's family in many ways. Alterations or loss of job, interference with spouse's employment, costs of medications, equipment, and structural modifications in the home all serve to strain household finances. In the US, annual costs plus lost earnings due to MS may average as much as $15000 per family (Inman, 1983). Financial as well as physical restrictions may interfere with leisure activities, vacations, children's education, and household activities. All family members are adversely affected by such factors. Relations between patient and spouse may be further stressed by complications such as depression, cognitive impairment, and sexual dysfunction.

The health care provider can best ameliorate these symptoms by ensuring that all potential sources of financial aid are tapped, through maintenance of a referral network to appropriate agencies and personnel. A knowledge of available community services, such as recreational programmes, support groups, transportation, and visiting nurse service, is quite important. The National Multiple Sclerosis Society and its local chapters are a valuable resource in this regard.

Certain problems are amenable to the therapies provided by psychologists and psychiatrists. Depression, loss of self-esteem, and difficulty coping with increased emotional, physical, and financial dependence, may all respond to individual and/or family counselling. Depression and related emotional disturbances are the psychological disturbances most frequently associated with MS (Whitlock and Siskind, 1980; Baretz and Stephenson, 1981). Realizing this, the primary physician should observe patients for signs and symptoms and maintain an atmosphere encouraging dialogue about emotional dysfunction, so that prompt psychological intervention may occur.

MS is a complicated disease with profound ramifications in all aspects of the patient's life. For this reason the multidisciplinary approach is the only one suitable. While the efforts of these health care professionals will not alter the natural history of the disease, they will prolong the lives and improve the quality of those so afflicted.

References

ALEXANDER, J. and ABRAMSON, A. S. (1984) Physical and surgical therapy. In *Multiple Sclerosis: a Guide for Patients and Families*, edited by L. C. Scheinberg, pp. 71–90. New York: Raven Press

BARETZ, R. M. and STEPHENSON, G. R. (1981) Emotional responses to multiple sclerosis. *Psychosomatics*, **22**, 117–127

BARRETT, M. (1977) *Sexuality and Multiple Sclerosis*. Toronto: Multiple Sclerosis Society of Canada

BARTLETT, J. G., GORNBACH, S. L. and FINEGOLD, S. M. (1974) The bacteriology of aspiration pneumonia. *American Journal of Medicine*, **56**, 202–207

BAUER, H. J. (1965) Prognostic criteria in multiple sclerosis. *Annals of the New York Academy of Science*, **122**, 542

BAUER, H. J. (1978) Problems of symptomatic therapy in multiple sclerosis. *Neurology*, **28**, 8

BLAIVAS, J. G. (1980) Management of bladder dysfunction in multiple sclerosis. *Neurology (NY)*, **30**, 12–18

BLAIVAS, J. G., HOLLAND, N. J., GIESSEV, B., LAROCCA, N. J., MADONNA, M. and SCHERNBERG, L. (1984) Multiple sclerosis bladder studies and care. *Annals of the New York Academy of Science*, **436**, 326–346

BLAIVAS, J. G., SINHA, H. P., ZAYED, A. A. H. and LABIB, K. B. (1981) Detrusor external sphincter dyssynergia. *Journal of Urology*, **125**, 542–548

BOYARSKY, S., LABAY, P., HANICK, P., ABRAMSON, A. and BOYARSKY, R. (1979) *Care of the Patient with Neurogenic Bladder*. Boston: Little, Brown and Co.

BUCKWOLD, F. J., LUDWIG, P., HARDING, G. K. M. *et al.* (1982) Therapy for acute cystitis in adult women. *Journal of the American Medical Association*, **247**, 1839–1842

CLIFFORD, D. B. and TROTTER, J. L. (1984) Pain in multiple sclerosis. *Archives of Neurology*, **41**, 1270–1272

COOPER, I. (1960) Neurosurgical relief of intention tremor due to cerebellar disease and multiple sclerosis. *Archives of Physical Medicine and Rehabilitation*, **41**, 1–4

DAVIDOFF, R. A. (1978) Pharmacology of spasticity. *Neurology (Minn.)*, **28**, 46–51

DAVIDOFF, R. A. (1985) Antispasticity drugs: mechanisms of action. *Annals of Neurology*, **17**, 107–116

DAVIDOFF, R. A. and SEARS, E. S. (1974) The effects of Lioresal on synaptic activity in the isolated spinal cord. *Neurology (Minn.)*, **24**, 957–963

DELWAIDE, P. J. (1985) Electrophysiological analysis of the mode of action of muscle relaxants in spasticity. *Annals of Neurology*, **17**, 90–95

DEVENPORT, J. K., SWENSON, J. R., DUKES JR., G. E. and SONSALLA, P. K. (1984) Fomaldehyde generation from methenamine salts in spinal cord injury. *Archives of Physical Medicine and Rehabilitation*, **65**, 257–259

DINSDALE, S. M. (1974) Decubitus ulcers: role of pressure and friction in causation. *Archives of Physical Medicine and Rehabilitation*, **55**, 147

DIOKNO, A. C. and CHILDS, S. J. (1985) Clean intermittent catheterization in UTI management. *Infections in Surgery*, **4**, 185–190

DIOKNO, A. C. and LAPIDES, J. (1977) Action of oral and parenteral bethanecol on decompensated bladder. *Urology*, **10**, 23–24

DOLEZAL, R., COHEN, M. and SCHULTZ, R. C. (1985) The use of clinitron therapy unit in the immediate post operative care of pressure ulcers. *Annals of Plastic Surgery*, **14**, 33–36

EDBERG, E. L., CERNY, K. and STAUFFER, E. S. (1973) Prevention and treatment of pressure sores. *Physical Therapy*, **53**, 246–252

FOX, S., KRNJEVIC, K., MORRIS, M. E., PUIL, E. and WERMAN, R. (1978) Action of baclofen in mammalian synaptic transmission. *Neuroscience*, **3**, 495–515

FREAL, J. E., KRAFT, G. H. and CORYELL, J. K. (1984) Symptomatic fatigue in multiple sclerosis. *Archives of Physical Medicine and Rehabilitation*, **65**, 135–138

FREEDMAN, L. R. and EPSTEIN, F. H. (1977) Urinary tract infection, pyelonephritis, and related conditions. In *Harrison's Principles of Internal Medicine*, edited by G. W. Thorn, pp. 961–962. New York: McGraw-Hill

HALD, T. and BRADLEY, W. E. (1982) *The Urinary Bladder Neurology and Dynamics*. Baltimore: Williams and Wilkins

HINMUN, F., JR (1973) Hydrodynamic aspects of urinary tract infections. In *Urodynamics*, edited by W. Lutzeyer and H. Melchior, pp. 14–22. Berlin: Springer

INMAN, R. P. (1983) Disability indices, the economic costs of illness and social insurance: the case of multiple sclerosis societies. *Vancouver Symposium of the International Federation of Multiple Sclerosis Societies*

KALB, R., LAROCCA, N. and KAPLAN, S. R. (1984) Sexuality. In *Multiple Sclerosis: a Guide for Patients and Families*, edited by L. C. Scheinberg, pp. 155–174. New York: Raven Press

KIRKLAND, L. R. (1984) Baclofen dosage: a suggestion. *Archives of Physical Medicine and Rehabilitation*, **65**, 214

KOLLER, W. C. (1984) Pharmacologic trials in the treatment of cerebellar tremor. *Archives of Neurology*, **41**, 280–281

KOSIAK, M. P. (1959) Etiology and pathology of ischemic ulcers. *Archives of Physical Medicine and Rehabilitation*, **40**, 62

KOSIAK, M., KUBICEK, W. G., OLSON, M., DANZ, J. N. and KOTTKE, F. J. (1958) Evaluation of pressure as a factor in the production of decubitus ulcers. *Archives of Physical Medicine and Rehabilitation*, **39**, 623–629

KUNIN, C. M. (1981) Duration of treatment of urinary tract infection. *American Journal of Medicine*, **71**, 849–854

LAPIDES, J. (1974) Neurogenic bladder: principles of treatment. *Urologic Clinics of North America*, **1**, 81–97

LAPIDES, J., DIOKNO, A. C. and LOWE, B. S. (1974) Follow up on unsterile intermittent self catheterization. *Journal of Urology*, **111**, 184–187

LAPIDES, J., DIOKNO, A. C., SILBER, S. J. and LOWE, B. S. (1971) Clean intermittent self catheterization in the treatment of urinary tract disease. *Transactions of the American Association of Genitourinary Surgery*, **63**, 92–96

LILIUS, H. G., VALTONEN, E. J. and WILKSTROM, J. (1976) Sexual problems in patients suffering from multiple sclerosis. *Journal of Chronic Disease*, **29**, 643–647

LOGEMANN, J. (1981) *The Evaluation and Treatment of Swallowing Disorders*. San Diego, Calif.: College Hill Press

LUNDBERG, P. O. (1978) Sexual dysfunction in patients with multiple sclerosis. *Sexuality and Disability*, **1**, 218–222

MALEK, R. S. (1977) Renal lithiasis: a practical approach. *Journal of Urology*, **118**, 893–901

MATTHEWS, W. B. (1975) Paroxysmal symptoms in multiple sclerosis. *Journal of Neurology, Neurosurgery and Psychiatry*, **38**, 617–623

MEDICAL LETTER (1983) An expanded pneumococcal vaccine. **25**, p. 90, 91

MEDICAL LETTER (1984) Influenza prevention for 1984–1985. **26**, p. 85

MEHROTRA, R. M. L. (1953) An experimental study of the vesical circulation during distension and in cystitis. *Journal of Pathology and Bacteriology*, **65**, 78–89

MOBLEY, D. F. (1976) Phenoxybenzamine in the management of neurogenic vesical dysfunction. *Journal of Urology*, **116**, 737–738

MOORE, D. C. (1971) *Regional Block: a Handbook for Use in the Clinical Practice of Medicine and Surgery*, 4th edn. Springfield, Illinois: Charles C. Thomas

MURRAY, T. J. (1984) The treatment of fatigue in MS. *Neurology*, **34**, 139 (abstract)

NARSETE, T. A., ORGEL, M. G. and SMITH, D. (1983) Pressure sores. *American Family Physician*, **28**, 135–139

NELSON, D. A., VATES, T. S. JR. and THOMAS, R. B. JR. (1973) Complications from intrathecal steroid therapy in patients with multiple sclerosis. *Acta Neurologica Scandinavica*, **49**, 176–188

NETTO, N. R. JR., RANGEL, P. E., DASILVA, R. P. and LEMOS, G. C. (1978) Relation between the vaginal introital and perianal flora in recurrent cystitis in women. *Urologia Internationalis*, **33**, 260–266

NGAI, S. H., TSENG, D. T. C. and WANG, S. C. (1966) Effect of diazepam and other central nervous system depressants or spinal reflexes in cats: a study of site of action. *Journal of Pharmacology and Experimental Therapeutics*, **153**, 344–351

PHILP, T., READ, D. J. and HIGSON, R. H. (1981) The urodynamic characteristics of multiple sclerosis. *British Journal of Urology*, **53**, 672–675

PONSKY, J. L., GAUDERER, M. W. and STELLATO, T. A. (1983) Percutaneous endoscopic gastrostomy: review of 150 cases. *Archives of Surgery*, **118**, 913–914

REULER, J. B. and COONEY, T. G. (1981) The pressure sore: pathophysiology and principles of management. *Annals of Internal Medicine*, **94**, 661–666

ROUSSAN, M. S., ABRAMSON, M. D., LEVINE, M. D. and FEIBEL, A. (1975) Bladder training: its role in evaluating the effect of an antispasticity drug on voiding in patients with neurogenic bladder. *Archives of Physical Medicine and Rehabilitation*, **56**, 463–468

SABRA, A. F. and HALLETT, M. (1984) Action tremor with alternating activity in antagonist muscles. *Neurology (Cl.)*, **34**, 151–156

SABRA, A. F., HALLETT, M., SUDARSKY, L. and MULLALLY, W. (1982) Treatment of action tremor in multiple sclerosis with isoniazid. *Neurology (Cl.)*, **32**, 912–914

SALTER, R. S. (1978) *Textbook of Disorders and Injuries of the Musculoskeletal System.* Baltimore: Williams and Wilkins

SCHEINBERG, L., HOLLAND, N. J. and KIRSCHENBAUM, M. S. (1981) Comprehensive long-term care of patients with multiple sclerosis. *Neurology*, **31**, 1121–1123

SCHEINBERG, L., HOLLAND, N., LAROCCA, N., LAITIN, P., BENNETT, A. and HALL, H. (1980) Multiple sclerosis: earning a living. *NY State Journal of Medicine*, **80**, 1375–1400

SCHEINBERG, L. and SMITH, C. R. (1985) Multiple sclerosis. In *Current Therapy in Neurologic Disease 1985–1986*, edited by R. T. Johnson. Philadelphia, Pennsylvania: B. C. Decker

SCOTT, F. B., BRADLEY, W. E. and TIMM, G. W. (1973) Treatment of urinary incontinence by implantable prosthetic sphincter. *Urology*, **1**, 252–259

SHAND, D. G., NIMMON, C. C. and O'GRADY, F. (1970) Relation between residual urine volume and response to treatment of urinary tract infection. *Lancet*, **1**, 1305–1306

SHEA, J. D. (1975) Pressure sores – classification and management. *Clinical Orthopedics*, **112**, 89–100

STAMM, W. E. *et al.* (1980) Antimicrobial prophylaxis of recurrent urinary tract infections. *Annals of Internal Medicine*, **92**, 770–775

STRAUSS, B. S. and BLAUFOX, M. D. (1971) Estimation of residual urine and urine flow rates without urethral catheterization. *Journal of Nuclear medicine*, **11**, 81–84

TILLOTSON, J. R. (1980) Bacterial pneumonias. In *Current Diagnosis 6*, edited by H. F. Conn and R. B. Conn., pp. 146–148. Philadelphia: W. B. Saunders

TURCK, M. (1981) New concepts in genitourinary tract infections. *Journal of American Medical Association*, **246**, 2019–2023

WEIN, A. J. (1980) Pharmacology of the bladder and urethra. In *Surgery of Female Incontinence*, edited by S. L. Stanton and E. A. Tanagho, pp. 185–199. Heidelberg: Springer Verlag

WHITLOCK, F. A. and SISKIND, M. M. (1980) Depression as a major symptom of multiple sclerosis. *Journal of Neurology, Neurosurgery and Psychiatry*, **43**, 861–865

YOUNG, R. R. and DELWAIDE, P. J. (1981) Spasticity. *New England Journal of Medicine*, **304**, 28–33, 96–99

Index